The Medical Interview:

MASTERING SKILLS FOR CLINICAL PRACTICE

● ● ● ● ●

The Medical Interview:
MASTERING SKILLS FOR CLINICAL PRACTICE

FOURTH EDITION

● ● ● ● ●

John L. Coulehan, MD, MPH
Institute for Medicine in Contemporary Society
Department of Preventive Medicine
State University at Stony Brook
Stony Brook, New York

Marian R. Block, MD, ABFP
Chairperson
Department of Family Medicine
The Western Pennsylvania Hospital
Pittsburgh, Pennsylvania

F.A. Davis Company • Philadelphia

F. A. Davis Company
1915 Arch Street
Philadelphia, PA 19103
www.fadavis.com

Acquisitions Editor: Margaret M. Biblis
Developmental Editor: Bernice M. Wissler
Cover Designer: Louis J. Forgione

As new scientific information becomes available through basic and clinical research, recommended treatments and drug therapies undergo changes. The author(s) and publisher have done everything possible to make this book accurate, up to date, and in accord with accepted standards at the time of publication. The author(s), editors, and publisher are not responsible for errors or omissions or for consequences from application of the book, and make no warranty, expressed or implied, in regard to the contents of the book. Any practice described in this book should be applied by the reader in accordance with professional standards of care used in regard to the unique circumstances that may apply in each situation. The reader is advised always to check product information (package inserts) for changes and new information regarding dose and contraindications before administering any drug. Caution is especially urged when using new or infrequently ordered drugs.

Library of Congress Cataloging-in-Publication Data

Coulehan, John L., 1943-
   The medical interview : mastering skills for clinical practice /
John L. Coulehan, Marian R. Block.— 4th ed.
      p. cm.
   Includes bibliographical references and index.
   ISBN 0-8036-0771-7
   1. Medical history taking. I. Block, Marian R., 1947-   . II.
Title.
   RC65 .C68 2001
   616.07′51—dc21

                                                                          00-065683

To Our Families

Acknowledgments

● ● ● ● ●

The Medical Interview includes numerous examples of clinician–patient inter-actions. Most are abstracted from taped interviews, although in every case we have removed personal references that might serve to identify the clinician or patient. In some cases we have altered the transcripts (mostly by shortening) in ways that serve to demonstrate specific points more compactly. We are grateful to the patients and clinicians who permitted us to tape and publish these conversations.

We wish also to acknowledge our debt to teachers and colleagues. Three outstanding physician-educators deserve special thanks. Eric J. Cassell, MD, taught us how to observe the clinician–patient interaction systematically and encouraged us in this work for many years. Alvan Feinstein, MD, taught us that the medical interview is a source of scientific data about the patient and in-spired us to find the science in the art of history taking. The late Kenneth D. Rogers, MD, gave us the wholehearted and sustained support we needed, first, to develop our course in medical interviewing and, later, to write this book.

In the years since the first edition of this book was published, we have continued to learn from our students, our patients, and our colleagues, as well as from the burgeoning literature on the analysis of clinician–patient interac-tions. A special thanks to our editor at F.A. Davis, Bernice Wissler, and to Marcy Cloherty and Heidi Campani, who provided invaluable help in preparing the manuscript and coordinating the endless mail, fax, and telephone interactions of two authors now working in offices 500 miles apart.

Although each of us had primary responsibilities for writing certain chap-ters, this book is a joint product; in a very special sense it is truly a collabora-tive effort, and we are both responsible for the entire text.

John L. Coulehan, MD, FACP

Marian R. Block, MD, ABFP

A Note to Learners and Teachers: How to Use this Text

● ● ● ● ●

This book teaches skills that manifest themselves as behaviors that clinicians display when they interact with patients. Our premise is that anyone can learn these behaviors, although some individuals will certainly have greater aptitude than others. Although these behaviors are fundamental to the clinician–patient relationship, this text is about behaviors, not relationships.

We use clinician–patient dialogue to demonstrate these behaviors. These dialogues are real; they are not perfect or ideal and they are meant to be criticized. They provide an opportunity for reflection and analysis, and teachers may find it useful to guide their students to answer such questions as:

- How would you have asked that question?
- How would you have responded?
- If this clinician had a second chance, how might these behaviors or words be changed to prevent the patient's angry response?
- What words convey that this clinician understands the patient's story?

Learners can immerse themselves in the clinical role by examining these interactions and developing skill in self-reflection. Learned in this non-threatening way, these techniques can be used in classroom situations with real or simulated patients, or to debrief videotapes or direct observation of patient interactions.

Beginners should read and experience Part One (Basic Skills: Understanding the Patient's Story) during their preclinical courses on communication and introduction to medicine and return to this section as they conduct their first interviews with patients. The chapters in Part Two (Basic Skills in Practice: Special Patients and Settings) may be added as learners move on to work with particular populations, such as the very young, the very old, and the ambulatory patient. Part Three (Challenges in Interviewing) is appropriate to the advanced learner with direct patient-care responsibilities, who is likely to encounter difficult interactions in that role. Newly trained clinicians will find it useful to return to this section as they develop their panel of patients.

Although we deal with the basic content of the medical history and emphasize data-gathering skills, our focus is on technique as opposed to content. Those searching for a cookbook of specific questions for specific content areas—what questions to ask about what symptom—will not find it in this text. Nor do we exhort clinicians to be kind and sympathetic or "patient-centered." That the patient is at the center of the interaction is assumed. Beginners worry about what question to ask next; this text is about listening and about observing the patient, oneself, and the interaction. Although they share the same core qualities and basic skills, we do not confuse history taking with counseling. But we also believe that allowing patients to tell their stories—and hearing them with empathy and respect—is a therapeutic goal in itself.

Contents

● ● ● ● ●

Introduction

● ● ● ● ●

THE POOR HISTORIAN

History-taking, the most clinically sophisticated procedure of medicine, is an extraordinary investigative technique: in few other forms of scientific research does the observed object talk.

Alvan Feinstein, *Clinical Judgment*

They cluster in the hall on rounds, eight of them—students, house officers, and attending physician—creating turbulence and obstructing flow. A medication nurse pushes a cabinet around them on the way down the hall, while the breakfast lorry closes in from the other direction. An intern begins the presentation with "Mr. Blank is a 52-year-old man who presents with abdominal pain...the patient is a poor historian...."

The attending physician learns that this sick person *claims* to have a number of symptoms and he is *apparently* taking several medications. The intern hastens to add that Mr. Blank is non-compliant, he doesn't seem to understand his illness, and he is, after all, a "poor historian." Having thus dispensed with preliminaries, the intern continues with the patient's physical findings and initial laboratory data. At this point the qualifiers disappear: the magnesium level does not *seem* to be 2.2, it *is* 2.2. Meanwhile, the attending physician reflects on the meaning of the term "poor historian," perhaps because of an unconscionable lack of interest in magnesium. The matrix of numbers vibrating among students and house officers takes on a life of its own, while the attending physician wonders about the nature of this patient's "poorness." The physician knows what the intern is trying to tell the group with the phrase "poor historian." She doesn't intend to imply that the patient is an impoverished history professor. Nor does she mean that the patient is a history student who is getting Ds and Fs. No, the intern is saying in precise medical shorthand, "I was unable to reconstruct a logical story of the illness in my conversation with this patient. We didn't communicate well." Reflecting further, the attending physician concludes that the term "poor historian" is appropriate, but perhaps it applies to the intern, who might be more correct in saying, "The clinical history is unclear because *I'm* a poor historian."

This vignette illustrates how data we obtain from speaking with patients and therapy we accomplish through the process of clinician–patient interaction are not often topics for discussion during medical rounds. While we consider information about serum magnesium, for which accuracy and precision are assumed, a fit topic for discussion, knowledge of the precise pattern of symptoms or the patient's beliefs about the symptoms appears less scientific and less relevant. Clinical students soon learn to spend less time listening to the patient's story and more time among their peers agonizing over the meaning of a magnesium value. Trainees learn to accept responsibility for how well (or how poorly) they perform a bone marrow aspiration, interpret an x-ray, or insert a flexible sigmoidoscope. As clinicians, we rarely blame the patient for an inadequate bone marrow aspirate, yet we believe the world is full of patients who perpetrate poor histories.

Stories of sickness and suffering—the kind of human stories that move us to enter a healing profession—gradually move to the background as we become socialized into the technical culture of health care. Students and professionals become preoccupied with quite different stories: technical tales in which organs and instruments rather than people are the main protagonists. Sometimes, in fact, the patient's personal narrative is entirely forgotten.

Nowadays it is not rare in clinical practice that investigations bring unexpected results to light and these, in turn, lead to more examinations along a side track. After a while the clinical team is interested in, say, the incidental finding of a renal cyst on an abdominal CT scan, while the cyst may have nothing to do with the patient's illness. The patient may have trouble getting anyone to pay attention to what he *feels* and *believes* and *experiences*. At some point, after multiple diagnostic tests and specialist consultations, the patient cries out, "But you haven't done anything about my fatigue!"

This narrow view that *real* medicine focuses only on "objective" data—numbers, graphs, and images—permeates clinical education. In this view, "subjective" data—the patient's story—lacks clinical value because it lacks quantification. In other words, what patients feel, the suffering they experience, and the disability that haunts them, all of which they describe through the medium of words, are secondary in importance to those physiologic quantities that can be observed directly. We clinicians, so this premise goes, address only the biochemical or physiological causes of suffering and pain. Our real work requires us to reduce persons and their illnesses to organs and diseases. If we correct bad numbers, suffering will go away. We don't need to pay attention to who the patients are, or to the fine details of their stories.

In fact, according to this view, patients and their stories often get in the way of "real" medicine. The patient "comes to function as a kind of translucent screen on which the disease is projected.... [But] the screen has opacities of its own which obscure the accurate perception of the underlying disease."[1] The poor historian, the patient with whom we have difficulty communicating, may be defined as having many such opacities. It is difficult to see through the person to observe the disease.

But should the patient be merely a screen that we try to work around, or to see through? A broader view of health care holds that the patient's narrative lies at the center of clinical practice. The great clinician and medical educator, William Osler, wrote, "It is a safe rule to have no teaching without a patient for a text, and the best teaching is that taught by the patient himself." In fact, experienced clinicians are aware that most diagnoses are made on the basis of patient interviews and that the clinician–patient interaction is an important therapeutic tool. Moreover, most health care professionals spend the bulk of their time interacting with patients.

Despite widespread lip service to this broader view of medicine, until 25 years ago medical schools generally did not include interviewing skills in their curricula. Medical educators did not consider history taking and talking with patients appropriate topics for serious study. These educators gave students "little black books" that included lists of questions about symptoms and past diagnoses. If the patient did not answer these questions clearly, concisely, and in a medically acceptable fashion, the patient was labeled a "poor historian." Clinicians told their students, "Talking with patients is important, but you'll pick up how to do it as you go along. The clinician–patient relationship is also important—crucial, in fact—but you'll pick that up as you go along, too. All you need is experience."

For a number of reasons, this attitude toward communication skills in medicine has changed in recent years. First, we have discovered that highly specialized, machine-intensive medicine is not necessarily the best medicine. Patients may find themselves doing better by the numbers, but feeling worse. They may undergo the most advanced tests and see the best specialists, but find themselves feeling just as sick, and often angry and confused when their high expectations are not met. At the same time, academic clinicians have begun to understand that pain, suffering, and dysfunction must be conceptualized in broad human terms as well as in biochemical terms if we are to be effective healers. Effective clinical practice requires a biopsychosocial or holistic model rather than a purely biological model.

Second, investigators have studied the process of interviewing and analyzed its individual components. This work, along with studies in fields as wide ranging as medical anthropology and clinical decision making, has shown that the "art of medicine" can be articulated and taught. It is not simply a matter of intuition and experience.

Third, patient-oriented studies have shown that good patient–clinician communication leads to better clinical outcomes and more satisfied patients. Poor communication leads to poor clinical outcomes, dissatisfaction, and malpractice litigation. In fact, when an adverse event occurs, clinician insensitivity and poor communication are major factors in a patient's decision to sue.[2,3] Finally, the pressing need to limit the costs of health care has led to a restructuring of our health care system around the concept of managed care. Managed care arrangements generally stipulate that each person must have a primary care professional to coordinate his or her health care. These generalists are expected to use resources rationally because they communicate well and understand their patients' problems, as well as understanding medical science.

This book is based on the premise that good patient–clinician communication is essential to good health care. Talking with patients is not a skill reserved for psychiatrists, psychologists, and social workers. It is essential for radiologists as well as internists, ophthalmologists, and pediatricians. Medical interviewing is a basic clinical skill. It is not a matter of common sense nor does it necessarily come with experience. It is a skill that can be broken down into component parts, and it can be learned. That is the subject of this book.

The Medical Interview is addressed primarily to students of medicine and other health professions who are about to begin their professional interaction with patients. It is designed to be a guide for those who are just learning to take a medical history and interact with patients, as well as a resource for those who are farther along in their education, including postgraduate trainees. Our particular emphasis is on microskills of the initial patient interview. Although we deal extensively with basic history taking, we also illustrate how these same skills serve as building blocks for all types of patient-clinician interactions. They lie at the core of the art and science of medicine, where the patient's experience is central.

The book is divided into three major sections. *The Patient's Story* presents fundamentals of clinical interviewing (Chapters 1 and 2) and various components of the medical history (Chapters 3 through 7). *Basic Skills for Special Patients and Settings* presents basic skills in different contexts: pediatric patients (Chapter 8), geriatrics and elder care (Chapter 9), cultural competence (Chapter 10), and the outpatient setting (Chapter 11). *Applying Basic and Advanced Skills: Challenges in Interviewing* includes guidelines for difficult interactions (Chapter 12), telling bad news (Chapter 13), interviewing the patient about complementary and alternative medicine (Chapter 14), avoiding malpractice litigation (Chapter 15), and patient education and negotiation (Chapter 16).

References

1. Baron RJ. Bridging clinical distance: An empathic rediscovery of the known. *J Med Philosophy* 1981; 6:5.
2. Beckman HB, Markakis KM, Suchman AL, Frankel RM. The doctor-patient relationship and malpractice. Lessons from plaintiff depositions. *Arch Intern Med* 1994; 154:1365–1370.

3. Vincent C, Young M, Phillips A. Why do people sue doctors? A study of patients and relatives taking legal action. *The Lancet* 1994; 343:1609–1613.

Suggested Reading

Hunter KM. *Doctor's Stories. The Narrative Structure of Medical Knowledge.* Princeton, NJ, Princeton University Press, 1991.
Lipkin M Jr., Putnam S, Lazare A. *The Medical Interview: Clinical Care, Education, and Research.* New York, Springer-Verlag, 1995.
Stuart MR, Lieberman JA III. *The 15-Minute Hour-Applied Psychotherapy for the Primary Care Physician,* ed. 2, Praeger, 1993.

PART 1

BASIC SKILLS: UNDERSTANDING THE PATIENT'S STORY

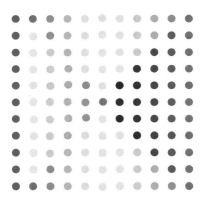

CHAPTER 1

I Attach the Same Meaning

● ● ● ● ●

INTERVIEWING AS A CLINICAL SKILL

*A very good way to find out how another person is thinking or feeling is to ask him.... At this point, however, a diffi-culty arises. If I am to acquire information in this way about another person's experiences, I must understand what he says about them. And this would seem to imply that **I attach the same meaning** to his words as he does. But how, it may be asked, can I ever be sure that this is so?*

A. J. Ayer, *The Problem of Knowledge*

Although medicine is based on a group of theoretical sciences, clinical medicine itself is a practical science: it is the science of helping ill people get well, rather than that of understanding disease. Like any other science, clinical medicine has basic units of observation, basic quantities of measure-ment, and basic instruments for obtaining these measurements. The units of observation are signs and symptoms, the quantities of measurement are words and sometimes numbers, and the most important instrument is the medical practitioner. Like any other scientific instrument, the clinician must be objective, precise, sensitive, specific, and reliable when making observa-tions about the patient's illness. In this text we examine interviewing and interactional skills as fundamental to the science of medicine. As we will show, interviewing skills are also at the core of the art of medicine. In fact, in medicine, art and science are synergistic.

OBJECTIVITY

What does it mean to be objective when interviewing a patient and taking a medical history? **Objectivity** means striving to remove one's own beliefs, prejudices, and preconceptions from observations; it involves eliminating bias or systematic distortion from one's observations. Other words for objectivity are **accuracy** and **validity**. The illness data should correspond to what the patient really felt and experienced. If, for example, you start with a preconceived notion of the illness and you discard or minimize ill-fitting items, you are not being objective. Consider this interview taken from an article by Platt and McMath.[1] The clinician here "knows" that the patient has severe lung disease and so is unable to hear the chief complaint:

Hello, I'm Dr. X, are you Mrs. Y?

Yes, I'm glad to know you.

What sorts of troubles have you been having?

I've been going downhill for 2 years. Nothing seems to be working right.

What is the worst part?

My legs. I have constant pain in my legs. It's gotten so bad I can't sleep.

What about your breathing?

Oh, that's all right. I can breathe fine. I just hurt so bad in my legs.

Are you still smoking?

Yes, with this pain, I've gone back to cigarettes for relief. But I'm down to half a pack or so a day.

Are you having pains in your chest?

No.

How about cough?

No, I hardly ever cough.

How much are you actually able to do?

Well, I was able to do everything until about 2 years ago, but now I can hardly walk half a block.

Why is that?

My legs. They hurt.

Do they swell up?

Well, they've been a bit swollen the last 2 or 3 weeks, but the pain is there whether they swell or not.

All right, I want to ask you some things about your medical history now.

The clinician in this case seems to ignore the patient's leg pain; when she complains about it, the clinician replies with questions about breathing. The clinician is undervaluing certain kinds of information—he isn't hearing what he doesn't expect—while overvaluing data related to a diagnosis that he "knows," namely, the patient's chronic lung disease. Failure of objectivity is unscientific and could lead to a missed diagnosis; it is also likely to make the patient feel ignored. When patients feel ignored, they tend to say less, and opportunities to obtain other important data may be lost.

How might the same doctor respond on a better day?

Hello, I'm Dr. X, are you Mrs. Y?

Yes, I'm glad to know you.

Thank you, I'm glad to know you too. What sorts of troubles have you been having?

I've been going downhill for 2 years. Nothing seems to be working right.

What is the worst part?

My legs. I have constant pain in my legs. It's gotten so bad I can't sleep.

Pain in your legs. Tell me more about that.

Well, it's gotten so bad I can hardly walk half a block.

You mean the pain forces you to stop?

Yes, that's exactly it. And, well, it gets better when I stop, but never really goes away. Even at night when I'm lying still it wakes me up, it's so bad.

The patient now is describing claudication, a symptom characteristic of severe peripheral vascular disease. The patient is now able to volunteer important details about the leg pain that not only aid the diagnostic process but also help her feel understood. **The skill of being objective requires, first, active listening, and second, effective feedback to the patient about what you have heard (see Chap. 2); in other words, you let the patient know that you understand.**

INTERPRETATION VERSUS OBSERVATION

It is easy to confuse interpretation with observation. When talking with a patient, your observation is what the patient actually says or does; the patient's words are primary data. Preceptors sometimes encourage students and other trainees to use terms that are really interpretations rather than descriptions. One example of such a term is "claudication," as in our example here; another is "angina," a certain kind of chest pain caused by coronary artery disease. These words are interpretations because they imply specific etiologies. The primary data of the symptom "angina" might be something like "substernal discomfort of a dull, pressing nature, lasting about 3 minutes, brought on by exertion, and relieved by rest." Interpretive terms are shorthand necessary for thinking and conversation in clinical practice; such terms are appropriate when the symptom has indeed been shown to be, as in this case, secondary to coronary artery disease. However, if you interpret the symptom prematurely, once you start using the word "angina," you may forget the patient's story and ignore data that point to the correct diagnosis. **Premature interpretation compromises objectivity.**

For example, here is a 68-year-old woman who lived for several years with the diagnosis of angina—that is, coronary artery disease—because her physician did not "hear" the primary data. Here is how she described her chest pain:

> Tell me about this chest pain.
>
> *It's a soreness in here, right through here [pointing to midchest] a lot. Some pain in my arm and a feeling here. And a burning in the middle here and a burning in my throat.*
>
> When does this pain seem to come on?
>
> *Oh, it can be any time, doctor. Sometimes I even get it in the middle of the night.*
>
> How about when you walk or are active in any way?
>
> *No, I can just be sitting.*

Despite the fact that the patient did not have and had never had exertional chest pain relieved by rest, the clinician ordered a complete cardiac workup, including coronary angiography. Even though the test results proved negative, she carried a diagnosis of coronary artery disease and lived a confined and limited lifestyle because of fear. Finally, a new clinician heard the story of burning and the nocturnal occurrence of pain and ordered endoscopy, which revealed massive esophageal reflux with esophagitis and spasm. Perhaps it would have been more serious to overlook coronary artery disease, but for the patient much was lost. Frightened that she might die at any moment of a heart attack, she persisted in her belief that she had heart disease and was unable to be rehabilitated to an active life.

Objectivity means avoiding premature interpretation on your part; it also means distinguishing between the primary data and the patient's interpretation of what it means. This is important to remember when a patient tells you, "My ulcer is acting up," or "My heart is giving me a lot of trouble," or "I'm here for my Hodgkin's disease." In such instances, the patient is interpreting certain symptoms as indicative of the presence of peptic ulcer or other known disease.

Here, for example, is the statement of a 78-year-old man who called his clinician with the following complaint:

> *I don't know what's wrong. Somebody said I must have had the flu but it's lasted so long and I've tried everything and I don't know what to eat, so I just had to call and find out what you thought because it's been*

going on now 2 weeks and—you know me—I don't call unless I really have to. And someone said I must have appendicitis or what's that thing that old people get?

This patient (like many patients) focuses on the etiology of his problem and does not tell the story of his symptoms. All we know is that, whatever has been going on, it has been going on for about 2 weeks and is probably related to the gastrointestinal (GI) tract. The clinician's next response might be:

Well, some people who get the flu do feel sick for quite some time.

Although this response shows that the clinician has heard the patient's theory, the clinician still would not know what is going on; worse, it shows acceptance of the patient's diagnosis without obtaining any primary data whatsoever. A better response might be:

Well, some people who get the flu do feel sick for quite a while, but I'm not sure you had the flu. What exactly were your symptoms?
Well, I had severe diarrhea—just like water—for a few days and I hurt low down in my belly. And weak, awful weak.

The clinician now has some primary data with which to start putting the diagnostic puzzle together.

Although the patient's interpretation should be considered separately from symptom data, the interpretation should not be ignored; it is important to acknowledge the patient's belief about etiology as legitimate, whether or not you agree with it. Such recognition of the patient's point of view is necessary in a therapeutic relationship and will maximize your opportunities for patient engagement and education (see Chap. 16). In this case, the clinician might well explain why the patient's appendicitis theory is unlikely, rather than simply ignoring it.

PRECISION

Precision is a characteristic of the scientific process that relates to the distribution of observations around the "real" value. Precise observations cluster around the mean, whereas imprecise observations are widely scattered. The basic units of measurement in a medical interview are words. In a medical history, words describe sensations perceived by the patient and communicated to the clinician. As verbal measurements, words should be precise. They should be sufficiently detailed and unambiguous to indicate the "real" data.

In the issue of precision we are dealing not with a systematic bias that leads purposefully in one direction or another, but rather with random, unsystematic error introduced by vagueness, poor listening, or lack of attention to detail. For example, if a patient complains of being tired, does "tired" mean that the patient has shortness of breath, muscle weakness, lack of desire for activity, or sleepiness? Although the clinician may correctly register the patient's words, he or she may have no idea what is actually being described unless there is sufficient detail to distinguish among dyspnea, muscle weakness, lack of motivation, and somnolence. To make this distinction, the next question might go something like, "What do you mean by tired?" or "Can you tell me more about this tiredness?" or "How would you describe this feeling without using the word 'tired'?" The good interviewer attempts to discover as precisely as possible what the patient is actually experiencing.

Here is an example of a physician trying to get a precise history about the patient's chief complaint of headache:

See, I get these migraine headaches.

What do you mean by migraine headaches?

The last two headaches—I had two headaches last week, one on Monday and one on Thursday. Now they weren't real, real bad but the ones that I had before that, I threw up. I got real, real cold.

How often do you get these headaches?

I had two real bad ones within 2 weeks' time, then I didn't have one for a few weeks. Now the ones that I had last week, I didn't throw up with them, but they were enough that I had to go to bed with them.

Are the headaches something that occur almost every week, almost every month, or every couple of months?

I get them all the time. It is just within the last few months that I have been getting them more frequently. But I have averaged maybe one or two a month.

When you get these headaches, where does it hurt?

They start here and they just go around [demonstrating on his head]. Sometimes they'll go on one side of my face, sometimes on the other side of my face. But they start in the back of my neck here.

Do you get any kind of problems with your eyes when these headaches are coming on?

Blurred vision. The light bothers me.

Both eyes or one eye?

I have to go, like, I go upstairs in my bedroom and like close everything up, and I just lay down with a blanket.

What kind of problem does the light give you when you have a headache?

It just bothers me, just the light itself, it's like a glare. The light itself bothers me.

What do these headaches keep you from doing?

Everything. I can't do a thing. When I get one, I have to go to bed. That's exactly what I do. Usually I throw up with them. I get real, real cold. It

*can be 90 degrees outside, I'm freezing. Mostly the throwing up is a light
vomiting.*

Is there anything you can think of that triggers these headaches?

*Nothing, it just starts. I can get up with a headache. If I get up with it,
I'm done for the whole day. I do nothing at all.*

Do these headaches scare you?

No, I'm used to them.

Okay, so they don't frighten you, it's just a matter of trying to....

To get rid of them.

There is no unambiguous test for the etiology of headache; only a careful
and precise history can distinguish between migraine and other types of
headache. By asking, "What do you mean by migraine headache?" this clinician does not accept the patient's or previous provider's diagnosis of "migraine" (an interpretation) and goes on to get many details (precision) about
frequency, location, visual symptoms, and other associated symptoms.

SENSITIVITY AND SPECIFICITY

Accuracy and precision are two criteria by which we judge medical data, including the medical history. Two additional criteria are **sensitivity** and **specificity**. The sensitivity of a test expresses its ability to "pick up" real cases of
the disease in question. The higher the sensitivity, the greater the percentage
of cases identified accurately by the test as being cases. Specificity, on the
other hand, refers to a test's ability to "rule out" disease in normal people. The
higher the specificity, the greater the likelihood that a negative test result actually identifies a person who does not have the disease. Few, if any, tests in
medicine approach 100% sensitivity and specificity; certainly the medical interview will not yield such definitive information.

A symptom may be very sensitive (most people with pneumonia have
cough) but not specific at all (dozens of diseases cause cough); it may be relatively specific (nocturnal midepigastric pain relieved by eating in cases of duodenal ulcer) but not very sensitive (most persons with duodenal ulcer do not
have that symptom). This relative lack of sensitivity and specificity for individual symptoms is one reason why clinicians often minimize the value of history taking and rush into more "scientific" tests. However, an individual symptom is rarely the appropriate unit on which to base decisions; we deal, rather,
with symptom complexes, patterns, or stories. We consider a detailed recon-
struction of the illness, rather than isolated statements about symptoms—not
just one symptom, but many; not just one point in time, but the whole story.

A complete symptom complex may well be quite sensitive and specific; it
may be adequate, in fact, to serve as the basis for diagnosis and therapy. Even
when the "complete" history does not contain enough information for a correct diagnosis, the history usually contains *most* of the needed information.[2]

Moreover, the history narrows the range of possible problems dramatically and yields a very small number of hypotheses to be ruled out, supported, or confirmed by physical examination and further studies. The well-conducted patient interview will yield a firm (and large) database on which to design an efficient (and small) diagnostic plan. To achieve this result, however, the clinician must approach the task objectively and precisely. The real sensitivity and specificity of a symptom complex are irrelevant in a given situation if the instrument through which the data are obtained—you, the clinician—lacks accuracy and precision.

RELIABILITY

Reliability or **reproducibility** is another important characteristic of scientific tests, including medical interviewing. Different observers should be able to obtain the same results. In the medical history, however, reproducibility must be tempered by several considerations about human nature and the interactive process. In caring for a patient in the hospital, three or four observers are likely to obtain three or four different versions of the patient's story. Much of the time, the differences may not be of great significance, but sometimes they will be crucial. Only one of four observers, for example, may note that the patient has had bright red rectal bleeding intermittently for the last 3 months. This fact might be lost in the review of systems because the patient actually came into the hospital for chest pain and was either too embarrassed to mention the bleeding or, perhaps, too concerned about his heart to mention a seemingly unrelated problem. It suddenly becomes an important issue when you find the patient has a stool guaiac test result that demonstrates occult blood or a hematocrit value of 32%. The health care team might have to shift gears from an ischemic heart disease workup to a lower GI bleeding workup.

Of course, just as in the laboratory, data that change from one "experiment" to the next are suspect. Reproducibility is a characteristic highly valued in testing; this apparent lack of reproducibility makes many clinicians question the value of medical history taking.

There are several reasons why various observers may get varying stories at different times.

First, every patient comes to the hospital or the office with a personal story that includes a series of symptoms, but most patients have no benchmark indicating which of these are more or less important in explaining their underlying condition. A severe headache may cause more pain than a sudden swelling of the left leg, but the latter could be secondary to lymphatic obstruction by metastatic cancer, whereas the former may have no pathologic significance at all. Each time a person is asked to relate the clinical story, the person learns, by virtue of the questions asked, what is of most importance to the interviewer. The patient learns, in a sense, to "package" the story and make it more efficient or relevant or interesting to the clinician. Therefore, it is likely that later observers will get a more clearly connected and flowing—and certainly different—history than will the first interviewer.

Second, a corollary to this "educational" process is that patients may learn to consider important some things that they had not bothered to mention originally. The person may have forgotten the first episode of syncope or considered an illness that occurred 3 years earlier to be entirely unrelated to the current illness. Repetition and focusing on specific symptoms not only will make the story more coherent but will also refresh the patient's memory or, perhaps, set the stage for some new insight. Therefore, it is reasonable to assume that later observers may pick up entirely new information that the patient neglected to mention earlier.

For example, here is how a first interview might go with a patient complaining of headaches. Knowing the importance to the diagnosis of differentiating new headaches from chronic ones, the clinician, a student, proceeds:

> Tell me about your headaches. When did they start?
>
> *Well, I started getting them about 3 months ago.*
>
> Is that the first time you ever had this headache?
>
> *Well, yes.*
>
> So headaches are really new for you.
>
> *Well, now that I think about it, I can remember one something like it about 2 years ago. I remember, we were on vacation and I had to stay in the hotel. I thought I had the flu or something.*
>
> That's interesting. When did you get the next one?

For the next clinician, the attending physician, who interviews this patient, the story may be revealed as follows:

> Tell me when these headaches started.
>
> *Well, I guess the first time I ever had one was about 2 years ago. But then I only had one every few months or so; they weren't frequent until about 3 months ago when I started getting them every week.*

Although both interviewers ask similar questions, notice how the patient's story is more organized and straightforward on the second telling. The first interviewer had to "dig" harder for the onset 2 years ago and could have missed it entirely.

Third, sick people may have already "organized" their illness in some way that makes sense to them before they see the doctor.[3] They may have tried getting rid of the symptoms on their own and perhaps may have asked for advice from family or friends. They may have read health columns in newspapers, seen a "TV doctor" discussing a problem similar to theirs, or searched the Internet for information. In addition, patients may have religious or cultural beliefs that "frame" their understanding of illness in general and their own symptoms in particular (see Chap. 10). In these ways, patients usually develop hypotheses or reasons for their problems and have ideas about what can or should be done about them. Consequently, they are likely to tell their stories in ways consistent with these hypotheses; they will emphasize symptoms that support their theories and minimize or forget symptoms that do not. The primary data—perceived symptoms—are filtered through the patient's own beliefs. In the process of being interviewed by several different people focusing on medical hypotheses, a patient's own hypotheses about the data may change. And when the story is filtered through a different set of beliefs, the story's elements—perceptions, symptoms, and attributions—appear to change.

Fourth, different histories may be obtained at different times because the patient simply and consciously changes the story. Clinicians often invoke this reason when they dislike the patient or are unable to account for the symptoms. The more the symptoms seem to be unrelated to "objective" findings or diagnostic tests, the more likely clinicians are to consider them exaggerated or even imaginary and, therefore, susceptible to change from one history-taking session to another. Although some patients, of course, do change their stories, the so-called unreliable patient is a much less frequent explanation for apparent inconsistencies than the other factors we are considering.

Fifth, interviewing skills play a part as well. An empathic clinician who lets the patient tell his or her story is much more likely to obtain an accurate picture than a clinician who asks a list of questions by rote. Interviewing expertise probably bears a general relationship to the person's experience level (student, postgraduate trainee, practicing clinician), but when one considers an individual interview of an individual patient, all bets are off. The inexperienced student who is able to spend time with a patient in a nonthreatening atmosphere may learn a lot more than a hurried attending physician. **In general, interviewing skills that maximize objectivity and precision produce more accurate data and reduce the rate of false-positive (making a diagnosis that is not there) and false-negative (missing the diagnosis) histories.**

SCIENCE AND ART AT WORK

As you develop clinical skills, you learn techniques to achieve objectivity and precision in gathering primary data from patients (see Fig. 1–1). These skills make good science and, what is more, allow the patient to "connect" with you in a therapeutic relationship. Thus, the basic skills of interviewing as an **art** serve also as preconditions for the **scientific** collection and analysis of clinical data. **Throughout this book you will find that our emphasis is on the interdependence of science and art in clinical practice.**

Is there a contradiction between a "just get the facts" interview and an empathic interview? There is no such contradiction; you cannot obtain all the clinically important facts without utilizing humanistic qualities like respect, "understanding exactly" (one definition of empathy), and suspending judgment.[4] If you try to do so, the "facts" that you get may be irrelevant, or worse, untrue. Active listening (Clinical Key 1–1), the first step toward achieving ob-

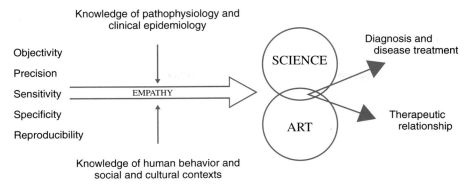

FIGURE 1–1   The art and science of medical interviewing.

jectivity and precision in the interview, is also the first step toward "connect-ing" with your patient and establishing a therapeutic relationship. The two are synergistic.

A patient says this best. The following is part of an interview in which the patient describes how it feels to be understood and not judged:

> *Aw, I'm not usually this able to talk to people like this. I don't really know you....*

CLINICAL KEY 1–1

 Active Listening Skills

- Remain quiet.
- Observe the patient.
- Let the patient talk.
- Listen for the primary symptom data. ("My head feels like it's caught in a vise")
- Listen to the words the patient uses.
- Listen to what's between the words: tone, pauses (paralanguage).
- Note discrepancies between *what* the patient says and *how* it's said.
- Listen for the patient's interpretation. ("I think I have a brain tumor")

but

- Do not confuse the patient's *theory* with the patient's *symptoms.*
- Do not form your own theory about the patient's illness until you obtain a precise description of the symptoms and a coherent narrative.

> That's true. I'm a total stranger.
>
> *And all of a sudden I have gone completely down the line and told you everything I could possibly think of to tell you. I've never been able to do that. I have very few people that I talk to personally or talk to about the way I feel ... um ... I talk to my family but there are only certain things that you can talk to your family about, and I have never had anyone I could talk to. I have always kept everything to myself. And now, all of a sudden, I've just flowed over like a broken toilet.*
>
> Was it helpful?
>
> *Yes, because I just learned something else about myself. The funny thing is, I have said all these things to you, and most times talking to people, I always think before I talk. I have said everything I have said to you without thinking about it first, and without wondering what you are going to think about what I am saying to you. And I can honestly say that I have never done that with anyone.*
>
> Uh huh.
>
> *I ... um ... have, maybe, I have a lot of friends but I mean, I even, I even think before I say what I say to them because there's always a chance that someone misinterprets.*
>
> Well, I'm glad. Because I like to think it's helpful.
>
> *It really is. I feel quite good about the whole thing.*

The patient here describes being able to say everything "without thinking about it first." He is describing his ability to reveal uncensored data that are vital to the diagnostic process; he was able to do this because he wasn't "wondering what you are going to think about what I am saying to you." This is precisely the aim of competent clinical history taking. Revealing uncensored data was crucial for this patient, who presented with a rash that proved to be secondary syphilis acquired in the course of multiple homosexual contacts. Had he filtered out the story of his sexual activity, about which he was embarrassed and ambivalent, the diagnosis would have been made less quickly or, perhaps, not at all. He later died of acquired immunodeficiency syndrome, and the need to communicate openly remained vital to his care.

SAGA OF THE FIFTH WHEEL

This section is an aside to address certain concerns of those who are just beginning to learn patient interviewing and physical examination. It is perhaps inevitable that the beginner sometimes feels like a spare part or a "fifth wheel." He or she has little or no responsibility for patient care. The patients may be sick, fatigued, and disgruntled at having to interact with a student. Besides their simple inexperience and the associated anxiety, students have several other realistic concerns about their first interviews. Three of the major concerns are:

- I don't know enough about pathophysiology to do a good history and physical examination, let alone to "get" the diagnosis.
- The patients have been worked over 10 times already and are generally tired of it all, and sometimes angry, by the time I come in to examine them.
- I have no responsibility for the patient, nor the ability to help, so I feel like an interloper—a fifth wheel.

Of course, each of these statements has an element of truth, but none of them need be a major constraint in your interviewing and physical diagnosis experience. Let us deal with each concern.

First, "I don't know enough pathophysiology." It is clear that you are not going to characterize patterns of symptoms as efficiently as an experienced clinician, nor will you be able to pick up subtle physical signs. You might, for example, examine a patient with gastroesophageal reflux disease before you study the GI tract in your pathophysiology course. You will complain, "I don't know what symptoms to ask about. I don't know what direction to take." As long as the content of the history (or physical examination) is all that interests you, there is no way to get beyond your lack of knowledge. However, the clinical art (and the point of this book) is to learn the process and method. Your goal is to learn to talk with patients in a way that maximizes both information gathering and therapeutic communication. The diagnosis (although interesting) is largely irrelevant at this point—you are not expected to make good diagnostic hypotheses without knowledge of relevant pathophysiology. Your goal is to characterize the symptoms and the person as precisely and objectively as possible and, more importantly, to create an interview situation in which this can occur. Unfortunately, some studies have suggested, at least in medicine, that the interviewing skills of clinical students actually decline as they progress through their training and learn more about disease.[5]

Second, "The patients have often had many other examinations and are sick and tired of it all." The anger your patient expresses (or just barely conceals) very frequently arises not from the mere fact of repeated examinations, but from the whole situation—being ill, having a backache that no one pays attention to, undergoing uncomfortable diagnostic studies, interacting with doctors who are rude or preoccupied and nurses who seem unsympathetic, and so forth. The anger is present even before you arrive on the scene.

How do you deal with this? It is crucial to clarify your role, not just as a student, but as a student learning to do an interview—someone who will not be taking care of the patient on the hospital unit. Then, make sure the patient has really consented to your interview and examination with a comment or question from you, such as "May I talk with you now about the problems that brought you to the hospital?" If he or she does not wish to talk with you and says so, let it go at that. For patients who are tired or in pain, suggest the possibility of your coming in later. If the patient seems angry, acknowledge the anger. This will give you a good opportunity to see how effective "interchangeable" responses can be in obtaining information and developing rapport (see "Levels of Responding" in Chap. 2).

Sick people, like anyone else, may have several mutually conflicting feelings at the same time. A given patient may want to be helpful to a student but simultaneously be angry about the situation, depressed about being ill, and simply exhausted. You can tip the balance in your favor: By being honest with the patient and really listening, you will avoid contributing to the patient's anger and will also tend to defuse it.

Third, "I can't help this patient." The issue of responsibility and helpfulness needs another look. The professional role is not something you put on overnight when you get your degree. You grow into it. As a clinical student, you are demonstrably more a clinician now than you were 2 years ago. Although still a learner, you are interacting with patients in a professional manner. The information you gather is important. Although the disease data you collect are only occasionally helpful, the personal data you collect will often contribute to the patient's well-being. If the patient has a specific request or complaint, you can discuss it with a unit nurse or resident. If the patient has a misunderstanding, you can clarify the problem or find someone else to do so.

Finally, simply listening to patients in an empathic manner is therapeutic. Listening might not repair the damaged myocardium or lower the blood sugar level, but it will make the patient feel better. That is, after all, what clinical medicine is all about, although the primary goal of helping another person feel better often becomes confused, or at least seems remote, in a busy office or hospital. The patient is in a strange environment with a potentially serious or life-threatening illness and is caught in a system—a health maintenance organization, an office, or a hospital—that is not always flexible or responsive to human needs. If you are willing to take the time to listen, you will be surprised at how therapeutic the encounter with you is for your patient, even though you are ostensibly "doing nothing."

SUMMARY ▪ SCIENCE AND ART IN INTERVIEWING

In this chapter we have stated one of the major themes of our approach to medical interviewing: the fact that conversation between clinician and patient is essential to both the science and the art of medicine. Because interviewing lies at the core of clinical science, we need to learn the following skills:

- *Objectivity* in clinician–patient interactions requires effective listening and responding skills.
  - Obtaining the primary symptom data enhances objectivity.
  - Jumping to premature interpretations compromises objectivity.
- *Precision* requires that the information we obtain be sufficiently detailed and unambiguous to use in diagnosis and treatment.

- *Sensitivity* requires that we use our interviewing skills to maximize our ability to identify "real" cases of illness.
- *Specificity* requires that we use our interviewing skills to maximize our ability to identify "real" cases of wellness.
- *Reliability* requires good interviewing technique to enhance reproducibility.

As shown in Figure 1–1, the science and the art of medicine are interdependent and synergistic. These fundamental skills enhance both.

Finally, a number of factors lead students who are just beginning to learn clinical interviewing to feel out of place, like fifth wheels. These factors, which may serve as barriers to learning and practicing new skills, include feeling as if you don't know enough, feeling reluctant to interact with patients who are tired and uncomfortable, and feeling awkward because you lack responsibility for the patient. In the next chapter, we explore the therapeutic core qualities, **respect**, **genuineness**, and **empathy**, which help overcome these barriers.

As we move on, basic skills used to obtain data from patients (objectivity, precision, sensitivity, specificity, and reliability) will enhance your ability to be empathic—that is, to *understand exactly* what patients are saying when they tell the stories of their illnesses.

References

1. Platt FW, McMath JC. Clinical hypocompetence: The interview. *Ann Intern Med* 1979; 91:898–902.
2. Rich EC, Crowson TW, Harris IB. The diagnostic value of the medical history. *Arch Intern Med* 1987; 147:1957–1960.
3. Kleinman A. *The Illness Narratives: Suffering, Healing, and the Human Condition.* New York, Basic Books, 1989.
4. Rogers C. *On Becoming a Person.* Boston, Houghton Mifflin, 1961.
5. Craig JL: Retention of interviewing skills learned by first year medical students: A longitudinal study. *Med Educ* 1992; 26:276–281.

Suggested Reading

Cassell EJ. *Talking With Patients. Volume 1, The Theory of Doctor-Patient Communication.* Cambridge, MA, MIT Press, 1985.
Cassell EJ. *Talking With Patients. Volume 2, Clinical Techniques.* Cambridge, MA, MIT Press, 1985.
Cohen-Cole SA. *The Medical Interview.* St. Louis, Mosby Year Book, 1991.
Feinstein AR. *Clinical Judgment.* Baltimore, Williams & Wilkins, 1967.
Rosenberg EE, Lussier MT, Beaudoin C. Lessons for clinicians from physician-patient communication literature. *Arch Fam Med* 1997; 6:279–283.
Smith RC, Hoppe RB. The patient's story: Integrating the patient- and physician-centered approaches to interviewing. *Ann Intern Med* 1991; 115:470–477.

CHAPTER 2

With Simple,
Kindly Words

● ● ● ● ● ●

RESPECT,
GENUINENESS,
EMPATHY

He longed to soothe her, not with drugs, not with advice,
*but **with simple, kindly words....***

Anton Chekhov, *"A Doctor's Visit"*

It is easy to agree that certain attitudes toward patients, such as genuineness and empathy, are praiseworthy. On first hearing this truism, you may think that these attitudes reflect the clinician's personality and value structure and are not immediately relevant to the medical history. You may not believe that these qualities are skills that can be learned and used. However, empathy and other qualities can, in fact, be understood as patterns of behavior. These behaviors can be practiced and learned.

In this chapter, we borrow some concepts from psychologists, particularly Carl Rogers and his followers, who first identified certain observable characteristics of the therapist that correlated with good therapeutic outcomes. They called them **therapeutic core qualities**, and the three most important were respect (or unconditional positive regard), genuineness (or congruence), and empathy.[1] They found that the content of psychotherapeutic intervention, such as the specific intervention dictated by a theory, was less important to outcome than the process of the interactions. Subsequently, other investigators defined specific skills evident in that process. They showed that qualities such as empathy, for example, could be broken down into a set of skills in listening to and responding to a patient.[2]

These therapeutic core qualities are important links between the art and science of medicine. They improve the interviewer's history-taking ability and the accuracy of the data obtained, and they lead to better therapeutic relationships in ordinary practice. In Chapter 1, we identified the goal of maximizing objectivity and precision in our communication with patients. In this chapter, we look at some generic concepts about how to do this before taking up the components of a medical history.

The following two examples serve to introduce these concepts. In one, the patient is a 50-year-old woman who, on her first visit to the clinic, complains chiefly of abdominal pain that becomes worse when she gets upset:

What happens when you get upset? What do you feel like?

Oh, I just feel right nervous, the stomach pains, my arm ... it pains, it seems like the strength is going out of my arm and hands.

How often do you get upset?

Quite frequently.

What's quite frequent?

Mostly every day it seems like I'm upset. I get something on my mind and that brings on the nauseated feeling.

So what's the usual sequence? You get upset first and then what happens? You get upset first or does the nausea come on first?

No. I get upset and then the nausea comes on.

Tell me about when you started being upset.

Oh really, right after my mother passed, really, in April, I've been mostly upset.

What happened when your mother passed away? I understand it must have been a very upsetting event; was she very close to you?

Yes, I was really close to my mother, and it seems like after she passed, I don't know, something just left out of me, I don't know what it was, you know.

In the second example, a new patient, a 40-year-old man, has come to the office for a checkup. The interviewer is inquiring about his family history and finds that the patient's father, who had divorced his mother, died of a ruptured brain aneurysm:

You don't know anything more about that?

Well, my understanding is, the context of this is, that my mother was raised in the Catholic Church, and divorce was a terrible scandal in her mind and she tried to forget about it as quickly as she could. It's such a painful subject that there was never any discussion about who he was and so forth. And as a consequence all I've really heard are niblets, and one of the things I understand is that my father was an alcoholic or at least he had a problem with alcohol, but really caused my mother a lot of problems. So, I don't know if that would be a complicating factor in terms of an aneurysm or not.

Not that I know of. How about brothers and sisters?

I have one full natural brother and then four half brothers.

Medical problems in any of them that you know of?

No.

And you work as?

An editorial writer for the Journal.

All we have are transcripts of the tape recordings, so we cannot reconstruct the tone or quality of the language or the nonverbal communication (e.g., head nods, eye contact, gestures). However, the clinician in the first example (who, by the way, is a student) appears to be connecting with the patient, acknowledging both the facts and the patient's feelings ("I understand it's a very upsetting event"). But in the second example, the practicing physician does not appear to be on the same wavelength with the patient; the physician's agenda has little regard for the other person. The patient has told the physician that his father died of a cerebral hemorrhage, but he does not know anything else about it because his parents were divorced. The divorce, the "painful subject," and the history of alcoholism that pour out are ignored by the physician, who abruptly answers the patient's overt question and moves on ("Not that I know of. How about brothers and sisters?"). The second excerpt gives us a feeling that (at least in this interview) the interviewer's history-taking skills lack the therapeutic care qualities of respect, genuineness, and empathy (Clinical Key 2–1).

RESPECT

Respect means to value an individual's traits and beliefs despite your own personal feelings about them and to see patients' feelings and behavior as a valid adaptation to their illness or life circumstances. Simply put, respect means being nonjudgmental. Some patients have irritating habits: smoking cigarettes, drinking too much, refusing to take medications, or even, at times, being antagonistic to their health care professionals. Other patients have beliefs about illness that try our patience: the man with severe emphysema might explain that his illness has nothing to do with his 100-pack-year smoking history but was caused by a cold he never got rid of in 1966. Another patient frustrates you with devastating migratory pains that refuse to go away, despite a normal examination and negative diagnostic tests. Some patients are obese or unable to keep themselves clean. Many have value systems different from yours or a healthy skepticism about the benefits of medical technology.

CLINICAL KEY 2–1
Therapeutic Core Qualities

Respect
The ability to accept the patient as he or she is.
Genuineness
The ability to be yourself in a relationship despite your
professional role.
Empathy
The ability to understand the patient's experiences and feelings
accurately, as well as to demonstrate that understanding to
the patient.

The skill in having respect is to separate your personal feelings about the patient's behavior or attitudes or beliefs from your basic concern—helping him or her get well. For example, the patient who believes that his emphysema is unrelated to smoking can still be guided to give a reliable account of his symptoms. Likewise, although the hostile patient makes you feel uncomfortable, you can still try to respect his or her reasons for being angry. Moreover, the emphysema patient's denial and the hostile patient's anger may actually be vital to their ability to tolerate their illnesses; such feelings should be accepted as part of the whole patient, not rejected as threats to the clinician's ego. When patients act in ways that make you anxious or angry, they ordinarily have good reasons—based in their beliefs—for doing so, although their reasons may be difficult for you to understand.

Respect involves valuing the patient as a person and as a historian. The following case example, taken from Platt and McMath,[3] demonstrates lack of respect in several ways:

> The interviewer failed to knock at the patient's door. He introduced himself in a hasty mumble so that the patient never had his name clearly in mind. He mispronounced the patient's name once and never used it again. The physician conducted the interview while seated in a chair about 7 feet from the patient. There was no physical contact during the interview. On several occasions, the patient expressed her emotional distress. On each occasion, the interviewer ignored the emotional content of her statements.

Exactly where is this pain?

It's so hard for me to explain. I'm trying to do as well as I can. [Turning to husband:] Aren't I doing as well as I can?

Well, is the pain up high in your belly, or down low?

I kept getting weaker and weaker. I didn't want to come to the hospital. I was so frightened [weeping].

Did the pain come before the weakness or afterward?

The physical examination was brusque; the examiner never warned his patient when painful maneuvers (for example, firmly stroking the sole of the foot) were to be done. At the end of the examination, the physician failed to comment on his findings or his plans. He said in parting, "We'll do some tests and see if we can find out just what's the matter with you," and left the room before the patient had an opportunity to question him.

Notice how the physician seems to have his own agenda, ignoring the patient both as a person, by not acknowledging her emotional distress, and as a historian, by not helping to clarify the nature of the pain and weakness. Clinical Key 2–2 presents a number of simple things you can do to demonstrate respect for your patient.

If the physician were demonstrating respect, the previous interview might have gone something like this:

Exactly where is the pain?

It's so hard for me to explain. I'm trying to do as well as I can. [Turning to husband:] Aren't I doing as well as I can?

I can see it's hard for you to explain and that you're trying hard. Perhaps you can show me where you are feeling it right now.

It's right about here [pointing] but what really frightened me was that I kept getting weaker and weaker and I didn't want to come to the hospital [weeping].

[Handing patient a box of tissues.] Here, do you need one of these? Was it the weakness that frightened you?

CLINICAL KEY 2–2

How to Demonstrate Respect for Patients

■ Introduce yourself clearly.
■ Do not use the patient's first name during an initial interview without permission ("May I call you John?").
■ Introduce yourself and explain your role.
■ Inquire about and arrange for the patient's comfort before getting started.
■ Continue to consider the patient's comfort during the course of your history and physical examination ("Would you be more comfortable if I lowered the bed?").
■ Warn the patient when you are about to do something unexpected or painful.
■ Respond to your patient in a way that shows you have heard what he or she has said.

Now the physician is focusing not only on the symptoms but also on the patient's feelings about the symptoms. In other words, the physician is communicating respect and, by so doing, is likely to acquire more accurate data in a more efficient manner.

GENUINENESS

Genuineness means not pretending to be somebody other than who you are; it means being yourself, both as a person and as a professional. The first time you encounter this concept of genuineness as a problem in medicine may be in your role as a student. How do you introduce yourself? Should you introduce yourself as a clinical student or as a clinician? Do you allow a patient to address you as "Doctor"? How do you respond when patients ask medical questions beyond your expertise or inquire about their own prognosis or care? Or when they say, "You look so young to be a doctor!" In all these cases, if you are to be genuine, you must acknowledge what you are: a student. You should introduce yourself as a student and, whenever appropriate, reaffirm to the patient your limited medical knowledge and limited responsibility (but not limited interest!) in the patient's care.

The terms "student doctor" and "student nurse," for example, represent useful concepts. They acknowledge the patient's need to perceive the clinical student in a professional helping role, while also genuinely describing what the student is. These terms also allow students to feel more professional and may facilitate a helping attitude toward the patient.

Interns, residents, physician assistants, nurse practitioners, and practicing physicians all experience situations in which patients ask for opinions or require procedures beyond the practitioner's capabilities. We may be required to call in consultants or refer patients to specialists. Genuineness requires you to be clear with the patient about what you do or do not know and can or cannot do, and to negotiate a plan for future care based on your capabilities. This aspect of genuineness is a component of being seen as trustworthy by your patients.

Being genuine also means being yourself in another way, that of expressing your feelings while staying within the bounds of a professional relationship. If a patient is in the hospital for a medical or surgical illness but has experienced a recent loss, such as the death of a spouse, it is desirable to respond to this fact with a statement such as, "I am sorry to hear that. How has it been going for you?" However, adding personal details (e.g., you too have lost a spouse or parent) may stress the limits of your comfort in a professional relationship. When patients say sad or comical things, it is appropriate to respond as a person and not just as a history taker. Demonstrating your interest in the patient as a person is another way of being genuine.

There are situations, however, when respect and genuineness may seem contradictory. Everyone has bad days, and you may happen to be at a low ebb yourself during your evaluation of the patient. You may have been on call and up all night with a patient in the intensive care unit. You may be having problems in your personal life or be eagerly anticipating a weekend of skiing when you leave the hospital. At other times, you may be outraged about the patient's behavior, such as canceling or coming late to appointments. What is the role of genuineness in these situations? Should you hide your feelings, disguise your bad day, or express them to the patient? Although genuineness means not pretending, it does not mean that you must share all your feelings with the patient. You must distinguish your genuine professional self from the vicissitudes, experiences, or interests of your personal self. As you go through training, you gradually develop your professional self into a well-integrated instrument of healing. It is this professional self that serves as the standard for genuineness. For example, the patient who makes you angry by continually not showing up for appointments can be told that you, as a person, are angry about that, but, as a professional, you try to confine your anger to that aspect of the relationship ("I know it's hard for you to get here, but when you're late I can't give you the time and the care that you need"). At the same time, you try to respect the patient by understanding his or her reasons for being late—chaotic lifestyle, three children younger than age 5, single parenting, the need to take two buses to get to your office, and so forth.

This discussion leads to two caveats:

- It is rarely helpful to share your personal anger or disgust with the patient in the name of being honest. You may confront the patient with inconsistencies (to you) in his or her story or point out the patient's erratic behavior, if you believe it will help therapeutically; this is not the same as sharing your own negative feelings.
- Sometimes clinicians are tempted to share their experiences and feelings as illustrations for the patient. This may range from statements like "I have young children too, and I know what you mean," to detailed personal anecdotes. Here again it is crucial to judge your personal revelations in the light of your professional judgment. Ordinarily, comments of rapport and connection are helpful. The type of car you own, the vagaries of parenting, or your opinions about a football team are not really self-revelations. On the other hand, it is rarely part of a genuine clinician–patient interaction to describe intimate experiences or specific moral values.

Here is an example of a genuine response by a medical resident who is seeing a woman with asthma, peptic ulcer, and numerous psychosocial problems. The patient has just related a personal history of abuse during her childhood, and continues:

> *I can write a book. Well, you know, I'm not any more, but I used to be atheist for awhile. God made me. I was a little girl, but I think about if you got children, you want the best for your children. If we are God's children, why did I go through what I went through? So that's why I feel the way I do.*

I think about that all the time when I see people who are sick. They didn't bring it on themselves. It makes you wonder. No answer to that one.

EMPATHY

Empathy is a type of understanding. It should not be confused with feeling sympathetic or sorry for someone. Nor is it the same as the virtue of compassion. Although compassion may well be your motivation for developing empathy with patients, empathy is not compassion. In medical interviewing, being empathic means listening to the total communication—words, feelings, and gestures—and letting the patient know that you are really hearing what he or she is saying. **Being empathic is also being scientific, because understanding is at the core of objectivity. The skill of empathy involves maximizing your ability to gather accurate data about the patient's thoughts and feelings.**

There are ways of responding to what patients say that will help you demonstrate to them that you understand. The data that the patient gives you about specific symptoms will be associated with feelings and beliefs. When you speak to patients, remember that you are speaking to a set of beliefs about the world. The elderly gentleman who gives you a detailed description of his abdominal pain may at the same time feel frightened because he fears that the pain means stomach cancer because his father died of stomach cancer. His description will be filtered through his fears and his belief; unless you attend to the worry, the patient may not give an accurate account of what he is actually experiencing. One such patient may magnify the symptom to ensure a complete workup that will not miss cancer; another may minimize the symptom in the hope of being reassured that it is not cancer. If the interviewer acknowledges the fear, it is easier to get an accurate idea about what is really going on.

An empathic response can also be important in helping patients clarify their feelings. At times, the patient will not be in touch with his or her own feelings. By checking within yourself—how would you feel, for instance, on finding blood in your stool?—you can formulate a response. Then, by checking back with the patient—by saying, for example, "That can be pretty frightening"—you as the interviewer can find out whether your assessment of what the patient might have felt is valid in that person's experience of illness.

LEVELS OF RESPONDING

It is useful to think of empathy as a feedback loop. You begin by listening carefully to what the patient is telling you, both cognitively and affectively. When you think you understand, you respond by telling the patient what you have heard. If you happen to be on the right wavelength, the patient will feel understood and be encouraged to reveal more of his or her thoughts and feelings.

If you do not get it right, but yet have demonstrated your interest by checking back, the patient is likely to feel comfortable in correcting your impression, thus giving you an opportunity to reassess and respond again.

Your assessment of the strength of the feeling that the patient is experiencing will influence what you say to the patient—in other words, your level of response. If the patient believes that you are picking up on everything he or she says and are listening attentively with a nonjudgmental attitude, not only will accurate cognitive data emerge, but also feelings and beliefs. In formulating a response, it is important first to assess the nature and intensity of a feeling that is expressed. For example, is the patient upset? If so, is he or she slightly concerned or furious? Your assessment will include not only what the patient says but also how it is said and how the patient looks when he or she says it.

In clinical interviewing, you must learn a professional way of responding, which is different from the way you might respond in social interactions. In social situations, we often ignore or minimize feelings. For example, when people say, "How are you?" or "How do you feel today?" they do not ordinarily expect you to reveal how lousy you are actually feeling. In the clinical setting, however, you really do want to know the slings and arrows of how the person is feeling. You acknowledge the intensity of any feelings expressed and demonstrate that you understand and accept them. Consider these four categories or levels of responding: **ignoring**, **minimizing**, **interchangeable**, and **additive**.

Ignoring

You either do not hear what the patient has said or act as though you did not hear. You give no response to either the symptom content or feelings. For example:

Most days my arthritis is so bad the swelling and pain are just too much.
And have you ever had any operations?

and

Do emotional problems at work seem to make it worse?
I think it's....
Do coughing, sneezing, bending, straining at stool, any of those things make it worse?
I never associated it with those things.

Minimizing

You respond to the feelings and symptoms at less than the actual level expressed by the patient. For example:

I was in agony with the pain and terribly frightened.
Well, I'm sure it wasn't that bad.

and

Most days my arthritis is so bad the swelling and pain are just too much.
What you need is something to take your mind off it.

Interchangeable

You recognize the feelings and symptoms expressed by the patient and assess them accurately, and you feed back that awareness at the same level of intensity. For example:

Most days my arthritis is so bad the swelling and pain are just too much. I can't seem to do anything at all any more and nothing seems to help.
It sounds as though the pain and disability are really getting to you.

and

I was in agony with the pain and terribly frightened.
Severe pain can be pretty frightening. Was it the pain that scared you or the thought of what might be causing the pain?

The interchangeable response is a good response in clinical history taking. It is usually a restatement in your own words of what the patient is trying to describe to communicate that you understand. When you give an interchangeable response, you are likely to find that it has a positive effect on the patient's ability to tell an accurate story. This kind of response is essential to being empathic.

In the following dialogue, the clinician responds to her patient's concerns even though she does not answer all the patient's questions right away:

But other than that I'm pretty good but it's my breasts I'm worried about. They started bleeding again, doctor. Why? I want you to take a look today. They're all bleeding in the inside. Is it anything to be concerned about?
Well maybe I can look and tell you.
Okay.
When did that start up again?
It seems like it will come and it will go, but now they're both all red and I noticed a whole lot of blood just drained out, especially this right one, it really hurts down there. This side don't hurt me, but this side hurts me [touches her breasts]. I don't know.
So you want me to take a look at your breasts [interchangeable response]. Is that what's worrying you most today, your breasts? Is there anything else?

No.

Okay, come and let me take a look. [Patient and clinician move to examination table, and she begins checking patient.] Okay, I can see why you're so concerned; it looks pretty raw here. Okay, this is pretty much like it was before.

Yeah, but it really does hurt.

Yeah, I can see that it hurts [interchangeable response]. This one is the worst, huh? Remember how well we were able to clear it up with medication the last time it got this bad?

Wonder what causes that. That's what worries me.

Yes, most women do worry about things that happen to their breasts [interchangeable response]. But this is not serious, although it's very annoying and painful. When bleeding comes from inside the breast, it is serious. But this is from the skin. It's more like a skin allergy. The skin is real sensitive.

Oh, is that what it is? Okay.

How does one achieve an interchangeable response? Two concise ways are through mirrors and paraphrases. A mirror (or "reflection") simply feeds back to the patient exactly what is said:

I feel really terrible.

You feel really terrible?

A paraphrase conveys the same meaning as the patient's statement but uses different words.

I feel really terrible.

So you're really not feeling well, are you?

Additive

In an additive response, you recognize not only what the patient expresses openly but also what he or she feels but does not express.[3] One common activity of clinicians that requires using additive responses is that of reassurance. This involves making an educated guess regarding what the patient is likely to be worried about and dealing specifically with those worries. Here is an example of an additive response during a follow-up visit by a young man with headaches:

Well, how are you? Are you still having headaches?

Saturday I had a bad one. I wasn't able to sleep for five nights; my system is so pumped up I can't sleep. The pills did work. I took one a couple of hours before I went to bed and one just when I went to bed.

You mean the pills I gave you before you went to the hospital?

> *Yeah. I took them two nights and last night was the first night I could sleep without them. I don't like to take a lotta stuff. I was having very strange effects from some of the medication.*

Like what?

> *Well, you know everything else about me, I might as well tell you this. Those green pills made me ... well, I can't describe the feeling it made me feel ... very strange. They also depressed me, believe it or not, even though you told me that they were antidepressants. I got depressed with them. For 2 days when I was taking them straight and in heavy doses, I found myself breaking into tears in situations ... I don't even cry when I want to [laughs]. It was very, very strange, so I stopped taking them.*

Okay. Can you tell me anything more about this strange feeling you had?

> *Ahhh.... [patient hesitates].*

Were you feeling like you were going to lose your mind? [additive response]

> *Yeah, I felt like I didn't have control over myself. I started to think I would get complications from the illness and how far behind it was making me get in my work because this is a very crucial time in my business. It really opened a lot of stuff for me. I never felt like this before.*

The ability to achieve an additive response comes with the experience of listening carefully to patients' stories over time and learning patterns from them. Note that in the previous example, the physician did not get it quite right. The additive response overshoots the patient's feeling, which was not so much "going to lose your mind" as it was "I didn't have control over myself." One of the benefits of an additive response is in facilitating this kind of correction, thereby improving accuracy.

An additive response also might be used for a patient with arthritis:

> *Most days my arthritis is so bad the swelling and pain are just too much.*

It sounds as though the pain is so bad that you think that things won't get much better.

If you have not gotten the sense of the statement quite right, the patient may respond:

> *Well, I do feel pretty bad, but I'm still hopeful.*

Here is another example of an additive response, this time in an interview with a 50-year-old woman describing her history of depression:

> *You know, sometimes I scare myself.*

You mean, you think about killing yourself?

> *Yeah, I do.*

USING WORDS TO IDENTIFY SYMPTOMS AND FEELINGS

Symptom Words

To increase your skill in responding appropriately, you need to pay attention to words, both your own and those of the patient. Professional education can sterilize your vocabulary. You become immersed in the language of medicine, which, although very precise in describing some attributes, leaves little room for feelings or emotions. Medical language is a language in which adjectives and adverbs carry little weight, and you are usually discouraged from using them in conversation. This socialization into the factual language of medicine can present real problems when you speak with patients. The world of the sick differs from the world of the well, but the difference does not include the sick learning the language of medicine. The most obvious problem you encounter with your medical vocabulary is that patients do not understand the words you use. When you say "hematemesis" rather than "vomiting blood," or "paresthesias" rather than "pins-and-needles sensations," your patient probably will not know what you are talking about.

Here is an example of a medical faculty member who was trying to ask a patient how much alcohol he drank:

> Okay. Do you use ethanol a lot, a little, weekends...?
>
> *Tylenol?*
>
> Daily?
>
> *Ethanol? Alcohol?*
>
> Drinks?
>
> *You mean ... alcoholic beverages? ... I usually have a drink every night.*
>
> Okay.

This doctor was thinking "use ethanol" rather than "drink alcohol," and the choice of words created some confusion, which in this case was temporary. Fortunately, the patient acknowledged the misunderstanding. Many times patients do not let on that they have not understood your statement. This is a particular problem with yes/no questions and with explanations or instructions in which no response is sought from the patient.

Feeling Words, Qualifiers, and Quantifiers

Another important result of medical language and thought patterns is our often-impoverished ability to describe feelings, qualities, and emotions with any accuracy or precision. Empathy requires both accurate understanding and feeding back this understanding to the patient. This skill demands that we identify not only symptoms but also feelings, not only quantities but also qualities. Patients use words to quantify many symptoms: how much pain, how

TABLE 2–1

DESCRIPTIVE WORDS FOR LEVELS OF FEELING				
Intensity	Anger	Joy	Anxiety or Fear	Depression
Weak	Annoyed	Pleased	Uneasy	Sad
	Upset	Glad	Uncertain	Down
	Irritated	Happy	Apprehensive	Blue
Medium	Angry	Turned on	Worried	Gloomy
	Testy	Joyful	Troubled	Sorrowful
	Quarrelsome	Delighted	Afraid	Miserable
Strong	Infuriated	Marvelous	Tormented	Distraught
	Spiteful	Jubilant	Frantic	Overwhelmed
	Enraged	Ecstatic	Terrified	Devastated

much blood, how much suffering, or how much vomiting. Although we are often more comfortable using numbers as quantities, patients frequently use analogies or comparisons to capture the intensity of their symptoms. For example, the patient who describes his pain as being as severe as a kidney stone is giving as precise a description as the patient who says that the pain is 8 on a scale of 1 to 10. Perhaps the former description is even more precise than the latter, because we may not know the patient's "10," but we do know that renal colic is one of the most severe pains a person can have.

Likewise, we must open up our windows to the world, and learn to use a broad vocabulary of feeling words. Table 2–1 presents examples of words that describe various emotions and their intensity. In giving an interchangeable response, you must "hit" not only the right feeling, but also the right intensity. The patient who says, "I am devastated by this pain" is not likely to believe you have really heard him or her if your response is, "So the pain upset you a little?" On the other hand, when the patient mentions that "I feel a little crummy today," the clinician is not sticking to his or her observations if the reply is "Sounds like you're feeling utterly hopeless." Once we accept the idea that medicine is about helping people to feel and function better, it is easy to understand how feelings reveal important data about the patient, which must be described as accurately as possible.

NONVERBAL COMMUNICATION

Nonverbal communication is the process of transmitting information without the use of words. It includes the way a person uses his or her body, such as facial expressions, eye contact, hand and arm gestures, posture, and various movements of the legs and feet. Nonverbal communication also includes paralinguistics—verbal qualities like tone, rhythm, pace, and vibrancy; speech errors; and pauses or silence. It is often through the nonverbal aspects of communication that we apprehend another's feelings. We recognize anger not so much by what a person says as by how it is said. Speech may slow down and get quiet in controlled anger, or the opposite may occur—with shouting and gestures such as pounding on a table. We can often tell when people lie unless they are good liars. They might look away, break eye contact, hesitate, or get "red in the face" (i.e., flush involuntarily). Common medical examples are the pressure of speech in the anxious or hypomanic person, or the flat voice tone of the very depressed. Patients who are ill often "sound" weak; we may gauge a person's state of health by how he or she sounds ("She's been through a lot of surgery, but she really sounds strong!").

Another component of nonverbal communication involves **kinesics**—that is, the use of personal space: how physically close we get to each other while talking to friends, business associates, lovers, patients. Other factors such as personal grooming, clothing, and odors (e.g., perspiration, alcohol, tobacco) also communicate information about the patient without words. For example, if a patient who is normally careful about personal grooming comes in disheveled and unkempt, you are alerted to the possibility of a problem even before he or she begins to speak.

Even though nonverbal communication may be obvious to you, the patient is likely to be unaware of it. This does not mean that nonverbal messages are invalid; in fact, they may be more accurate than the verbal message, precisely because they are usually unintentional and uncensored. Although it is interesting to note various aspects of nonverbal communication, you may wonder what to do with your observations. Look for consistency: note nonverbal behaviors, and determine whether they are congruent with the patient's verbal message. When congruence exists, the communication is more or less straightforward. However, when there is a discrepancy, an effort must be made to ascertain which is the "real" message.

Here is an example of a patient who came in for a routine follow-up of abdominal pain and reported first that her husband, from whom she was separated, died recently of some sudden and unknown cause (he was 27 years old). David is the child they had together.

> *I want to tell you something before we start.*
>
> OK.
>
> *David's dad died. And now, it's like every week it's something new.*
>
> Oh my. [Note the genuine response.] What happened?
>
> *I don't know. He just went to sleep and never woke up.*
>
> My goodness, when did that happen?
>
> *Last Friday, right before the ninth.*
>
> Oh, I am so sorry to hear that. Ah, how is David doing?

The clinician went on to explore how the patient and her son were reacting to this event, but the patient was discussing these usually sad issues with a bright smile on her face. Although she was separated from her husband, they had remained close because of David, and her cheeriness seemed inappropriate. What did the smile mean here? What kind of problem did this discrepancy suggest? Indeed, the clinician seemed more upset about this news than the patient. It later came out that the patient was having great difficulty, particularly in communicating to her son appropriate ways to mourn and remember his father. Although the clinician did not confront the patient early in the interview, he was alerted to a possible problem and later helped guide her toward a more appropriate response.

Often the nonverbal message is more accurate than the verbal statements. You may choose in some situations, especially early in the interview, simply to note a discrepancy and use it to help you understand the patient. Or you might use the nonverbal communication to modify your own nonverbal behavior, your conversation, or both. For example, if the patient seems tense, as evidenced by facial flushing or fidgeting, you may modify your voice tone and the way you are sitting in response to the patient's discomfort by speaking in a more soothing way and leaning forward to demonstrate your interest.

At the same time that you are observing the patient's nonverbal behavior, the patient is, perhaps unconsciously, observing your nonverbal behavior as well. As a result, your job is twofold: You should be aware of your own nonverbal behavior as well as the patient's. For example, if you seem uninterested, never looking at the patient or looking often at your watch, the patient may be unable to provide the details you need. Likewise, if you stand by the door rather than sit by the bed, patients may assume you are in a hurry and, respectful of your time, leave out critical data they decide are unimportant. Attention to your own nonverbal behavior requires a high level of self-awareness and discipline. It is particularly important to be conscious of how you respond to distractions during the interview, such as an emergency across the hall. You need to demonstrate your focus on the patient by maintaining eye contact, an attentive posture, and a seeming lack of awareness that all hell is breaking loose somewhere else.

Gestures

Although specific gestures have been the subject of study and suggested interpretations, their meanings must always be judged in context. When the gesture or facial expression appears to imply something different than the words, an effort must be made to ascertain which—the gesture or the words—is delivering the real message. Interpretation is no problem when a gesture "confirms" the patient's statements or the doctor's hypothesis based on those statements. Consider this example in which a patient is suffering from headaches. The physician learns that the patient has been under much stress recently.

So you have a lot of things on your mind.

Yes. About them, about some of the members of my family, and, um, mostly it's money worries, mainly money. [Patient puts her hand on the part of her head that has been painful.]

> It's funny, when you say "money worries," you know where you point to?
>
> *Huh?*
>
> You point right where it's hurting.
>
> *Yeah, aha.... That's mostly it, you know.*

In this situation, pointing out the relationship between financial stress (verbal) and tension headaches (nonverbal, pointing to head) might well be effective both in demonstrating your empathic understanding and in making explicit a connection the patient may already experience implicitly.

Table 2–2 presents a list of common gestures and some of their suggested interpretations. Two of these deserve comment. The helplessness or hopelessness gesture is typically biphasic. Both hands are raised briskly to face level, with elbows fixed, palms facing each other; they are rotated slightly outward, fingers spread, and thumb and fingers slightly flexed as though preparing to grasp. This position is held briefly, and then the hands fall limply down to the lap. This gesture suggests that the patient feels helpless about the problem or situation. The first part may represent reaching out for assistance, while the second part (hypotonia and withdrawal) emphasizes the futility of receiving any help.

TABLE 2–2

GESTURES AND POSSIBLE INTERPRETATIONS	
Gesture	**Possible Interpretation**
"Steepling" of hands involves joining them with fingers extended and fingertips touching, like a church steeple	Confidence or assurance of what is being said
Slight raising of the hand or index finger, pulling at an earlobe, or raising the index finger to the lips	A desire to interrupt the speaker
Helplessness or hopelessness gesture (see text)	Feeling of hopelessness; a request for help is futile
Respiratory avoidance response (see text)	Rejection of or disagreement with what is being said
Raising a finger to the lips	An attempt to suppress a comment
Crossed arms (note the manner in which the arms are crossed and muscular tension, especially in the hands)	A defensive gesture indicating disagreement, a sign of insecurity, or simply a comfortable position
Increased muscle tension, "white knuckle syndrome"	Fear or tension
Crossed legs	An attempt to shut out or protect against what is going on in the interview, or simply a position of comfort
Uncrossed legs, shifting forward in the chair	Receptivity to what is going on in the interview

The respiratory avoidance response includes frequent clearing of the throat when no phlegm or mucus is present. A variation of this is the nose rub, which involves a light rub of the nose with the dorsal aspect of the index finger. These gestures indicate rejection or disagreement with statements being made. For example, the clinician asks, "How are things at home?" The patient answers, "Fine," clears his throat, and lightly rubs his nose. He may actually be saying, "Things aren't really going very well at home."

Paralanguage

When you hear a patient's speech, you hear pauses, tone, and modulation, in addition to words. Likewise, the patient hears the pitch and rhythm of your conversation. Table 2–3 lists the elements of **paralanguage**. Paralinguistic cues can contribute significantly to your understanding of the patient and to the patient's perception of you as a helping person.

Let us deal briefly with just one aspect of paralanguage: pauses. The patient pauses a moment before answering your question, or before making her next statement. Why does she pause? The functions of pausing include:

- Absolute recall time
- Language formation time
- Censorship of material
- Creating an effect (timing)
- Preparing to lie

People rarely need to pause before recalling a place, age, or date fixed in time. For example, a person readily remembers the age at which a parent died, but might have to think a moment before remembering a living parent's current age. It is easy to answer a "yes/no" question without pausing, even if giving the incorrect answer: "Do you drink alcohol?" Yes. No. This has little meaning. Alternatively: "How much alcohol do you usually drink in a day?" or "Tell me about your use of alcohol." These questions demand some thought

TABLE 2–3

COMPONENTS OF PARALANGUAGE	
Component	**Examples**
Speech rate	Slow, fast, deliberate
Pauses	Long, short, inappropriate
Pause/speech ratio	Mechanical, halting, flowing speech
Tone or voice quality	Whiny, flat, nasal, bright, breathy
Pitch	High, medium, low
Volume	Loud, soft, wide variations
Articulation	Clear, precise, slurred

SOURCE: Adapted from Cassell EJ. *Talking With Patients. Volume 1, The Theory of Doctor–Patient Communication.* Cambridge, MA, MIT Press, 1985, with permission.

and integration. Listen carefully. How much of a pause occurs before the answer? How much stumbling or backtracking?

In general, it is helpful to listen to the number, quality, and placement of pauses. Frequent long pauses associated with low amplitude and a "dead" tone suggest depression. Frequent pauses over factual answers throughout the history suggest dementia or organic brain dysfunction. Pauses over answers in selected areas may indicate sensitive topics, with time required for censorship of material. We return to this aspect of medical interviewing later in this book, in the sections on truth telling and difficult interviews.

CHALLENGES TO UNDERSTANDING EXACTLY

Some history-taking situations present unavoidable technical difficulties. These include, for example, language barriers, the patient's state of consciousness (comatose, delirious, psychotic, or demented), and the patient's educational level, culture, or language skills. We review specific issues related to language and culture in Chapter 10 and interviewing elderly patients, who may have cognitive impairment, in Chapter 9.

With patients who do not speak our language or who are demented, we ordinarily dismiss the possibility of a useful interview and seek information elsewhere. We may arrange for an interpreter or elicit information from a family member. Other challenges to acquiring accurate symptom data are more subtle: language barriers may involve just a few crucial words or the patient's anger (see Chap. 12) may result in an inaccurate response.

Listen carefully for responses that seem inappropriate or confused. It is useful early in the interview to detect problems that lead to faulty data collection. Only then are you ready to proceed with eliciting the chief complaint and history of the present illness.

SUMMARY ▪ CORE THERAPEUTIC SKILLS

In this chapter we presented three fundamental skills of clinician–patient interactions:
- Respect
- Genuineness
- Empathy

Respect means to be nonjudgmental, and genuineness means being yourself—although a professional self—in the interaction with the patient. Empathy means understanding exactly what the patient is saying and letting the patient know that you understand. To enhance empathy in the clinical encounter:
- Strive for interchangeable responses.
- Develop and use a good vocabulary of descriptive words.

- Pay attention to nonverbal communication, especially paralinguistics.

Armed with an understanding of these fundamental skills, you are now ready to begin the interview, as we move on to Chapter 3.

References

1. Rogers C. *On Becoming a Person.* Boston, Houghton Mifflin, 1961.
2. Ivey AE, Authier J. *Microcounselling.* Springfield, IL, Charles C Thomas, 1978.
3. Platt FW, McMath JC. Clinical hypocompetence: The interview. *Ann Intern Med* 1979; 91:898–902.

Suggested Reading

Cassell EJ. *Talking With Patients. Volume 1, The Theory of Doctor–Patient Communication.* Cambridge, MA, MIT Press, 1985.

Cassell EJ. *Talking With Patients. Volume 2, Clinical Techniques.* Cambridge, MA, MIT Press, 1985.

Coulehan JL. Being a physician. In: Mengel MB, Holleman W (Eds.). *Fundamentals of Clinical Practice. A Textbook on the Patient, Doctor, and Society.* New York, Plenum Medical Book Company, 1997, pp. 73–101.

Coulehan JL, Platt FW, Egener B, Frankel R, Lin CT, Lown B, Salazar WH. "Let me see if I have this right . . .": Words that build empathy. *Ann Intern Med,* 2001, in press.

Lavasseur J, Vance DR. Doctors, nurses, and empathy. In: Spiro H, Curnen MGM, Peschel E, St. James D (Eds.). *Empathy and the Practice of Medicine.* New Haven, CT, Yale University Press, 1993, pp. 76–84.

More ES. "Empathy" enters the practice of medicine. In: More ES, Milligan MA (Eds.). *The Empathic Practitioner. Empathy, Gender, and Medicine.* New Brunswick, NJ, Rutgers University Press, 1994, pp. 19–39.

Platt FW, Keller VF. Empathic communication: A teachable and learnable skill. *J Gen Intern Med* 1994; 9:222–226.

Suchman AL, Markakis K, Beckman HB, Frankel R. A model of empathic communication in the medical interview. *JAMA* 1997; 277:678–682.

CHAPTER 3

Why Should You Come to Consult Me?

● ● ● ● ●

THE CHIEF COMPLAINT AND PRESENT ILLNESS

*"Never mind," said Holmes, laughing; "it is my business to know things. Perhaps I have trained myself to see what others overlook. If not, **why should you come to consult me?**"*

Arthur Conan Doyle, "A Case of Identity"

from *The Adventures of Sherlock Holmes*

In the next four chapters we discuss the traditional parts of a complete medical history—that is, the chief complaint, present illness, other active problems, past medical history, family history, social history or patient profile, and review of systems. In each section we introduce, describe, and illustrate skills or techniques useful for that part of the interview—skills particularly appropriate to the content or medical objective (e.g., the review of systems requires a different approach than the history of the present illness). This division of the interview is for simplicity of illustration only and does not imply that open-ended questions or interchangeable responses, for example, are useful only in the "present illness" section. Remember, too, that one does not necessarily proceed in this order or, for that matter, in one sitting. Sometimes you learn the family history in the opening moments of the encounter ("My mother had breast cancer, so I thought I'd better come in for a checkup"); or the patient profile evolves over several encounters with the patient.

This chapter deals with (1) the setting, (2) getting started, (3) the chief complaint, and (4) the present illness. When patients share their stories, they begin to make sense of their illnesses both cognitively and emotionally; and for the clinician, gathering the database helps to establish the etiology of the symptoms and the relationship with the patient.[1]

THE SETTING AND GETTING STARTED

In the past, clinicians usually first learned their interviewing skills with hospitalized patients. Although the emphasis is now on ambulatory care, students still frequently begin their experience in the hospital setting. The hospital is an unnatural habitat; as a result, the patient, who is "dis-eased," may not feel "at-ease." Patients may be similarly uncomfortable, although perhaps less so, in the clinic or emergency room or physician's office. When you see a patient for the first time, his or her blood pressure and pulse are often elevated, the face flushed, the handshake cool and damp, and the gestures clearly nervous. These characteristic signs indicate the autonomic response to the stress of illness, seeking help, meeting a new clinician, and the possibly unknown procedures and outcome. If you appear hurried, indifferent, or unsympathetic, the patient is likely to feel even more uncomfortable; this discomfort creates a barrier to effective communication.

The beginning of the interview sets the atmosphere for the rest of your history and physical examination. Quickly show your respect with a friendly greeting and begin by establishing a sense of privacy for the interview. For example, if there is another patient sharing the hospital room, draw the curtain around the bed. Even though this obviously does not provide a soundproof barrier, it provides the patient with a psychologic sense of privacy. If the patient can walk comfortably, it may be better to do the interview in a convenient lounge or waiting area, if this would be more private. If the patient has visitors, you might suggest that they wait outside or, if possible, that you will return later to see the patient. Before beginning the history, check to see that the patient is as comfortable as possible. Try to seat yourself in a way that will facilitate communication. People have spheres of "personal space": Get close enough for a person-to-person interaction, but do not intrude on the patient's intimate space.

In a small hospital room it may be difficult to place yourself comfortably so that you strike a balance between being halfway across the room and sitting on top of the patient. If necessary, move your chair. Try to sit at the same level as the patient; this helps establish good eye contact during the interview. Often it is most comfortable to sit at an angle to the person, rather than facing him or her directly: This allows you to maintain good eye contact, but also provides natural opportunities to look away at times. Good eye contact does not mean staring fixedly, which will only make the patient feel uncomfortable; there are always natural breaks in eye contact. You can also use your body to demonstrate interest: lean slightly toward the patient rather than lounging back in your chair.

Consider these guidelines:

- **Introduce yourself and explain your role.** Although local policies differ, if you are a student, we strongly suggest you introduce yourself as such. Besides being genuine and not using a professional facade, you will also be defining your limited **contract** with the patient. When the patient asks your opinion about his or her diagnosis or treatment, asks for pain medication, or requests anything outside your capacity to respond, you can comfortably remind the patient of the boundaries of your contract. You can tell the patient that you will convey the question to the resident or nursing staff, or suggest that the patient do so.

- **Don't begin by saying, "I've been asked (or sent) to take a history and do a physical."** Such a statement is likely to make the patient feel that you have no real interest in him or her and may set the interview off on the wrong track. A better start would be to say, "I'd like to talk to you today to get some information about why you're in the hospital, and then to examine you. Will that be all right?" As part of this introduction, you obtain permission (the contract) to do the history and examination; by so doing, you demonstrate respect for the person.

- **Taking notes is essential** because you will be writing up the information you obtain. As you begin, inform the patient of your need to take notes and the reason for it; this will also let the patient know what will happen to the information you are obtaining. However, don't let your note taking control the interview. If you attempt to record the conversation verbatim—with the exception of the chief complaint— the process of taking so many notes will interfere with the flow of the conversation. Eye contact will be limited if you are mainly concerned with note taking, and you are likely to miss the nonverbal communication, thereby interfering with rapport and missing useful data about the person. While you are making notes, look up frequently; this will demonstrate your interest. You will find with more experience that only an occasional word or phrase needs to be written down to help you remember, synthesize, and later reconstruct the story in complete written form.

THE CHIEF COMPLAINT

The **chief complaint** in a standard medical history is the main reason why the patient sought medical help. **It is usually recorded verbatim in the patient's own words.** The chief complaint is often elicited by such questions as:

- "How can I help you today?"
- "Can you tell me about your trouble?"
- "What symptoms made you decide to see a doctor/come to the emergency room?"
- "Can you tell me about your problem?"
- "Tell me about the main thing you feel is wrong."
- "What brought you to the hospital?" (Although this question may be subject to concrete answers like, "A taxi.")
- "Tell me why you came today."

Consider this example of how one medical resident began an interview with a new patient in an outpatient clinic:

> I guess the best place to start is to ask you what brings you here today.
> *Well, I haven't had a physical really for 6 years now, since my daughter was born.*

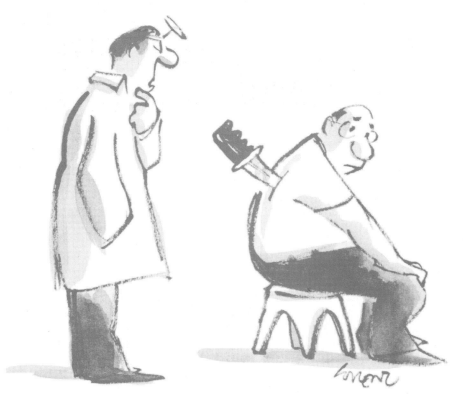

"It's got to come out, of course, but that doesn't address the deeper problem."

> I am going to be writing some things down on paper here, okay? Is there any particular reason why you chose now to come in?
>
> *I figured I kept putting it off and putting it off. I'd make appointments and put them off. There is no particular reason. I just felt as though it was time, I suppose.*
>
> Nothing is bothering you at this point?
>
> *No, it's just that I am overweight, that's all. I go up and down, up and down.*
>
> So that was your major concern, the weight problem?
>
> *Yeah.*
>
> Can you tell me about that?

The chief complaint, stated verbatim, is "It's just that I am overweight." It took a little digging to clarify that; the physician was appropriately not satisfied with "There is no particular reason."

Sometimes an opening question leads to a clear-cut chief complaint, as in this example:

> What can I do for you?
>
> *Um, the reason why I'm here is, since the latter part of July up to now, my bowels wouldn't move and I'd have to, in like 4 and 5 days, I'd have to take either milk of magnesia or a bulk laxative, and I just thought it was maybe something that I was eating, and this still continues until now, and it's the reason why I'm here to see you.*

In other cases, the same opening question might lead to a much more complex and rambling answer:

> Now what can I do for you, Mrs. P?
>
> *Well, first of all, I'm here mainly because I've been experiencing that tired, worn-out feeling most of the time. I can go to bed, say 9:00 in the evening, and get up at 8:00 or even later and I still feel very tired. And, I don't know.... I've still been experiencing hot flashes and sometimes now.... I don't experience them as often as I used to, but I still do, especially towards the evening or at night, and it awakens me when I do experience something like that. Maybe that's part of the reason why I felt so tired, I don't know. Anyways, now in the evening when I experience this kind of hot feeling, I just get that craving—I want to eat, you know, or sometimes it works just the opposite where I feel kind of nervous, I get that nervous feeling, and now last week I had headaches just about every day on arising; I had a little runny nose, so maybe, I don't know, maybe I could attribute that to a cold, but I'm just mentioning those things to you. And, sometimes you know my head just feels as though ...*

it feels stuffed ... when you have a head cold; that's just the way it has felt many times. And I had a hysterectomy, let's see, about 1992 or '93 and since then I just have had no sexual desire or anything. I mean, as far as I'm concerned that doesn't mean a whole lot. I know it upsets my husband a bit.

What is the chief complaint? Ostensibly, it is her first statement, "mainly because (of) that tired, worn-out feeling...," but in context the situation is less clear. What is really bothering her most? Why did she come here today, as opposed to last month or next week? This patient rambles on and on, presenting a challenge to the interviewer that we will discuss near the end of this chapter (see p. 55). The clinician permits this lengthy response, and, in so doing, acquires a wealth of useful information about the patient's symptoms and concerns. The clinician will later establish more structure for the patient to clarify her complaints. In contrast to this example, Marvel and colleagues[2] found that physicians often do not allow patients to complete their opening statements. Rather, they interrupt and steer the discussion toward a specific topic, thereby diminishing the chance of getting to the patient's real chief complaint.

The discursive patient is not the only one who presents problems in identifying the chief complaint, however. Often, the actual reason why the person comes to see the physician lies embedded somewhere else, far from the patient's initial statement (see cartoon on p. 41). Here is an example of a patient who presents with chest pain that he has had for some time:

I'm glad you came in today. Tell me why you came in.

Okay. I been having some problems with my chest; you know it's, it's like pressure and plus I have a knot under my arm, under my armpit.

Okay. You have pressure.

Yeah, I have pressure, and I don't know if it's because I smoke a lot of cigarettes, or I don't know what it is.

Um hum.

All I know is it's pressure across my chest. It's not what you call a pain or anything—it hurts; it's pressure all across here.

Um hum.

And, then, I have this knot under my, under my armpit.

Okay.

About the size of a half-dollar.

Okay, let's talk about the chest pain first; when would you say it started?

Um, I'd say about a month ago; maybe it might have been longer but I didn't pay it any attention.

> Um hum.
>
> *You know but I can't jog because if I just start jogging, it bothers me in my chest.*
>
> What made you decide to get it checked?
>
> *Well, two things actually, I want to get back in shape and I got a note from the Health Department that this test came back positive. See I'm a barber and they test for tuberculosis.*

By asking "What made you decide to get it checked?" this physician not only has the answer to why the patient came in now, but also an important new piece of data—namely, the positive tuberculin test result. We also learn that the patient may believe there is a relationship between his symptoms and the positive tuberculin test result. He really came to the doctor because of the test result, perhaps simply to fulfill a legal requirement for his license, and perhaps, in addition, because the test result made him reinterpret his chest problems as being more serious than he thought they were. In any case, if the workup for tuberculosis is negative, the physician knows that the patient will need reassurance that the cause of his trouble does not lie in the positive tuberculin test result.

When you consider why a person might come for medical help at a certain time, it is not enough simply to elicit the symptoms. The symptoms, as in the previous example, may have been present for some time. Although the answer to a question like "How can I help you?" frequently contains the core of the patient's problem, sometimes it does not. The **ostensible reason for coming**, as initially stated by the patient in the chief complaint, may not be the same as the **actual reason for coming**.[3] This is most often true with:

- People who have chronic diseases
- People with vague, chronic, or recurring symptoms
- People who say they just want a checkup

Alvan Feinstein[4] used the term **iatrotropic stimulus** ("iatrotropic," toward the physician) to indicate why the patient decided to seek care today rather than yesterday, tomorrow, or last year. If you can answer the question "Why now?" you have probably uncovered the iatrotropic stimulus or the actual reason for coming. Despite the fact that the person has an "acceptable" disease or symptom (congestive heart failure or shortness of breath), it may not satisfactorily explain why the patient is here today, as described in Clinical Key 3-1. If you really listen, the iatrotropic stimulus will come out during the interview. Sometimes it arrives only at the last moment, when you are about to walk out of the room and the patient says, "Oh, by the way, Doc, I'm sure this has nothing to do with it, but...."[5] We will touch on the "Oh, by the way" or "hand on the doorknob" phenomenon later, in Chapter 11. However, basic respect, empathy, and open-ended questioning early in the interview go a long way toward minimizing or avoiding that phenomenon. The earlier in the in-

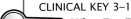

CLINICAL KEY 3-1

Why Do Patients Seek Care at a Particular Time?

- First, the symptoms of the illness may increase to the point that they become unbearable and the person simply realizes he or she needs medical help.
- Second, anxiety about the meaning of the symptoms may, for one reason or another, reach the point where the person seeks medical help, even though he or she may have been sick for quite a while, or may even have had a decrease in symptoms.
- Third, the symptom in the chief complaint is sometimes a "ticket of admission" to the physician's office or emergency room; the actual problem may be an entirely different symptom that the patient is at first afraid to mention, or it may be some life stress or crisis.

terview you ascertain the patient's reason for coming, the more efficient you will be, wasting less time digging for data. For example, the patient with the rambling "chief complaint" whom we met earlier in this chapter actually provides all of her concerns within the opening 2 minutes of the interview. The clinician can take notes and come back to each in turn, prioritizing for maximum efficiency. We will return to this technique in Chapter 11, when we discuss primary care interviewing.

THE PRESENT ILLNESS

The **present illness** is a thorough elaboration of the chief complaint and other current symptoms starting from the time the patient last felt well until the present. The best strategy for this part of the interview is often, first, to let the patient talk, then to use a variety of nondirective and directive questions to clarify and embellish. Generally you move from open-ended questions to more specific "Wh" questions (who, what, when, where, why, and how), laundry list questions (menus), or closed-ended questions, as appropriate, to achieve precision in symptom description.

Open-Ended Questions

Examples of open-ended questions are:
- "Can you tell me more about that?"
- "Did you notice anything else?"
- "What was the pain like for you?"

Another version of these open-ended questions is to restate them as gentle commands, requesting the patient to elaborate:

- "Tell me more about that."
- "Tell me what else you noticed."
- "Tell me what the pain was like."

Nondirective or open-ended questions are always a good way to start, allowing the patient freedom to talk and the examiner time to sit back and "size up" the patient. They are especially good for eliciting the less structured data of the present illness and the psychosocial aspects of the patient's problem. These questions allow the patient, who, after all, is the one who knows the story, to choose the most important symptoms and to point the way. The most nondirective of all statements are **minimal facilitators—** queries like:

- "Yes?"
- "Uh huh?"
- "And?"
- "And what else?"

Nonverbal cues, such as nodding your head in agreement or smiling, also may serve as minimal encouragement for the patient to continue talking.

Wh Questions

Nondirective questioning usually just sketches the picture, without giving precise detail. Patients only rarely spontaneously volunteer all the needed details; a rambling, vague patient may take too much time and still not provide the information you need, whereas a shy, reticent patient may say little or nothing. In a medical interview you move from the general to the more directive, but still open-ended, **Wh questions**. These describe the attributes of the patient's symptoms and specify the story. They are described in Clinical Key 3–2.

Directive and Closed-Ended Questions

Patient disclosure of relevant clinical information is most strongly correlated with open-ended questions, but other types of questions are usually also necessary to develop the patient narrative. **Laundry list questions**, or **menus**, are sometimes useful when a patient cannot find words to express a certain characteristic. For example, "How would you describe this pain—sharp, dull, burning, or tight?"; "Would you say it lasted a few seconds, a minute, 10 minutes?" Such questions obviously exclude other descriptive words and should be used only when a nondirective approach ("Can you describe the pain?") and Wh questions ("What is the pain like?") have both failed.

Directive, or **closed-ended, questions** provide detail; they are good for emergency situations ("What's your name?"; "How old are you?"; "Are you allergic to any drugs?"), for reticent patients, and for structured data, such as the past history and the review of systems. They are also useful as focused questioning when you have already generated hypotheses in the interview and are

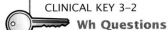

CLINICAL KEY 3–2

Wh Questions

WHERE
Exactly where is it on your body? *or* Show me where it is.
WHAT
What does it feel like? *or* Tell me what it feels like.
WHEN
When did it start? Does it come and go, or does it stay?
When does it occur (episodic, inception and duration,
    fluctuation, and frequency)?
HOW
How is it altered by season, by time of day, by sleep, by food,
    by exertion, and so forth? Describe how your daily activities
    affect it.
WHY
Why do you think it occurs? Why do you think you have this
    problem?
WHO
Who is affected by it? (consequences to patient and other
    people)

trying to build a case for one particular diagnosis. However, a "high control" interview in which the interviewer asks one directive question after another will produce false or incomplete evidence, not to mention a discontented patient. Some other examples of closed-ended questions are:

- Are your parents still living?
- Did you actually pass out?
- Have you ever been anemic?
- Does this pain occur when you take a deep breath?
- Is there any trouble with your vision?

One does not ask yes/no questions in situations in which information may be sensitive, because a lie will close off all access to that information. For example, it is not useful to say, "Do you drink alcohol?" if one suspects alcohol may be a problem; try, "How much alcohol do you usually drink in a day?"

Finally, there are at least two types of questions to avoid.

- **Avoid leading questions**, which encourage certain responses from the patient to fit the interviewer's own hypothesis, such as "You're feeling better now, aren't you?" or "That pain wasn't on the left side of your chest, was it?" This type of query suggests to the patient what you want (or don't want) to hear.
- Likewise, **avoid multiple questions**, such as: "Do you have any trouble sleeping and how about coughing?" Sometimes these slip out,

TABLE 3–1

TYPES OF QUESTIONS IN THE MEDICAL INTERVIEW	
Start with ↓	Open-ended questions (general) Open-ended questions (topical) Minimal facilitators
Proceed to	Wh questions Laundry lists or menus Closed-ended questions "Yes/no" questions
Avoid	Leading questions Complex/multiple questions

because your mind is working too quickly and dragging your tongue along with it. Slow down; wait. Table 3–1 summarizes the various types of queries employed in taking the medical history.

Symptom Description

Throughout the history of the present illness, it is important to describe the patient's symptoms as carefully as possible without jumping to conclusions. For example, "I'm having trouble breathing" does not necessarily indicate dyspnea on exertion; it could indicate stuffy nose or the chest sensation of a pregnant patient at term. It is also important to avoid jumping to conclusions about the meanings of words. Many words popularly used to describe symptoms mean different things to different people. Examples are "diarrhea," "constipation," "tired," "dizzy," "my side," "sick," "weak," "high blood," "low blood," "insomnia," "gas," and "heartburn." The novice has a tendency to establish quantitative aspects of symptoms ("How many times a day?") before establishing the qualitative aspects. The expert interviewer attempts to establish what he or she is dealing with ("Are the stools soft or watery?") before measuring it. You want first to make sure that you and the patient mean the same thing by, say, the word "diarrhea"; then you can fill in the quantitative data. Table 3–2 presents examples of patient statements, followed by either quantitative (prematurely specific) or qualitative follow-up questions.

The symptom called "dizziness" presents a prime example. A patient comes in and says, "My main problem is dizziness. It just came on me about a month ago, and it's been getting worse now. I'm so dizzy I can hardly stand up sometimes. What's wrong with me, Doc?" The first thing wrong is the word "dizziness." There are at least four symptoms commonly labeled with this word:

- Vertigo, a definite sense of rotation or environmental motion
- Presyncope, the sensation that loss of consciousness is about to happen
- Disequilibrium, the sensation that balance, especially during walking, is impaired
- Lightheadedness, a vague head sensation that is not vertigo and not presyncope

TABLE 3–2

REPORTED SYMPTOMS: EXAMPLES OF QUANTITATIVE AND QUALITATIVE CLINICIAN QUESTIONS		
Complaint	**Quantitative Questions**	**Qualitative Questions**
I've been having chest pain.	How long have you had it? How often does it come?	What does it feel like? Where exactly is it located?
My side hurts.	How long have you had it?	Show me where.
I have diarrhea.	How many times a day?	What do you mean by diarrhea?
I vomited blood.	How much?	What did it look like?
I can't walk as far as I used to without getting tired.	How far can you walk?	What do you mean by "tired?"

Some people also idiosyncratically label weakness, fatigue, or anxiety as dizziness.

The following exchange, adapted from Reilly,[6] shows an example of a clinician trying to find out precisely what a patient means by dizziness:

> Can you describe what you mean with words other than dizzy?
>
> *I feel out of balance. I feel like I might fall down even. I haven't yet, but I get awful woozy when I walk.*
>
> Is it mainly when you walk that you have trouble, or do you get this feeling sometimes when you are sitting or resting?
>
> *I guess it is mainly when I am up and around.*
>
> Can you tell me, then, how you feel bad when you walk? Try not to say dizzy.
>
> *Well, I feel I'm unsure of myself. I can't trust my walking.*
>
> Does everything around you spin or move, or do you feel like you're spinning?
>
> *No, not exactly.*
>
> Do you feel like you are going to faint?
>
> *I feel like I will fall, not faint.*

Notice the mixture of open-ended and directive questions that the clinician uses to characterize as precisely as possible what the patient is experiencing. There is much more to find out about this symptom, but from the exchange so far the patient appears to be describing disequilibrium rather than vertigo, presyncope, or lightheadedness.

Consider another example in the following interchange with a patient who indicated the need to come in because of cough. Note how the clinician begins with an open-ended question, but specifies that she wishes to hear about the cough, then follows up with Wh questions until the symptom is characterized.

Tell me about the cough that you've been having.

It's just worse at night, I can't get no sleep.

What happens?

I'm up on three pillows. I'm just miserable, that's all.

You go up on three pillows to try to prevent the cough?

Yes.

How is it miserable?

Well, if I lay flat I can't breathe, and then I start gasping and gasping for breath, and the only way I can stop is when I sit up and watch TV or something.

The patient in this example actually suffered from congestive heart failure with orthopnea: she became short of breath when she lay flat in bed. She experienced tightness in her chest and a sense of "gasping" for breath that she chose to call "cough." Later in the conversation, the clinician learned that she had chest pain and dyspnea on exertion as well as these nocturnal symptoms.

In this next, longer example, the clinician wants to pin down the exact timing of the onset, duration, periodicity, and pattern of chest pain because he is concerned that this 62-year-old smoker may have coronary artery disease and knows that only precise symptom description will guide the diagnostic process. Each time the patient gives a somewhat vague statement, the clinician follows up with an attempt to clarify.

... and a little bit too fast, it might just be my imagination though, I don't know.

Uh huh. When did this all start? [Wh question]

Well, just since the weather has been hot, like it is, you know.

Several weeks it's been going on, would you say? [clarification]

Uh huh, just—now the chest pain is not continuous, like, during the day, I don't have to be doing anything, I can just be sitting.

And where do you feel it? [Wh question]

It's in here. And like full, just too full, it's fullness in here.

And then how long does it last when it comes? [Wh question]

Not too long.

Minutes, hours? [clarification, laundry list]

Not hours, just maybe a half hour, or something—you know, it doesn't last.

Do you do anything that seems to relieve it? [Wh question]

No, I don't take anything, just sit and be quiet, or either I'll rest.

Uh huh. [minimal facilitator]

And rest seems to help, when it starts acting up, whenever I could or would be doing around the house, I let it go and just rest.

Does it sometimes come on while you are doing something? [closed-ended question]

Yeah, mostly, if I'm doing something like trying to sweep or clean in the house, or something like that.

How about with walking? [clarification, closed-ended question]

With walking sometimes, and like mostly. I'll go up to the mall every day and that way I am inside walking and they have benches, I'll sit ... when it starts acting up.

And then how long does it take to go away once you sit? [Wh question]

Once I sit, oh, I'll say, half an hour to an hour.

And it will take a half hour or an hour to go away?... [clarification]

...Uh huh.

Or do you sit for that long even though it's gone before that? [clarification]

Uh huh. I just sit for that long until it eases.

And it takes a half hour to an hour for it to ease up? [clarification]

Uh huh.

Notice how the clinician in this example tries to establish a pattern of chest pain brought on by exertion and relieved by rest. Perhaps the most critical detail to establish if one suspects coronary artery disease is the length of time it takes for the pain (in this patient, a "fullness" in the chest) to ease with rest. In typical angina, the pain ceases after several minutes or less. This patient is not typical. It is likely that had the response been "Less than 5 minutes" to the question "And then how long does it take to go away once you sit?" the clinician would not have requested further clarification.

Summarization, Confrontation, and Clarification

Summarization is a technique by which the clinician feeds back to the patient the main points of what has been said thus far. Frequent summaries help (1) ensure that the interviewer has the story straight, (2) provide focus, (3) serve as transitions from one topic to another, and (4) keep the interviewer organized. A summary may be as simple as repeating a particularly important statement to see if you have it right, such as "Okay, as I understand it, the pains you had in 1998 were exactly like the ones you're having now...." In other cases, a brief summary helps you get back on track if the patient is wandering and switching topics, such as "Okay, we'll get to the cough in a minute, but I need to understand your chest pain better. You said it was like a heavy pressure right in the center of your chest, and it lasted about 5 minutes...."

Summaries are also very useful as transitions from one part of the interview to another. Here is an example of a summary that segues from history of the present illness to the past medical history:

> *So that's about how it happened.*
>
> Okay, let me see if I have it straight. You felt perfectly well until 2 days ago when you began to notice an uncomfortable feeling right in the middle here around your belly button, and this has gradually gotten worse, and you are now also having diarrhea. [Patient nods.] OK, I think I understand pretty well what's been going on the last 2 days. How about in the past, have you had any problems with your health in the past?

Sometimes as you try to summarize, you note discrepancies in the story; and because you want to know exactly what happened, it is usually necessary to point out those discrepancies. When you do this, you are using **confrontation**. This rather dramatic word has connotations of pointing out falsehoods, rationalizations, or neurotic conflicts, and in its everyday usage often implies opposing sides. In the medical interview, however, confrontation is simply an attempt to clarify inconsistent statements; you heard one thing and now it appears that the patient is describing the experience differently, or contradicting an earlier statement. Which version is right? For example:

> Now let me see if I can understand this. You said before that you were coughing up some bloody stuff with that heavy cough last year. But just now you said, when this cough developed yesterday, it was the first time you ever saw blood come up. Did I misunderstand you?

In other words, confrontation is a device to clarify the data. You say what you heard, but ask for more detail, perhaps to resolve ambiguities in the story, as in the earlier example of our patient with chest pain.

A FEW EXAMPLES

Here are three examples of beginnings of interviews. In each case, we have labeled the clinician's statements or questions with the technique being used. Note the importance, in this part of the interview, of social greetings, nondirective questions, minimal facilitators, clarification, and summarization.

EXAMPLE 1

> Okay, hello again. I'm Dr. Block. Tell me what I can do for you today. [social greeting, nondirective question]
>
> *Well, I have a terrible vaginal itch, and I don't know whether it's the vaginitis or whether it's the urine, urinary tract infection. My regular doctor treated me for vaginitis.*
>
> That was Dr. Hill? [clarification, facilitation]
>
> *Uh huh. Then I got, um, a urinary tract infection and then the vaginitis came back. But during the whole ordeal, I've never got any relief.*

During the treatment for the vaginitis, during the treatment for the urinary tract infection, you still had this terrible itch? [summary, clarification]

EXAMPLE 2

Good morning. [social greeting]

[Patient is seated on end of exam table.] Good morning.

Why don't you have a seat back over here, and we can talk a little bit first. Tell me why you came today. [attending to the patient's comfort, nondirective question]

Um, to get my blood pressure checked.

To get your blood pressure checked? What do you know about your blood pressure? [reflective response, nondirective question with topic specified]

Well, I have heard various things over the past couple of years, really, that it has been high, and um....

For several years? [clarification and facilitation]

[Nods] And I went about, oh, it was quite a while ago, maybe 5 or 6 months ago to the health center, um, and the doctor told me it was high, but he could not treat me until I lost approximately 38 pounds, so I haven't been able to take the weight off and I was kind of, well, he did not give me any special diet to follow or you know, what I should cut out of my diet, and I was very discouraged by it, so when I went to the emergency room because I cut my finger, um, the nurse told me that my blood pressure was very high and I should have it checked, and since I don't have a family doctor, she suggested I come here.

EXAMPLE 3

It's nice to see you again. What brings you here today? [social greeting, open-ended question]

Doctor, I'm not well.

I take it you have not been feeling really well for a while. [summary based on previous knowledge of this patient]

No, well, I haven't been feeling very good for about the last, oh, I'd say about a week, about a week now.

Uh huh. [facilitation]

About a week now, I haven't been feeling good.

What have you noticed? [nondirective question]

Oh, some soreness in here right through here, and some pain in my arm and a, a, a strangulating feeling right in here and a burning in the, in the middle, right here and a burning in my throat, a little bit, and dizzy—I felt real dizzy when I was on the scale out there, you know, and I called you and the nurse, and she helped me and I wasn't real bad and you know, I told her to open a window and she said first "Do you want me to open a window?" and I said "Yeah and I want to get near the air."

Does that help? [clarification]

Oh yeah.

CHALLENGES TO ELICITING THE CHIEF COMPLAINT AND PRESENT ILLNESS

The patient's style of speaking may present challenges in getting a coherent story. The profoundly depressed patient may not have enough energy to give a detailed, logical story, whereas the anxious and talkative patient may embellish his or her story with unnecessary details. Some patients are so reticent that you find yourself asking a series of narrow, closed-ended questions until the interview comes to a distressing stop. Other patients have so much to say that you feel as though you are losing control in a confusing quagmire. You worry that, when the interview is over, you may know a lot about the patient but very little about the illness.

The Reticent Patient

The Problem

The reticent patient simply says nothing, or almost nothing. When only a limited amount of information is needed (e.g., a patient with an acute laceration or a sore throat), this may not be a problem. There are other times, however, when lack of detail seriously compromises history taking, such as for the patient on p. 50 with chest pain, in whom a detailed and unambiguous history is essential for making the diagnosis.

The Remedy

The trick here is to guide the reticent patient without asking leading questions; sometimes one way of asking an open-ended question works where another way does not. Consider this example:

Can you tell me what the problem is?

Uh, that's what I came to see you about, Doc.

What have your symptoms been?

Tired, awful tired.

It almost appears as though the interview will come to an end with the first question, but the interviewer simply asks another open-ended question that, this time around, elicits the chief complaint. A "laundry list" or menu is another useful technique. This interview went on:

> Can you tell me more about it?
>
> *No, just tired.*
>
> When you say tired, do you mean a feeling of not being rested or a feeling of weakness in your muscles? Or do you have trouble doing things you used to do because you get short of breath?
>
> *That's it, Doc, just not rested.*

The physician uses a menu to clarify the symptom without leading the patient. Notice the difference between asking the patient to choose from several possibilities and raising the same possibilities in a sequence of yes/no questions. In the latter case, you can never be sure that the patient is not simply saying what he or she thinks you want to hear.

Patients may be reticent because of depression, dementia (simply cannot remember the symptoms), anxiety, denial, a taciturn personality style, or cultural distance from the physician. Some patients expect to be interrogated like witnesses. These persons may have trouble with an open directive like "Tell me what happened," and respond better to more structure: "Tell me what happened first," and then, "What happened next?" They may need frequent reminders demonstrating your open, relaxed attitude, such as "It is important for me to know exactly how you felt when that happened—tell me as best you can."

The Patient Who Rambles

The Problem

Some patients embellish their problems with numerous seemingly unrelated details. In other settings such persons might be considered exquisite story-tellers, but you have a limited amount of time for the interview, and entertainment is not your goal. Sometimes the details seem connected to the story, as with our patient on p. 42; at other times it is difficult to see any connection at all. At times the details are related to the medical history but are unnecessary, such as the patient who has an attack of diarrhea and describes in great detail his or her attempt to find a bathroom.

The Remedy

The trick is to direct the patient back to the task at hand without appearing to be rude or disinterested. One way to do this is to acknowledge your own confusion and feeling of being lost in the details, as well as your need to accomplish the task at hand. Most patients accept this kind of direction very well. For example, you might say to the patient with diarrhea:

> It certainly sounds as though you had a hard time with that episode; since our time is limited, though, perhaps you can tell me more about the diarrhea itself. Tell me what it was like.

In this instance the physician uses a summary statement ("sounds as though you had a hard time") and a reminder of time constraints, followed by a question that directs the interview back to the characterization of the illness.

In the case of the patient on p. 42, an interviewer's open-ended question ("Now what can I do for you, Mrs. P?") leads to a deluge of disconnected information that would leave most clinicians feeling totally bewildered and wondering where to go next. Although this patient may have stated most of her medical history in one fell swoop, it is difficult to sort it out. Many clinicians are reluctant to ask open-ended questions because they fear receiving precisely this kind of rambling response. In reality such responses are infrequent. When they do occur, it is best to acknowledge your confusion and try to direct the patient to one topic at a time. One possible reply might be:

> Okay, I'm getting a bit confused. Let's see if we can take one problem at a time. You mentioned tiredness even though you seem to get a lot of sleep. Other than the hot flashes, is there anything else that seems to wake you up at night?

Either during or after the interview, you will have a chance to think about why the patient talks this way. Among the causes are anxiety, loneliness, histrionic personality style, thought disorder, or a particular set of beliefs about how symptoms and events are related. Sometimes this kind of response is simply the person's conversational style, which is less appropriate in the context of a professional relationship than it is in a social interaction. Sometimes the associations are so bizarre that you must consider psychiatric illness as the cause.

The Vague Patient

The Problem

With the vague patient, the interviewer cannot figure out exactly what the patient is describing. You may wonder whether the symptom itself is vague or whether it is simply the patient's description of it that is vague. Some sensations are difficult to describe, such as dizziness or poorly localized abdominal pain. When you know the patient, it is easier to judge the source of the problem. The patient who, in the past, has always given a precise history is probably experiencing a vague sensation, whereas a patient who has a vague conversational style may well have a precise symptom that simply requires more work to translate into medically useful words.

The Remedy

One technique for the vague patient is to provide a choice of useful descriptors without leading the patient. For example, you might use a menu such as, "Was the pain sharp, dull, or burning?" or "Was it all over, or in just one place, or did it move from place to place?" Alternatively, you can ask if it resembles a symptom with which both the patient and physician are familiar, such as (for lower abdominal or pelvic pain in a woman), "Does it feel anything like menstrual cramps?" Another approach is to ask the patient if he or she has ever felt anything like this particular symptom before, and then to ask, "What's different about it this time?" To find the location of a vague symptom, you can ask the patient to point to where it hurts.

In this example of a vague opening, the clinician simply indicates that vague terminology such as "cold" or "flu" (… tell me more about what you mean") is unacceptable, and the patient begins to describe the symptoms in more detail.

EXAMPLE 1

What can I do for you?

[Clearing throat] I think I've got, um, a cold or flu or something … yesterday I felt terrible, so I feel I just need some kind of a prescription.…

OK. Tell me, you say you have a cold; tell me more about what you mean.

Um [Clearing throat] fatigue is the most.…

Fatigue?

Just kind of drained.

Aha.

Kind of scratchy throat, not really sore. Ah, a lot of drainage.…

Coughing?

A little bit, but not getting anything up.

Just sort of dry?

Dry coughing, I don't feel as though there's anything collected down there yet. And, that's another thing that worries me, having had a history of asthma, I have a fear of bronchitis.

EXAMPLE 2

Sometimes the patient does not respond to simple requests for more precision:

Well, doctor, well, I got the dizziness, I'm getting more, looks like I'm, looks like I'm getting tired and more tired, I go up the steps and I just, just like dizziness, I, I go like this, I just go dark, I, and I can't see.

> What do you mean by dizziness?
>
> *When I go up the steps and when I get up in the morning, I got that dizziness again, I'm just falling back.*
>
> What happens to you when you're dizzy?
>
> *Well, when, when I drink water, if I drink cold water, that's when I get it, then I start having chills, I get real cold, just like I'm shaking.*
>
> But how do you feel when you're dizzy?
>
> *I just go back, like this, and then sometimes I, I can't see, I, I have to close my eyes like that and then open my eyes up like that and I still can't just like....*

In this example, we are left wondering whether the patient's description is vague or the symptom is vague. The clinician could have tried asking, "Tell me what you mean, but try not to use the word 'dizzy.'" Another possibility would be to provide a menu:

> When you say dizziness, is it a feeling that you may pass out or that you may lose your balance?
>
> *No, not exactly.*
>
> Could you describe it as a spinning sensation as though you or the room is moving, or is it more of a lightheadedness?
>
> *That's it, lightheaded, just lightheaded.*

Whether the patient is reticent, rambling, or vague, the clinician's goal is to obtain a story that is clear, internally consistent, logical, and not fictional. Most patients share these goals but may not necessarily share with the clinician the same criteria for judging the story. Your first approach is to clarify, teach, or demonstrate the kind of story that will be helpful. If this approach does not work, you are probably faced with one or more of three issues:

- The patient's personality style, perhaps stressed by the illness, interferes with telling an adequate story.
- A strong emotion gets in the way of the patient's telling a clear, logical story.
- The patient's beliefs are sufficiently different from yours that a story that appears incoherent is actually quite logical once you understand the basic premises from which the patient reasons.

We examine these issues in Chapters 10 and 12.

SUMMARY ▪ CHIEF COMPLAINT AND HISTORY OF THE PRESENT ILLNESS

In this chapter we discussed, first, how to set the stage and get started:
- Establish a sense of privacy for the interview.

- Introduce yourself appropriately and establish a contract.
- Maintain an attentive body position.
- Minimize distractions.
- Take notes, but maintain enough eye contact so as not to "lose" the patient.
- Use language the patient can understand.

The next step is to obtain the chief complaint:

- Record the chief complaint in the patient's own words.
- Consider the possibility that the iatrotropic stimulus, or actual reason for coming, is different from the ostensible chief complaint.

With regard to the history of the present illness, we presented the following facilitative techniques:

- Move from the general to the specific, using open-ended questions to introduce each topic.
- Use nonverbal encouragement, like silence and head nods; and minimal facilitators, like mirrors, paraphrases, and saying "Uh huh," "And?" or "Yes?"
- Proceed to Wh questions to characterize symptoms.
- Employ menus or direct questions when necessary for specification or efficiency.
- Strive for interchangeable responses to show that you are listening and to encourage disclosure of accurate information about thoughts and feelings.
- Avoid leading questions that reveal the answer you expect or desire, or multiple questions that confuse the patient.
- Give the patient time to answer in his or her own words.
- Clarify and maintain direction for both the patient and yourself by using summaries, clarification, and, when needed, confrontation.

Among the challenges to obtaining a good narrative are various interactive styles, including those involving patients who are reticent, rambling, or vague. Various techniques may help you overcome these challenges.

References

1. Adler HM. The history of the present illness as treatment. Who's listening and why does it matter? *J Am Board Fam Pract* 1997; 10:28–35.
2. Marvel MK, Epstein RM, Flowers K, Beckman HK. Soliciting the patient's agenda: Have we improved? *JAMA* 1999; 281:283–287.
3. Bass LW, Cohen RL. Ostensible versus actual reasons for seeking pediatric attention: Another look at the parental ticket of admission. *Pediatrics* 1982; 70:870–874.
4. Feinstein AR. *Clinical Judgment.* Baltimore, Williams & Wilkins, 1967.
5. White J, Levinson W, Roter D. "Oh, by the way ..." The closing moments of the medical visit. *J Gen Intern Med* 1994; 9:24–28.
6. Reilly BM. *Practical Strategies in Outpatient Medicine.* Philadelphia, WB Saunders, 1984.

Suggested Reading

Lipkin M Jr. The medical interview and related skills. In: Branch WT (Ed.). *Office Practice of Medicine,* Philadelphia, WB Saunders, 1987, pp. 1287–1306.
Platt FW. *Converstaion Failure. Case Studies in Doctor-Patient Communication.* Tacoma, WA, Life Sciences, 1992.

CHAPTER 4

Transforming Experience into Memory

● ● ● ● ●

OTHER ACTIVE PROBLEMS, PAST MEDICAL HISTORY, AND FAMILY HISTORY

To hold a true belief about an event in one's past experience is not sufficient for remembering it. There is still a distinctive factor lacking.... Now it sometimes happens that a belief ... **transforms itself into a memory.**

A. J. Ayer, *The Problem of Knowledge*

Once you have elicited the chief complaint and present illness, other parts of the history, although tedious at first, are, in a sense, easier because they deal with structured data and specific questions about predetermined topics. The trick is to emphasize the relevant features of past health and medical care experiences without getting too overwhelmed with a mass of detail. Feinstein[1] has cautioned us to avoid the "Scylla of overdirection" and the "Charybdis of digression." By this he means the ability to keep your inquiry open-ended enough to avoid missing the important events without getting bogged down in endless details about unimportant events.

This chapter and the two that follow cover parts of the medical interview that fill in the total picture of your patient's health and illness experience. These aspects of the interview provide important details that enhance your evaluation of the person's current illness and your response to it. In this chapter, we discuss the search for other active problems, the past medical history, and the family history. These components provide you with information about the context or setting in which the illness occurs, including the previous state of the patient's health, as well as the presence of risk factors that have implications for both the current diagnosis and the prevention of future ills.

OTHER ACTIVE PROBLEMS

You have just made it through the history of the present illness, working hard to maintain the narrative thread (what happened first, what happened next) without getting sidetracked by distractions, such as a too-early preoccupation with what the diagnosis is. You begin to build the themes of the interview: what the story of the illness is, who the patient is, how the interview is going. You progressively narrow your focus to delineate a single problem or condition that you hope will explain the patient's symptoms and findings. At this point, however, you should step back and ask yourself: What am I missing here? What else could be going on with this patient? In other words, what are the patient's **other active problems** (OAPs)?

Patients often have a number of chronic conditions that may affect their current distress. The notion of a singular "present illness" that is quite distinct from "past medical history" is not tenable: the patient who comes to the emergency room because of fever and productive cough may at the same time be under treatment for diabetes, hypertension, coronary artery disease, and osteoporosis. In this case, the patient has several active medical problems, any of which may contribute to the current syndrome or must be considered in responding to it. Thus, it is crucial to differentiate these problems from the traditional items in past medical history (e.g., appendectomy in 1986, motor vehicle accident in 1994, allergy to amoxicillin noted in 1989).

The search for OAPs may be accomplished by asking nondirective questions at the end of the present illness segment of the interview. For example:
- "Okay, I think I've gotten the story straight so far. Has anything else been bothering you?"
- "Can you think of other symptoms or problems that you've had recently?"
- "Do you have any other illnesses that have been acting up lately, or that you see a doctor for?"

In this way other problems that relate to, or influence, the present illness may be uncovered early, thereby avoiding last-minute surprises during the review of systems. A patient may be admitted to the hospital with pneumonia but may also suffer from chronic renal failure, diabetes, and hypertension. These chronic illnesses are also current problems and clearly affect the situation at hand.

Another good screening question for OAPs is, "What medications do you take?" ("Insulin shots" may be the response of the patient who forgot to mention diabetes.) Regardless of how the patient responds, always broaden your inquiry to include any regularly used drugs, such as oral contraceptives (which the patient may not consider a *medication*), aspirin, cold preparations, pain relievers, herbal remedies, and over-the-counter laxatives. Remember also to ask about vitamins or mineral tablets. Because many people consider these "natural" products and not medications, they may not mention them unless specifically asked.

Here is an example of an interview in which a 62-year-old retired metal worker came to the office for a complete checkup "because I've never really had one." The clinician picks up on other active problems at the end of the present illness segment:

> Okay, so the main concern you have, aside from wanting a checkup, is this pain in your left side. Are you having any other problems with your health?
>
> *No, nothing really. As I said, the main thing is to establish a relationship with a family doctor.*
>
> Okay, that's good. Let me find out a little more about you. Do you take any medications?
>
> *Yeah, well, Dr. Gold has had me on that Vasoretic for a few years for my pressure.*

Notice how this patient, like many people, requires repeated open-ended prompts to reveal continuing and obviously important details about his health. What is going on here? Certainly, the patient is not trying to hide the fact that he takes medication for hypertension; indeed, it may have become so routine to him that he doesn't initially label it as a health "problem." Most likely, the clinician would have stumbled on this information later in the interview during an extensive past medical history or an exhaustive review of systems, but it is an important feature to know up front: in a routine checkup, chronic hypertension makes a difference.

The past medical history sometimes also presents opportunities to explore OAPs. If the patient reports serious, chronic, or ill-defined symptoms in the past, it is a good idea to ask if these or similar symptoms are occurring now.

THE PAST MEDICAL HISTORY

Clinical Key 4–1 presents some good ways to begin the past medical history. Patients may respond in general terms such as, "I've always been sickly," or "Well, I used to have stomach problems," or, alternatively, begin to discuss particular symptoms. Adult patients frequently have one or more chronic illnesses, and each of these may have had several exacerbations or have required hospitalizations at different times. They may or may not be relevant to

CLINICAL KEY 4–1

Good Ways to Begin the Past Medical History

- "How has your health been in the past?"
- "Tell me about how your health has been in the past."
- "Tell me about any serious illnesses you have had in the past, starting from when you were a child."
- "Now I'd like to ask you about any illnesses or medical problems you've had in the past. How has your health been?"
- "Okay, I think I understand what's been happening in the past few weeks, how about your health in the past?" and then, progressing to more specifics, for example:
- "Have you had any emotional or psychiatric problems in the past?"

the current illness. You should focus the inquiry on discrete episodes that caused substantial disability or a difference in the usual health pattern, and attempt to determine the diagnosis they, or their clinicians, have given to these illnesses.

You should never simply assume that a diagnosis the patient relates is, in fact, the correct medical diagnosis. For example, a patient might tell you that he or she has had "four or five heart attacks" in the past when, in fact, the patient has never suffered an acute myocardial infarction; this problem arises because the term "heart attack" means different things to different people. A good question to ask is "What exactly were your symptoms that made your doctor think that?"

There is no point, however, in trying to confirm every item of the past history by grilling the patient on obscure details. Your time and energy and those of the patient are limited. Here is how one clinician, who himself became a patient, expressed his feelings about being asked "ancient history":

> It's bad enough that I don't know all my family's medical diseases or what my grandparents, whom I never knew, died of, but I begin to feel positively stupid when at the mature age of 44 I do not know whether as an infant I had measles or chickenpox. I may do a little better with more recent conditions, but the feeling sinks again when it comes to medications I've taken that have given me trouble. "Those little red pills" seems an insufficient answer, and the recording physician's dubious look does not help much.... By this point in the interview, when I am asked questions about the specific timing and location of my varying symptoms, I begin to answer with a specificity born more of desperation than accuracy.[2]

After you acquire general information about the person's past health, you fill in important categories of past medical history (as shown in Table 4–1). Old records can and should be obtained when, based on your evaluation, you believe the information will be relevant to caring for the patient. A couple of pointers on specificity:

TABLE 4–1

PAST MEDICAL HISTORY

Serious illnesses, beginning in childhood
Hospitalizations
Surgical procedures
Accidents or injuries
Gynecologic and obstetrical history (women)
Allergies
Current medications
Immunizations

- **Dates.** The exact date or year of an illness, if remote, is generally not important. Inquiry that is too precise will lead both to frustration and to falsely precise answers ("specificity born of desperation"). A "hysterectomy in the early 1970s" is usually adequate; it does not matter whether it was 1972 or 1973.
- **Allergies.** You should clarify what your patient means by the term "allergy." A person may tell you he is allergic to flu shots because, after having one, he had several colds that winter, or another may tell you that she is allergic to aspirin because it gives her stomach discomfort. The first case is a personal attribution of a poor outcome, and the second case illustrates a side effect rather than a true allergy to aspirin. Be sure to ask specifically about allergies to medications.

Here is an example of a past medical history obtained from a 39-year-old woman at her first office visit for evaluation of headaches. She was found to have elevated blood pressure. Note the ease with which the clinician prepares the patient for each new topic:

Okay, let's talk about your past health. Did you have any unusual childhood illnesses, problems at birth or as an infant?

Bronchitis.

Bronchitis. What do you mean by bronchitis?

Well, I'm not sure. That's what my mother told me. I guess I used to get sick a lot when I was a kid.

Were you ever hospitalized? Any serious illnesses or operations?

Well, I've had D & Cs done, and I had my appendix out with part of my ovary.

Part of your ovary came out and...?

Well, I have a history of cysts growing on my ovaries. My gynecologist says I'm okay now.

Now, you mentioned you have two children. Any problems with your pregnancies or with childbirth?

With my little girl, yes. I had a lot of water, plus I had a bladder infection.

> **Did you have high blood pressure with that?**
>
> *No, but I was sick a lot, nauseated a lot. It was like morning sickness but I had it for 8 months with her.*
>
> **Doctor put you to bed at all?**
>
> *No.*
>
> **Any other hospitalizations, any other medical problems in the past that you had that you can remember?**
>
> *No, just the D & Cs and the children and that one operation I had.*
>
> **Do you have any allergies?**
>
> *I am allergic to goldenrod.*
>
> **To what?**
>
> *Goldenrod. Wool. I have hay fever. Anything like flowers—I get around them, I constantly sneeze my head off or get stuffed up. Roses, stuff like that. Right now, I'm having a time because we went up to the lake and we have a lot of goldenrod growing wild.*
>
> **Do you take anything for it?**

This is an example of a fairly typical and complete past history that demonstrates how "old" news is relevant to the present problems. Notice how the interviewer asks exactly what the patient means by bronchitis. Although the patient is not sure, she later reports symptoms of allergy. Symptoms of allergy plus a childhood history of bronchitis suggest atopy, with the "bronchitis" perhaps representing episodes of childhood asthma. The patient has now "outgrown" her asthma but still has an atopic disposition, as evidenced by the hay fever symptoms. The clinician also uncovers the history of fluid retention during pregnancy. This symptom could indicate pre-eclampsia, which may be relevant to her hypertension now. Notice how the interviewer asks specifically if the patient had high blood pressure. He also tries to determine if she was treated for hypertension without realizing it by asking, "Doctor put you to bed at all?" Another way to ask would be, "How was that treated?" The question regarding whether the patient takes anything for her hay fever is relevant for at least three reasons: (1) to avoid the embarrassment of recommending something the patient has already tried, (2) to help ascertain symptom severity, and (3) to learn if medications that can raise blood pressure in susceptible persons were used.

FAMILY HISTORY

The **family history** is the systematic exploration of the presence or absence of any disease in the patient's family that may influence the patient's health or risk of particular diseases. What illnesses and conditions are relevant? They include:

- Frankly hereditary diseases, such as sickle cell anemia or osteogenesis imperfecta
- Familial illnesses, such as coronary artery disease, adult-onset diabetes mellitus, or carcinoma of the breast, in which genetic factors play a significant role
- Family traits, such as short stature
- Illnesses such as manic-depressive disorder or alcoholism, which may not only be familial, but may also profoundly affect the patient's psychosocial environment
- Current illnesses in the family that *may* suggest an infectious process or toxic exposure in the environment

And what do we mean by "family"? To determine the risk of hereditary disease, we generally mean the patient's parents, siblings, and children. The patient's grandparents, cousins, aunts, and uncles are of somewhat lesser importance. The spouse is a vital member of the patient's family but is of no importance to familial disease. In dealing with contagious disease and toxic exposures, however, we might expand the concept of "family" to include the whole household, perhaps in this instance even including coworkers.

The family history always enriches our understanding of the patient, whether in making a diagnosis or in managing the illness, but because time and energy are limited, the potentially enormous amount of information must be tailored to the specific situation. How much we want to know depends on the patient, the type of problem, and the ability of the patient to give the information. For example, a family history of breast cancer is obviously of less relevance to a 10-year-old boy with tonsillitis than to a 45-year-old woman with a breast mass. A seriously ill patient may have a very relevant family history but be too sick to give it. This might be the situation, say, in a seriously ill patient with an acute myocardial infarction whose father died of a heart attack at age 44; the family history can wait until the patient feels well enough to remember and discuss the details. Clinical Key 4–2 presents good ways to start the routine family history.

CLINICAL KEY 4–2

Good Ways to Begin the Routine Family History

- "I'd like to know a little about your family."
- "Are there any illnesses that seem to run in your family?"
- "Has anyone in your family been seriously ill?"
- "How about your parents? Children?"
- "Has anyone in your family had heart attacks?"
- "Do you have any concerns about problems that you think run in your family?"

Although not strictly speaking "family history," in the case of acute, possibly contagious disease, you must inquire about possible family exposures. For example:
- "Has anyone else at home or work been sick lately?"
- "Have you come into contact with anyone who has similar symptoms?"

Here is an excerpt of a routine family history that will give you a sense of the flow of this part of the medical interview. Notice how the clinician first introduces the new subject area (a transition) and then goes on with a specific question:

Okay. I think I understand the symptoms. Now I'd like to find out a little about your family. How about your parents, are they still living?

They're deceased.

Do you recall what they passed away from?

My mother had a heart attack 2 months ago.

How old was she at that time?

63, I think.

How about your father?

About 7 years ago.

What did he pass away from?

Lung cancer.

How old was he?

Oh, I'd say 57.

Brothers or sisters?

Yes, I have nine brothers—I mean I have five brothers and three sisters.

Do they have medical problems that you are aware of?

No.

Is there any history of high blood pressure in the family?

My mother.

Your mother, okay. How about diabetes?

No.

The clinician begins with a general question about problems or illnesses, then follows up with some specific yes/no questions about illnesses that one tends to see in families, such as hypertension and diabetes, or illnesses of particular relevance to this patient, who has hypertension.

But we observe something else here. Notice that the patient's mother is *recently* deceased. The clinician here faces a choice about how to proceed, given this information. Should she explore the patient's feelings, or continue with the family history? In this instance, the interviewer proceeds with the history and this approach appears to be useful. Had the patient's mother died at an advanced age after increasing illness or disability, the clinician would expect the patient to feel differently than if she died suddenly at a relatively young age. A potential problem here is that the clinician accepts the stated diagnosis of "heart attack" and learns little more. There are many possibilities: Was it a sudden event? Were there many previous attacks? Was she sickly for years, perhaps with rheumatic heart disease and a final deadly "attack"? And what of the resulting effects on this person—the patient—with a sickly mother? The clinician will, later in the interview, return to her recent loss and deal with it more effectively and compassionately. Information about diseases in the family has social, as well as medical, dimensions. Everyone has feelings about his or her close relatives, especially parents and children. We must acknowledge, be prepared for, and deal with these feelings in a compassionate way during the interview.

Knowledge about family history shapes the patient's beliefs and worries about health, health risks, and current symptoms. A patient with chest pain may believe that she has a bad heart like her mother, even though she is young and suffering from a totally different type of problem. A patient approaching the same age at which a parent died may have special concerns about his or her own health. Consider this family history in a 41-year-old woman who came because "it's been a while since I had a good checkup":

Your parents still living?

My father is living. My mother died when she was 42.

How is your father? Is he in good health?

Uh huh.

How old is he?

He was born in 1930.

So he's 71.

Yes.

Any brothers or sisters?

Two sisters. Both are in good health as far as I know. I don't keep very good contact with them, because I live here and they live out of state.

Any medical problems? You said there are some medical problems that run in your family. What are they again?

My mother had a bad heart. Most of it is in my mother's family. Like my grandmother died, she had cancer. She had diabetes too. When my mother died, she had had a plastic valve put in, then slowly deteriorated. She had sclerosis of the liver and a bad heart. She lived about a year after she had the plastic valve put in.

A woman who dies at the age of 42 after having an artificial valve probably had rheumatic, or possibly congenital, heart disease. Although there is some chance that the daughter may suffer from a similar problem, of more relevance is the daughter's beliefs about the matter. Note that she is 41 years old and her mother died at age 42. If she is found to have no signs of heart disease, it will be important to reassure her that her symptoms are totally unrelated to what went on with her mother.

Even the most straightforward questions sometimes lead to double-edged answers:

> You said you've been pregnant five times?
>
> *Yes.*
>
> Do your children live at home with you?
>
> *Yes.*
>
> Five of them?
>
> *Yes.*
>
> How old are they?
>
> *20, 15, 13, 10.*
>
> That's four children.
>
> *Oh, I lost one.*
>
> Did he die of disease?
>
> *No, he died—he had a little growth on his eye and he died in surgery.*

The interviewer dedicated to using a mechanical set of family history questions could have simply ignored the fact that she gave only four ages. Although the death of her child seems to have no strictly "medical" bearing whatever, a parent who has lost a child will certainly have feelings attached to the memory of the event and also may have negative feelings about the medical system, which, she may believe, caused her child's death.

In some cases, discussion of family history may cause the patient to become anxious. In asking about family diseases, you imply that they may be related to the patient's current medical problem. It is helpful to be reassuring and to emphasize the "routine" nature of the inquiry. Here is an example of a clinician who stumbles on anxiety-provoking information in asking a routine family history question:

> Yeah, Okay. Very good. Now your mother and father, what did they....
> Are they still alive?
>
> *Um, my mother is alive, my....*
>
> Age?

Notice how the clinician hesitates over the initial question, realizing that the first thing he needs to know is if the parents are living; then, barely listening to the response, he asks another question. The dialogue continues:

> *She is 64.*
>
> She have any illnesses you know of?

Uh....

Heart disease, lung disease, anything?

No, nothing of that sort; she's had a well-known skin cancer and uh, and she seems to have a recurring, it's a problem with her back, but actually it's a nerve that has to be blocked every once in a while.

Okay. Your father?

I never really knew that much about my father, but as I understand it he died of a cerebral hemorrhage.

How old was he?

Oh, he must have been in his early 40s.

Was an autopsy done or anything to find out....

There was so little ... there was a bad occurrence, bad divorce between our mother and father when I was real young and I never saw him after age 9 months really. So I'm very hazy on the particulars of this.

The clinician here stumbles on two kinds of loaded information: (1) that the father died of a cerebral hemorrhage at about the same age the patient is now, and (2) that the patient does not know much about it because of a "bad occurrence." The clinician ignores the "bad occurrence" and goes after a possible cause of the hemorrhage, a cerebral aneurysm being relevant here because this condition can be hereditary.

But nobody knew whether it was traumatic; did he get hit or anything?

I don't know the details, to tell you the truth. He had, well, I just don't really know enough to talk about it.

Cerebral hemorrhage at a young age would be an unusual thing. No other causes being known.

I could find out more, my mother may know more about it.

If she knew, it would be important to you—if she would know, for instance, if he had an aneurysm in his brain that burst, which is one of the ways you can have a cerebral hemorrhage at a young age. I think that would be very important, for instance, for your general health information, so perhaps you can find out. Okay? Do you know anything more in terms of other problems?

Note the interviewer's graphic description of "an aneurysm in his brain that burst" and the statement that this "would be very important to you" while quickly moving on to "other problems." The patient, whom we first met in Chapter 2, now goes on to talk about the "painful subject" while the clinician completely ignores the affective content of the interview.

Well, my understanding is, the context of this, that my mother was raised in the Catholic church and divorce was a terrible scandal in her mind, and she tried to forget about it as quickly as she could. It's such a painful

> *subject that there was never any discussion about who he was and so forth. And as a consequence, all I've really heard are niblets, and one of the things I understand is that he was an alcoholic, or at least had a problem with alcohol, but really caused my mother a lot of problems. So, I don't know if that would be a complicating factor in terms of aneurysm or not.*
>
> Not that I know of. How about brothers and sisters?
>
> *I have one full natural brother and then four half brothers.*
>
> Any medical problems in any of them that you know of?
>
> *No.*

This example demonstrates insensitivity to the patient's feelings and self-disclosure. It also shows that, by pursuing an item of family history, the clinician can increase the patient's anxiety and raise new questions in the patient's mind about his or her own health. A person who tells you that his sister had breast cancer, that his father (who smoked two packs of cigarettes per day for all of his adult life) developed lung cancer, or that his uncle (an asbestos worker) died from mesothelioma may feel that he is at high risk for developing the same diseases, or at least some form of cancer. The more you press for details, the more your patient may feel that there is a connection with his or her present illness. Such a patient who does not have the environmental exposures may need reassurance that he or she is not at special personal risk.

Another source of anxiety arises from the psychologic bias called **availability.** An unusual illness that happens to occur in a family member is highly visible and "available" to the patient. Therefore, it has a greater impact on his or her fears than we, as medical practitioners, might feel is justified. We look at the disease statistically and understand that it is not familial and that the chance of its occurring twice in a small number of people is extremely remote. However, as a clinical student, resident, or practicing clinician, you will find that availability plagues you all the time, just as it plagues your patients. After you diagnose your first case of glioblastoma multiforme, you are likely to overreact to your next group of patients who complain of headaches. For the same reasons, you must be especially sensitive to the anxieties of the dizzy patient whose sister has multiple sclerosis, or the mother of a child with vomiting and recent varicella infection whose nephew had Reye's syndrome.

You can avoid creating anxiety by being clear about why you need the information, sensitive to the patient's responses, and informative in your explanations:

- Make it clear that taking a family history is a routine part of your complete medical interview
- Listen carefully for any emotional overlay or any connections made by the patient between family illnesses and his or her own.
- Demand no more detail than is required for your care of the patient.

- If the patient does become anxious, direct your attention to the anxiety by allowing the patient to express his or her concerns directly. In some cases, you may have to give an additive response (see Chap. 2) to relate the patient's free-floating anxiety to some unconsciously held causal belief (e.g., the coincidence of the patient's current age and her mother's age at the time she died).

SUMMARY ▪ Other Active Problems, Past Medical History, Family History

In this chapter we discussed the importance of searching for other active medical problems (OAPs) in addition to the present illness:

- When you've completed the history of present illness, open up the interview again with nondirective questions to search for OAPs.
- A question about current medications or other conditions under treatment is a good method of screening for OAPs.

The information you gather about the patient's past medical history helps to fill in the context of the present illness:

- Introduce the past medical history with a general question or statement, such as "I'd like to know a little more about how your health has been in the past."
- The level of detail you request about past illness should be dictated by present needs.
- Identify what the patient means by "allergy." Be sure to distinguish true allergy from side effects.

The family history is helpful for frankly hereditary diseases, family traits, and polygenetic conditions like heart disease, diabetes, and cancer:

- Be sensitive to the social and psychological or emotional dimensions of the information you obtain, particularly in the family history.

Recording the family history with the use of a genogram is described in Chapter 7.

References

1. Feinstein A. *Clinical Judgment*. Baltimore, Williams & Wilkins, 1967.
2. Eisenberg L, Kleinman A. Clinical social science. In: Eisenberg L, Kleinman A. (Eds.). *The Relevance of Social Science for Medicine*. Dordrecht, Holland, D. Reidel, 1980.

Suggested Reading

Waters I, Watson W, Wetzel W. Genograms. Practical tools for family physicians. *Can Fam Physician* 1994; 40:282–287.

CHAPTER 5

Gaining Richness and Reality

● ● ● ● ●

THE PATIENT PROFILE

*Dialogue...can exhibit the object from each point of view,
and show it to us in the round, as a sculptor shows us
things, **gaining in this manner all the richness and
reality** of effect that comes from those side issues that are
suddenly suggested by the central idea in progress, and
really illumine the idea more completely, or from those
felicitous after-thoughts that give a fuller completeness
to the central scheme, and yet convey something of the
delicate charm of chance.*

Oscar Wilde, *The Critic as Artist*

The patient profile, also called the **social history,** is the part of the medical interview in which we attempt to learn something about the patient as a person. Illness is not simply disordered pathophysiology; illness happens to a person and involves changes in the person's feelings and abilities. Moreover, getting sick, seeking care, getting well, and staying well all have social determinants, sometimes only an influence but sometimes a direct cause, as with accidents or domestic violence. Therapeutic decisions require knowledge of the patient as a person.

The importance of the social history may not be readily apparent in the acute hospital setting, where the diagnostic and therapeutic objectives are set on an hour-to-hour (if not minute-to-minute) basis. In this artificial setting, knowing what the illness is like for the patient or what the patient's lifestyle is like seems much less important than knowing about the disease process. Yet this artificial view becomes irrelevant when it is time to discharge the patient, and the social environment and family support system become critical. For example:

- How many stairs will my patient have to climb?
- Who will prepare her food?
- How will he or she juggle the complicated medication schedule?
- How much will his employment allow changes in lifestyle necessitated by the illness?
- What about disorders that are clearly occupational, such as back injuries in a young mother or carpal tunnel syndrome in a heavy-equipment operator?

Patients now leave the hospital earlier than they used to, so they tend to be sicker when discharged and require more support in the home environment. Moreover, most medical care does not occur in the hospital. Office visits involve chronic and recurrent conditions that interact continuously with the patient's life circumstances.

Traditionally, we place the patient profile in a separate section of the written case history as if the social history were a self-contained aspect of the interview, but this is an arbitrary separation for the sake of organization only. The social history sometimes is critical to making the diagnosis (sexually transmitted diseases and personality disorders are excellent examples); at these times the social history may actually be part of the history of the present illness.

You are continually acquiring social information throughout the interview from "small talk," the patient's manner of dress and speech, and demographic information that may appear on the chart. Another important aspect of your interaction is assessing educational level and intelligence, both of which are critical to your ability to communicate successfully; much of this assessment is done automatically as you converse at your patient's level of comprehension and in a manner appropriate to his or her life experience.

WHAT GOES INTO THE PATIENT PROFILE?

Just as it is a mistake to believe that there is such a thing as a "complete" review of systems, it is also a mistake to believe that there is a "complete" patient profile. You have time constraints. How do you limit the inquiry so as to avoid a lengthy assessment? What is relevant in the limited time you have? What information must be obtained when the patient is first admitted to the hospital or on the first office visit, and what can be developed over the course of a hospital stay or a long-term relationship with the patient? Unless the situation is an emergency, your goal is to learn enough, at least, to answer three questions. How do the patient's personal characteristics or lifestyle:

- Contribute to the etiology of this illness?
- Aggravate or limit the severity of illness?
- Interfere or help with getting well?

A good way to begin the patient profile is with general questions such as:

- "Can you tell me a little about yourself? Your family? Your work?"
- "How have things been going for you otherwise? At home? At work? In your marriage?"
- "Tell me what else has been going on in your life."

Often one of the most useful parts of an entire history is a detailed description of what the patient usually does on an ordinary day and exactly how this is modified by the illness. For example, for a person who may be suffering from dementia, the description of a typical day may be more revealing than a mental status test would be, particularly when the dementia is mild. The description also may be more clinically important, because what really counts is how the patient functions in the environment, not how the patient performs on a mental status test.

The degree of completeness needed depends on the situation. Some information may emerge in the course of the interview without specific questioning, and often data are acquired not on the first day of hospitalization or during the first office visit but over time as you get to know the patient and understand what is relevant to his or her care. Keep in mind that the idea is to find out the patient's strengths and weaknesses and the nature of his support system, if any. How has this person coped with illness or other stress in the past? How does she or he keep distress within manageable limits? Remember that more intimate data are more easily and reliably obtained when you know the patient better, whether later in your initial history, later in the interview, later in the hospitalization, or years later. Tailor what you need to know to the situation at hand.

DEMOGRAPHICS AND OCCUPATIONAL HISTORY

The patient's age, education, race or ethnic background, religion, and residence are among the most fundamental data about the person. These characteristics affect the risk of various diseases, beliefs about the causes of illness, and the ability to participate in recommended therapy. Often this information is provided for you on the "front sheet" filled in by office or hospital personnel when the patient registers or is admitted.

Data about employment, school, or retirement are vital to understanding the patient and to building an understanding of the patient's support system. Are there financial problems related to the patient's job or lack of a job? Is the retired person actively involved in hobbies or volunteer work? How does the patient cope with being a single parent? How does the patient unwind from the rigors of daily living?

Clinical Key 5–1 presents essential points of a quick occupational survey that should be included in any medical history. Describe what the person actually does on the job. For example, a patient who "works for the phone com-

CLINICAL KEY 5–1

Essentials of a Quick Occupational Survey

- "Do you work outside your home?"
- "What kind of work do you do?"
- "Tell me what that job is like for you."
- "Is that what you've always done? What other jobs have you held in the past?"
- "Do you now—or did you in the past—have exposure to fumes, chemicals, dust, loud noise, radiation?"
- "Do you think anything at work (or at home) is affecting your symptoms now? How about stress at work?"

pany" may be a manager, a telephone installer, or a maintenance person who works out-of-doors on telephone lines. Similarly, a steelworker may operate heavy equipment, drive a truck, or work in an office. Each job exposes the patient to different risks, ranging from chronic stress to serious accidents. By not considering occupational exposures, clinicians miss the opportunity to diagnose certain acute and chronic illnesses.[1] Table 5–1 presents various examples of occupational and environmental causes of medical problems.

TABLE 5–1

EXAMPLES OF OCCUPATIONAL AND ENVIRONMENTAL CAUSES OF MEDICAL PROBLEMS		
Condition	**Industry/Occupation**	**Agent**
Pulmonary tuberculosis	Medical personnel	*Mycobacterium tuberculosis*
Encephalitis	Animal handlers	Rabies, B-virus
Toxic encephalitis	Battery manufacturing, smelters	Lead, solvents
Viral hepatitis	Day-care staff, medical personnel	Hepatitis C, hepatitis B
Toxic hepatitis	Cleaners, plastics industry	Carbon tetrachloride, chloroform
Malignant neoplasm of the respiratory system	Woodwork, radium processing, nickel smelting and refining, insulators, construction workers, plumbers, coke oven workers, uranium and fluorspar miners	Wood dust, radium, nickel, asbestos, coke oven emissions, radon, chromates, nickel, arsenic, bis(chloromethyl)ether
Malignant neoplasm of bone	Chemists	Radium
Malignant neoplasm of bladder	Rubber and dye workers	Benzidine, naphthylamine, auramine, 4-nitrophenyl
Malignant neoplasm of kidney	Coke oven workers	Coke oven emissions
Leukemia	Radiologists, rubber industry, occupations with exposure to benzene	Ionizing radiation, benzene

Continued

TABLE 5-1

EXAMPLES OF OCCUPATIONAL AND ENVIRONMENTAL CAUSES OF MEDICAL PROBLEMS—cont'd		
Condition	**Industry/Occupation**	**Agent**
Agranulocytosis or neutropenia	Explosives, pesticides, pharmaceuticals	Phosphorus, arsenic
Inflammatory and toxic neuropathy	Pesticides, pharmaceuticals, refinishers, degreasing, plastics	Arsenic, hexane, methyl butyl ketone, copper disulfide, other solvents
	Battery or smelter workers	Lead
	Dentists, battery workers	Mercury
	Paper industry	Acrylamide
Extrinsic asthma	Jewelry and alloy workers; paint, plastic, insecticide, foam, latex manufacturing; bakers; wood and furniture workers	Platinum, isocyanates, phthalic anhydride, formaldehyde, flour, dust
Coal worker's pneumoconiosis	Coal miners	Coal dust
Asbestosis	Asbestos industries and users	Asbestos
Silicosis	Quarriers, sandblasters, ceramic work	Silica
Talcosis	Talc processors	Talc
Chronic pulmonary beryllium disease	Beryllium alloy workers, nuclear reactor workers	Beryllium
Byssinosis	Cotton industry	Cotton, flax, hemp
Acute bronchitis, pneumonitis, and pulmonary edema due to fumes and vapors	Bleach industries, silo fillers, arc welders, oil industries, plastics industry	Chlorine, nitrogen oxides, sulfur dioxide, trimellitic anhydride
Renal failure	Battery makers, plumbers, solderers, electrolytic processes, smelting	Lead, arsine, mercury
Contact and allergic dermatitis	Leather tanning, poultry, adhesives and sealants, boat building and repair	Irritants (cutting fish oils, solvents, acids, alkalis), allergens

SOURCE: Abbreviated and adapted from Landrigan PJ, Baker DB. The recognition and control of occupational disease. *JAMA* 1991; 266:676–680, by Wajdy Hailoo, MD, Chief, Division of Occupational and Environmental Medicine, Department of Preventive Medicine, State University of New York at Stony Brook, Stony Brook, NY.

LIFESTYLE

Nutrition and Diet

Your patients may have strong beliefs about the role of diet in their health and illnesses and many will have tried popular weight-reduction plans and vitamin supplements. Often you will recommend dietary changes, such as reduction in fats or increase in dietary fiber, for both primary prevention and treatment of disease. To give appropriate advice, you will need to understand the person's eating habits. Specific food intolerance (e.g., lactose intolerance), food allergies, the condition of the patient's teeth, the ability to shop for and prepare food, income, and ethnic and cultural influences (which may be resistant to change) all affect dietary habits.

Clinical Key 5–2 presents an approach to an efficient nutrition and dietary survey. **The question "Tell me about your diet" may be misinterpreted if the patient is not on a weight-reduction diet.** Details are important. If the patient has toast for breakfast and a sandwich for lunch, find out what goes on the toast and between the two slices of bread.

Daily Activities and Exercise

How your patient spends a typical day reveals additional factors that contribute to illness or facilitate getting well. For example, the sedentary retired salesman will need an explicit and graded exercise program with frequent monitoring of his progress as he recuperates from a heart attack. People who

---

CLINICAL KEY 5–2

An Efficient Nutrition and Dietary Survey

A. Initial screen:
- "Are you happy with your (present) weight? Any recent gain or loss? What did you weigh a year ago?"
- "Tell me what's been happening with your weight."
- "Are there any major food groups that you either eat a lot of or don't eat at all?"

B. Then, depending on the answers and the clinical situation: (e.g., is the patient's weight normal? Are there drug–food interactions?)
- "Tell me more about your eating habits."
- "How many meals do you eat each day? What about snacks? What about eating in the evening, after dinner, or at bedtime?"
- "Do you have any trouble taking your pills because some of them need to be taken with food? or on an empty stomach?"

C. Then, more specific depending on the clinical situation:
- "Tell me about your intake of:"
  salt (for patients with congestive heart failure or hypertension)
  fiber (for patients with chronic constipation, hemorrhoids, or diverticulosis)
  dairy products (for patients with possible lactose intolerance or patients who need calcium)
  fat (for patients who are overweight or have hyperlipidemias)
  caffeine (especially for patients with palpitations, tremors, or anxiety symptoms)
- "Tell me what you've eaten over the last 24 hours, beginning with just before you came to the office and working back."
- "Is this a typical day for you? How is it different?"

are constantly on the go, eating on the run and rarely preparing their own food, may need to undertake major and difficult changes in lifestyle to treat obesity and hyperlipidemia.

Exercise is a major feature in the patient profile. Vague answers such as "I like to play tennis" or "I have a rowing machine at home" are not necessarily indicators of regular aerobic exercise. Perhaps the patient has not had time for tennis since the summer of 1997 or the rowing machine has sat unused for years in the basement. To monitor health effects, you must inquire specifically about regularity and duration, as well as manner, of exercise. As you do this, you can also assess the potential for various types of trauma that result from sports and exercise programs (e.g., stress fractures in joggers, major knee injuries in skiers).

Use of Tobacco, Alcohol, and "Recreational" Drugs

You should ascertain the amount, frequency, and context of these behaviors. Assessing truthfulness is a common problem when eliciting smoking, alcohol, and drug histories because these are loaded topics, and most people (both patients and health care professionals) feel that there are "right" and "wrong" answers to questions about them. For example, when asked, "How much do you smoke?" many smokers reply, "Too much." Notice how there is no quantification in this answer; the reply is colored by the patient's awareness that it is "wrong" to smoke. It may be easier for such patients to talk more neutrally about what age they started to smoke or how many times they have tried to quit.

Here is a smoking history obtained from a 40-year-old man presenting with shortness of breath. The interviewer tries to find out exactly how much is "not too much" and also tries to determine whether the patient's current respiratory symptoms caused him to cut down and whether the cumulative smoking history is sufficient to cause medical problems like chronic bronchitis or perhaps carcinoma of the lung:

Okay. How much do you smoke?

Oh, not too much.

How much is not too much?

Oh, umm, not half a pack a day.

Is that as much as you've always smoked? Have you ever smoked more than that?

Uh, when I was barbering, I would smoke more, sometimes a pack. You know, but they would burn out. You know, because when I was doing a customer or something, they'd burn out, so I'd just light up another one.

Uh hmm. How old were you when you started?

Thirteen.

Similarly, use of "recreational" drugs or excessive intake of alcohol is seen by most patients as a habit of which the clinician will disapprove. Some will deny the use of these substances, particularly if asked a yes/no question. Here is an example of a interviewer (who can smell alcohol on the patient's breath) trying to elicit the history of alcohol use in a 28-year-old woman presenting for evaluation of hypertension:

> ...You are using some aspirin and Tylenol?
>
> *Every once in a while. It's not regular, but that's the only drugs I take.*
>
> And are you a pretty steady drinker?
>
> *I have one or two drinks at work, you know. After work I....*
>
> ...Okay. Do you have any more than that?
>
> *Sometimes it's more than that but basically....*
>
> Is that something that would be hard for you to give up?
>
> *Well, it's a very social type thing for me, I guess ... so ... yeah, I'd have to think about it, ha ha.*

A Digression on Truth Telling

Often in this situation it is not so much what the patient says, but how she says it. This patient paused and looked away, and began to use phrases such as "you know" and hedges like "basically." She also displayed some nervous laughter. These are often clues that a person is telling less than the truth. You may notice pauses (time to censor material), shifts in position, eye aversion, and hedges in the verbalization, such as "not really" instead of "no." The most

---

CLINICAL KEY 5–3

Screening Your Patients for Problem Drinking

The CAGE questions:

C Have you ever felt you ought to *cut down* on your drinking?
A Have people *annoyed* you by criticizing your drinking?
G Have you ever felt bad or *guilty* about your drinking?
E Have you ever had a drink first thing in the morning *(eye opener)* to steady your nerves or get rid of a hangover?

If all answers are negative, problem drinking is not likely. If one or more are positive, explore further the role of alcohol in the patient's life.

Or ask both:

- Have you ever had a drinking problem?
- Was your last drink within the last 24 hours?

These two questions together have a high predictive value. If the patient answers both in the affirmative there is a high risk of a drinking problem; those who answer both in the negative have a low risk of having a drinking problem.[2]

revealing question in this example is the indirect one ("Is that something that would be hard for you to give up?"), to which the patient's answer ranges from denial ("Well, it's a very social type thing ...") to agreement ("I guess so, yeah ...") to ambivalence ("I'd have to think about it"). It is rarely useful to tell a patient that you doubt the accuracy of his or her story, especially when you have not already built a relationship. You should make a mental note of the behavior, however, in the hope that in the future you will be able to use the information to help the patient. Clinical Key 5–3 presents questions widely used to screen patients for alcohol problems.

Another patient with a history of narcotic addiction, when asked about his current drug use, replied, "No, not much. I mean some. Yeah, I'm using." Illicit drug use and narcotic addiction, particularly when the clinician is potentially the patient's source of drugs, is a difficult situation that demands careful attention to both the substance and style of the patient's statements.

SPIRITUALITY AND BELIEFS

The existential or spiritual dimension of life includes a person's deepest beliefs and values. Who am I? Where do I come from? Where am I going? What gives meaning to my life? Spirituality is often expressed as a religion or a relationship with God, but it may mean other forms of experience or belief such as a passionate love of nature, a sense of oneness with the universe, or a deep commitment to helping others. For many people, spiritual values influence their experience of illness, especially their understanding of what the illness means, how they should respond to it, and what the outcome will be. Although spirituality is potentially an important component of any patient's well-being, the more progressive, prolonged, and threatening an illness becomes, the more likely it is that the patient will turn for strength and support to spiritual values. As discussed further in Chapter 13, spiritual assessment is crucial in the care of dying patients and is often a factor in discussions about living wills or advance directives.[3] Clinical Key 5–4 presents FICA, a useful acronym for asking about spirituality as part of the complete patient profile. The first three steps (faith, influence, and community) can be accomplished quickly. For example, here is a clinician interviewing a new patient who has come in for an "executive physical":

> Now I want to ask a couple of questions about what means most to you. Do you see yourself as a spiritual person?
>
> *Uh, I don't know ... I don't think I've ever been asked that [pauses]. I was raised a Catholic, you know, but haven't practiced, not since the kids were young.... We don't usually go to church. [Another pause] But, you know, I feel that God is everywhere in nature, all around....*

With a single question, this clinician has learned that the patient comes from a Catholic tradition (F), but is not a part of a practicing community (C).

CLINICAL KEY 5–4

An Approach to Spiritual Assessment

F Faith   Do you consider yourself a spiritual or religious person?
Tell me more about that.
What things do you believe in that give meaning to your life?

I Influence   Are these beliefs important in your life?
Does this belief influence how you take care of yourself?
How has your belief influenced your behavior during this illness?
What role do these beliefs play in regaining your health?

C Community   Are you part of a spiritual or religious community?
Is this community a support to you? How?

A Address   How would you like me, your clinician, to address these issues in your health care?

SOURCE: Adapted from Pulchalski CM, Romer AL. Taking a spiritual history allows clinicians to understand patients more fully. *J Palliat Med* 2000; 3:129–137.

It is unclear how much influence (I) the Catholic tradition has in his life, although he has suggested another deeply felt faith or experience (God-in-nature) that might be of importance to him in coping with illness. It seems unlikely that the clinician will need to go further at this point. However, when patients express strong spiritual commitment, it is important for the clinician to ask whether (or how) they wish to have their spirituality addressed (A) in their health care.

We consider sociocultural aspects of illness and the impact of the patient's health beliefs and expectations in Chapters 10 and 14.

RELATIONSHIPS

Support System

You have begun to develop an idea of the patient's support system when you know the answers to questions such as the following:
- Who lives in the household?
- Are there family members nearby who are willing and able to help in time of crisis?
- Has there been recent bereavement? (Widowed persons have higher rates of illness and death, particularly during the first year of widowhood.)
- What kind of help does the young mother have with her new baby?
- Who will care for the elderly, demented woman when her husband (who normally cares for her) has his hernia surgery?

For patients with chronic illness or disability, especially when there is no family or the family has limited financial or emotional resources, part of the clinician's role is to arrange for needed health services (e.g., transportation to the office, home care, Meals-on-Wheels), usually with the help of social agencies.

Marital and Other Significant Relationships

As you begin to understand the patient's lifestyle, you also develop a sense of the patient's relationship with the spouse or significant other. You may not need to ask direct questions about it. Because patients may regard this information as intimate and possibly unrelated to their illness, it is best to ask questions in a somewhat indirect and open-ended manner, which permits patients to reveal as much or as little as they wish. You may begin, for example, with questions relating the patient's illness to the current state of the relationship: "How has your being on chemotherapy affected your husband?" Such questions allow the patient to say anything from "Okay" to "Well, we've had our rough spots but things are pretty good right now" to "To tell you the truth, I keep wanting to leave him, but I'm too sick now." Once the patient has indicated an interest in discussing the relationship, more specific questions are useful:

- "What are some of the good and bad things about your present relationship?"
- "What would you change?"

In addition to the impact of illness on relationships and of relationships on illness, certain diagnoses or clues to diagnoses reside in the story of the patient's relationships. For example, the criteria for diagnosing certain personality disorders lie in the patient's history of difficult relationships with family, friends, and employers.

Domestic Violence

Domestic violence, also known as *intimate partner violence*, was long considered a strictly "private" matter by both health professionals and law enforcement. Now it is recognized as a serious public health problem, sufficiently prevalent to justify screening in the medical setting. Detecting relationships that are physically or emotionally abusive is an important function of the patient profile. Clinical Key 5–5 outlines an approach to screening for domestic violence that begins with less threatening and somewhat general questions, and progresses to more specific queries that focus on the patient's safety.[4,5] Note how each question allows patients to answer from their own point of view, avoiding judgmental wording and remaining open ended.

Here is an example of a 52-year-old college professor with a history of breast cancer and recent treatment for clinical depression:

> *The other thing I wanted to talk about is going back on the Zoloft because it works for me but I'm not sure I need it.*

> **CLINICAL KEY 5–5**
> **Detecting Domestic Violence: The "SAFE" Questions**
> **Stress/Safety**
> What stress do you experience in your relationships?
> Do you feel safe in your relationships?
> Should I be concerned for your safety?
> **Afraid/Abused**
> Are there situations in your relationships where you have felt
>   afraid?
> Has your partner ever threatened or abused you or your
>   children?
> Have you been physically hurt or threatened by your partner?
> Has your partner forced you to have sexual intercourse that you
>   did not want?
> **Friends/Family**
> If you have been hurt, are your friends or family aware of it?
> Do you think you could tell them if it did happen?
> Would they be able to give you support?
> **Emergency Plan**
> Do you have a safe place to go and the resources you need in
>   an emergency situation?
> If you are in danger now, would you like help in locating a
>   shelter?
> Would you like to talk with a social worker (a counselor, me) to
>   develop an emergency plan?

Tell me more.

Well ... my husband and I may be separating so things are stressful. In the morning I feel pretty low and I don't want to get out of bed but then once I get to work I feel okay and I feel okay for the rest of the day.

Any sleep problems?

No.

Any problems with your energy, concentration, being irritable?

No, no, I'm okay that way.

[Knowing the past history of an abusive relationship] You know, with this going on at home, how are you feeling about your safety?

...[slowly] Okay, right now.

Do you know what to do if you don't feel safe?

Yes, I have to leave. I have friends I can go to, and I have the number of the women's shelter.

Notice how the clinician asks in an open-ended and nonjudgmental way about the patient's safety and ensures that she has a plan. This interview also includes a quick screen for depression.

SEXUAL HISTORY

Sexual functioning is an essential part of most patients' life experience and may be an important factor in caring for patients. Clinicians deal every day with issues related to contraception, infertility, sexually transmitted diseases, rape, or incest. A sexual contact may be the source of illness (human immunodeficiency virus [HIV], hepatitis B, human papillomavirus), and knowledge of the patient's sexual orientation and behavior drives your diagnostic hypotheses and informs your plans to screen and educate the patient. Depression, anxiety, and anger may relate to underlying sexual problems; conversely, many physical diseases or medications lead to sexual dysfunction.

Despite its importance, most of us find sexuality a difficult topic in the interview. We live in a sexually repressive culture characterized by lack of information and secrecy, and questions about sexual orientation and behavior are difficult for us to ask and for patients to answer. You have feelings and attitudes about this topic and so do your patients; a young person may accept your question about sexual preference whereas an elderly person may think you are way off the mark for asking.

Here's how one patient describes the reaction of her physician:

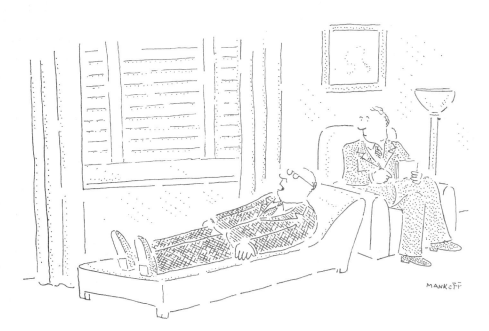

"Frankly, I've repressed my sexuality so long I've actually forgotten what my orientation is."

There's something I need to talk to you about, it's from last time and I thought I could set it aside but I can't.... This is really hard. Okay, when I started to talk about my sexual relationships you sat back and went like this [patient demonstrates folding arms across chest] and it made me feel like I had done the wrong thing bringing it up. And then when I called you, I felt that you really rushed me off the phone and I figured you were mad at me because of what I had said about my sex life. Because I used to jump into bed with every guy and I feel so ashamed. Now I think, what's the point?

And consider this not uncommon example of how an outpatient, whose chief complaint is a sexual problem, dances around the issue, digresses, and finally gets to the point with open-ended prompting:

Hi, good morning. Long time no see, it's good to see you. Why did you decide to get a physical now?

Well, it's just that, well [patient seems anxious] you know, I'm getting older and I kinda figured it's been a while.

Yeah, it has, it's been almost 5 years since I last saw and did a physical on you.

Well, I've been in more recently than that and saw someone else. Actually I wanted to mention that to you because you see I have this way of clearing my throat [patient demonstrates a kind of half cough] and I do it constantly and your associate put me on Claritin for it and I thought that was a lazy approach, without actually figuring out what's causing it. I mean, shouldn't I have been tested for allergies or something?

Well, I'll make that a part of our evaluation today. Let me get an idea, first, what else is on your list?

Well, this is embarrassing to talk about. But my sexual performance, I'm concerned about my sexual performance.

Tell me more. How long has it been going on?

Well, it started about 18 months ago [patient having difficulty going on]....

And is it that you're having trouble maintaining an erection?

Well it's the strength and the duration. Maybe I'm just getting old, it's an age thing. I didn't tell my wife I was going to talk to you about this.

What are some techniques to make this part of the interview easier? First, there is no requirement to get a "complete" sexual history from every patient. Sometimes a couple of screening questions ("Are you having any sexual problems?" "Are you concerned about your risk of any sexually transmitted diseases?") suffice, and these questions may be asked as part of the review of systems. If the patient answers in the negative, no more need be said; you have, however, indicated that sexual concerns are legitimate fare for discussion, for either you or the patient to initiate. You may continue with other aspects of the history, at the same time building rapport, and return to the sexual history, if necessary.

Second, knowing something about the patient as a person facilitates asking more specific questions about sexuality. For example, once you know whether the patient is married or is living with someone, it is easier to ask about sexual preference and activity. When in doubt, you should use the term "partner" rather than gender-specific terms such as "boyfriend" or "wife." If you ask only about opposite-sex partners, the patient may infer that you accept only heterosexual activity and a homosexual patient may avoid relating his or her actual sexual preference. (On the other hand, the married 75-year-old may well be offended by the use of the term "partner.")

Third, delaying this part of the history until later in the interview also allows you to become familiar with the patient's language and makes it easier to use words that he or she can understand. As with other intimate bodily functions (voiding and defecating), patients may describe their sexual functioning with words conditioned by their age, level of education, and cultural background. Other descriptions may be idiosyncratic and obscure. What do words like "relationship," "birth control," or "safe sex" mean? Open-ended questions permit the patient to use his or her own words. In your follow-up questions, you then can use the patient's own words, thereby ensuring a common basis for understanding.

Clinical Key 5–6 presents some useful ways to initiate the sexual history. If the patient indicates problem areas, then proceed with more detailed questioning. The history should be more extensive, for example, when a patient requests birth control, fears a sexually transmitted disease, or has a sexual problem as a presenting complaint. Consider this example of a 41-year-old male whose chief complaint is "no desire":

Hi, I haven't seen you for a while. How can I help you?

Well, doc, I just have no interest in sex at all. I thought maybe I needed to work out so I started going to the gym. I thought maybe it was that and I started a dietary supplement, I've been taking GNC men's formula. I'm playing racquetball. And then I started reading stuff and read something about testosterone levels so that's why I'm here.

Okay. How long has this been going on?

Well it started maybe a year, year-and-a-half ago. My wife's afraid it's her but our relationship is better than it's ever been. We're going to church together now, we have these two great kids, our jobs are good; we're so lucky.

Uh huh.

We are pretty tired, I'm really tired. I get home from work and all I want to do is eat supper and get into bed.

When you do have sex, do you have any problems?

CLINICAL KEY 5–6
Beginning the Sexual History

- Introductory statements ease the transition to a potentially difficult topic.
  "I always include questions about sexual problems in my routine history because they're so common. Have you had any problems?"
  "I know sexual concerns can be hard to discuss, especially with a total stranger, but it sounds as if you have some concerns. Tell me more."
  "It's important that I ask about your sexual partners and about when you first started having intercourse so I can help you avoid certain illnesses. Is that okay?"
- "Are you having any sexual problems?"
- "Do you have any questions or concerns about sexuality or sexual functioning?"
- "Many people who are ill experience a change in their sexual function. Have you noticed any change?"
- "Has your interest in sex changed recently? Since you've been ill?"
- "A lot of men have sexual problems when they take blood pressure medicine. Have you noticed any problems?"
- "It sounds as though your marriage has been a good one. How about your sexual relationship?"
- "Many girls (boys) your age have questions about sex and birth control. How about you?"
- "Many people these days worry about AIDS. Do you have any concerns about being at risk for AIDS?"

Well, that part is fine, at least it was until about a month ago and that's when I made this appointment because I couldn't keep my erection. But that was the first time that happened.

Have you noticed anything else? You know, sometimes when a person loses their desire, it's part of some physical or emotional problem. Have you felt sick in any way? Weight loss? Headaches?

No, nothing like that. Overall, I feel good.

Any feelings of depression, or loss of interest in other things? Any trouble or change in enjoying things you've always enjoyed?

No, that's what's funny about this.

Notice how the clinician observes good basic interviewing technique by using open-ended questions and facilitation, making it unnecessary to ask very specific questions. The clinician also discloses the reasoning behind certain questions.

With more reticent patients you may need to ask specific questions about change in libido ("Do you feel like making love—having sex—as much as you used to?") or pleasure ("Do you feel satisfied when you make love?"). Choose words that the patient can understand. If you are not sure you are being understood, ask ("Do you understand what I am asking?"). As much as possible, you should ask questions that permit patients to answer from their own point of view and in their own way (e.g., "Do you feel satisfied?" as opposed to "Do you have an orgasm?").

When you suspect a sexually transmitted disease, it will be necessary to know about sexual preference and number and regularity of sexual partners, and to ask if the partners have had any sexually transmitted disease symptoms. These are difficult topics because a sexually transmitted disease or same-sex partner may embarrass the patient, and he or she may not want to acknowledge that a partner may have gone outside the relationship. Patients may feel anger and guilt or may perceive the clinician as accusatory. Consider this example of a 54-year-old married financial consultant who presented to his doctor (of many years) with a rash on his palms and soles:

> *So what do you think this is?*
>
> Well, most likely it's a virus of some sort. But because it's on your palms and soles the list of possibilities is rather short, but it includes syphilis.
>
> *Syphilis?! Isn't the only way you can get that by sexual contact?*
>
> That's correct. And I'm not jumping to any conclusions here, but you need to know it's on the list. [Pause] Let me get the requisition for some lab work for you and I'll be back. [The clinician decides not to ask a direct question and, instead, gives the patient some time to absorb this information by stepping out for a moment.]
>
> *[When clinician returns] I feel terrible, I have to deal with the consequences, but I did have unprotected intercourse with someone not my wife. Can we figure out what this is as fast as possible?*

You should express your questions in the same neutral way that you talk about other illnesses or infections: "Are you concerned that you might have gotten this from someone?" or "Is there any chance that you have been exposed to someone with a similar infection?" Sometimes it helps to introduce a difficult question with a statement, such as "I think you may have an infection that is acquired only during sexual intercourse, but I don't want to make any assumptions about your sexual relationships. Is it possible that you've been with someone who has the same thing?" If the patient says, "That's impossible," accept that statement as representing the patient's belief. You can still add, "If you do think of anybody who might have this, it would be good if you could tell them to get checked." Do not argue with the patient. If the diagnosis is uncertain, say so and outline the plan for making the diagnosis clear. In the case of reportable venereal diseases, the clinician might say, "By law, I am required to report this illness, and someone from the health department may talk to you about who else might have it."

Here is an example of the kind of sexual problem that arises frequently in medical patients. You should determine if the problem is the result of medication side effects, difficulties in the relationship, or some combination of factors:

> ... Are you living at home now? Living with your boyfriend?
>
> *He's like 16 years older than me and we've been together for about 15 years, but see there's a, a little bit of a problem when we have to, 'cause see since I've been on those steroids, you know it messes with your sex life, too. I don't have any.*
>
> You don't have any desire?
>
> *No, and uh, that creates a problem. I just have no desire. It was like if he put his hands on me, I might get real evil, you know, like "get your hands off of me," you know.*
>
> I see. How are things between you and him otherwise? Are things strained in general?
>
> *I wish he would get out of my life.*

One final note: Many people also want to know what is "normal" in sexual matters and discern whether they fit the normal standard. They may ask your opinion. Do not confuse being genuine (see Chap. 2) with giving personal details of your own life. Some questions that patients may put to you are clearly inappropriate ("What would you do? Would you have an abortion?" or "Did you have sex before you got married?"), and it is best to answer in a polite and straightforward manner, "Well, we're not here to discuss what I think. I'm more interested in finding out how you feel about this pregnancy (or about learning that your son is gay)." In this way, you will help the patient explore his or her own feelings and symptoms as opposed to yours, which are not the focus of the interview.

THE PATIENT PROFILE AT WORK

Here are two examples that demonstrate the importance of the social history or patient profile in the diagnosis and management of medical problems. In the first example, a 61-year-old woman with diabetes and hypertension urgently scheduled a visit to her family physician, complaining of chest pain, headache, and increasing concern about her blood pressure. The physician, confused about which problem was really the chief complaint (because the symptoms were chronic and the blood pressure under control), asked the patient to clarify her concerns:

> Uh, what, what would you say is the thing that's worrying you the most right now?

Well, mostly, is how, getting those bills paid. See, I'm on, I'm on assistance.

Oh, I see. Tell me more about this worry. Did something new happen?

Mostly it's a gas bill and then, um, see I own a house. I have the taxes, keeping up with them, and, ah, just finances generally.

Did you recently get your gas bill?

Yes, I did.

When did that come?

Yes, ah, it came the other day.

In this instance, the social problem was *the* problem. Notice how the physician looked for positive or confirmatory evidence that it was her inability to pay the gas bill that was really bothering the patient. This doesn't mean that her chest pain, headaches, and high blood pressure weren't "real," but it was very helpful in answering the "why now" question—that is, why the patient sought care at this particular time for symptoms that had not changed.

The final example is a patient in whom a variety of lifestyle factors contribute to his illnesses, which include obesity, headaches, and secondary syphilis:

The thing that is interesting to me is I am busy and I am constantly on my feet and I must put in at least 4 miles each day, but it doesn't affect my weight because of the types of things I eat. I don't eat heavily, it's just the things I eat.

How do you mean?

When I have not eaten for a whole day, I go to some deli and grab a creampuff and go to bed. That gives me sugar, and sugar helps me. Sugar really helps me keep elevated. I have a terrible—well, I have to drink orange drink. I don't eat breakfast, as a matter of fact, I only eat one meal a day, but it's a junk meal. And I'm very hooked on, I have to have a sugar-type drink in the morning to get elevated. Could use one now!

Now that you know all these things, is there any way you can change something? Like when you go to New York, you can find some time for yourself, even if it's sitting down for 10 minutes, instead of 10 seconds?

I lived there for 2 years, and when I started the business, I didn't realize at the time that the business was going to grow as quickly as it did, and I found out I was going to New York more and staying in hotels. Hotel living is disgusting. This is the part where it gets into the personal part of it. My lifestyle changed quite a bit; a lot of things changed for me. I have always felt that I had very strong religious convictions and things like that. When I moved to New York, my lifestyle totally changed. I went to parties where everybody was having sex with everybody else and you really didn't even get to know the person. You may never see them again and that type of thing. Well, all these things happened to me in this period. And I have to be honest with you, they frightened me, but I enjoyed them. I knew they were wrong, but there was a part of me that enjoyed them. So I was getting very confused. I felt that it was time for me to come back.

You felt that this was a way of coming back home?

Exactly. What happened to me recently was that because of me going back to the way I wanted to be and things not working out the way I thought they should, so I figured why should I make sacrifices and be this person. You know, and not getting the results I want from it. I'll go back to being the other person. And I went back to being the other person and I got [laughing loudly] a social disease! Now you know my life story. That's it in a nutshell.

Note how the clinician skillfully uses open-ended questions ("How do you mean?") and interchangeable responses ("You felt this was a way of coming back home?")

This patient (whom we met briefly in Chapter 1) acquired syphilis, probably at a party at which he had multiple sexual partners. He was finding his obesity difficult to control and was experiencing constant fatigue and stress-related headaches. The rash caused by his secondary syphilis became public evidence of what he saw as religious transgressions. He was dreadfully afraid that he had been exposed to HIV during his semianonymous gay sex. His anxiety and guilt made it difficult for him to work as hard as he felt he needed to in order to keep his business going. This patient did, indeed, develop acquired immunodeficiency syndrome (AIDS) and died about 2 years later.

SUMMARY • The Patient Profile

We close this chapter with Table 5–2, which displays key elements of the patient profile and some typical questions you might ask to begin to explore these elements. These questions are by no means a screening algorithm; they are simply examples of how one might choose to screen for these elements on an initial visit with the patient.

References

1. Landrigan PJ, Baker DB. The recognition and control of occupational disease. *JAMA* 1991; 266:676–680.
2. Cyr MG, Wartman SA. The effectiveness of routine screening questions in the detection of alcoholism. *JAMA* 1998; 259:51–54.
3. Pulchalski C, Romer AL. Taking a spiritual history allows clinicians to understand patients more fully. *J Palliat Med* 2000; 3:129–137.
4. Ashur ML. Asking about domestic violence: SAFE questions [letter]. *JAMA* 1993; 269:2367.
5. Neufeld B. SAFE questions: Overcoming barriers to the detection of domestic violence. *Am Fam Physician* 1996; 53:2575–2580.

TABLE 5-2

ELEMENTS OF THE PATIENT PROFILE	
Topics	**Typical Screening Questions**
Demographics and Occupation	
Age, gender, race, ethnic group, religion, marital status, education, occupation	Now that I know something about your symptoms, tell me a little about yourself. All I know is that you're 53 years old and married.
	What kind of work do you do? What exactly does that job involve?
Lifestyle	
Nutrition and diet	Tell me a bit about yourself.
Daily activities and exercise	What is an average day like for you?
Cigarette, alcohol, and drug use	What's your diet like? Tell me what you eat on an average day.
	Do you have time for regular exercise?
	Do you smoke cigarettes?
Relationships	
Family and household composition	Now tell me about your family. You've been married how long? Children?
Support system	
Marital and other significant relationships	Any stresses or problems with your family?
Sexual history	Any problems in your marriage?
Spirituality	Do you consider yourself a spiritual or religious person? Tell me more about that.
Health Beliefs and Expectations (see Chap. 10)	What are you hoping to get out of this visit today?
	Do you have any concerns about taking medication?
	Do you have an advance directive or living will?

Suggested Reading

Eisenstat SA, Baucroft L. Domestic Violence. *N Engl J Med* 1999; 341:886–892.

Elliot BA. Screening for family violence: Overcoming the barriers [editorial]. *J Fam Pract* 2000; 49:137–138.

Feldhaus KM, Koziol-McLain J, Amsbury HL, Norton IM, Lowenstein SR, Abbott JT. Accuracy of 3 brief screening questions for detecting partner violence in the Emergency Department. *JAMA* 1997; 277:1357–1361.

Maurice WL. *Sexual Medicine in Primary Care.* St. Louis, MO, Mosby-Year Book, 1999.

Mazonson PD, Mathias SD, Fifer SK, Buesching DP, Malek P, Patrick DL. The mental health patient profile: Does it change primary care physicians' practice patterns? *J Am Board Fam Pract* 1996; 9:336–345.

Miller TA. Diagnostic evaluation of erectile dysfunction. *Am Fam Physician* 2000; 61:95–104, 109–110.

Newman LS. Occupational illness. *N Engl J Med* 1995; 333:1128–1134.

Rodriguez MA, Bauer HM, McLoughlin E, Gruneback K. Screening and intervention for intimate partner abuse: Practices and attitudes of primary care physicians. *JAMA* 1999; 282:468–474.

Ross MW, Channon-Little LD, Rosser BRS. *Sexual Health Concerns: Interviewing and History Taking for Health Practitioners.* Philadelphia, FA Davis, 2000.

Rovi S, Mouton CP. Domestic violence education in family practice residencies. *Fam Med* 1999; 31(6):398–403.

White J, Levinson W. Primary care of lesbian patients. *J Gen Intern Med* 1993; 8:41–45.

Zink T. Should children be in the room when the mother is screened for partner violence? *J Fam Pract* 2000; 49:130–136.

CHAPTER 6

No Air of Finished Knowledge

● ● ● ● ●

REVIEW OF SYSTEMS, PHYSICAL EXAMINATION, AND CLOSURE

*A physician of this kind never gives a servant any account of his complaint, nor asks him for any; he gives him some empirical injunction with an **air of finished knowledge** in the brusque fashion of a dictator, and then is off in hot haste to the next ailing servant....*

Plato, *The Laws*

THE REVIEW OF SYSTEMS

The **review of systems** (ROS) demonstrates your responsibility for the total patient and may uncover significant symptoms or problems not otherwise elicited. Clinicians who feel uncertain about how to conduct an interview, or about their ability to integrate data, sometimes take refuge in a long, detailed ROS. They ask in great detail about every possible symptom, as if it were possible to get all the information simply by asking a comprehensive set of questions. Others look upon the ROS as a pro forma detail of little value—in other words, a burden.

What, then, are the goals of the ROS? First, to uncover any additional active medical problems not yet discussed; and, second, to identify additional symptoms that may be related to the symptoms for which the patient is seeking help, or may influence them. The interviewer may ask questions to address these ends at any time. The ROS as a specific segment may be "emptied" when the relevant information is obtained elsewhere.

Platt and McMath[1] observed more than 300 clinical interviews conducted by medical residents and delineated five syndromes of "clinical hypocompetence." They called one of the syndromes "flawed database" and illustrated it with this vignette:

> The clinical interview took 44 minutes to complete. Time allocation was as follows: introduction = 1 minute; definition of chief complaint (cardinal symptom) and development of present illness = 15 minutes; major past medical events, health hazards (smoking, alcohol, medications), and family illnesses = 8 minutes; and review of systems = 20 minutes.[1]

In this case, the interview was structured in such a way that its efficiency in generating data was very poor. A large portion was devoted to the ROS; this is generally unnecessary when one uses earlier parts of the interview to develop an understanding of the patient's life, habits, interests, and other active medical problems, as well as to skillfully explore the current illness. Clinical Key 6–1 presents a more functional allocation of time.

As you gain experience, much of the ROS may be conducted while you perform the physical examination. As you examine the patient's ears, you might ask if he or she has had any problems with hearing, ear infections, and so forth; as you examine the eyes, you might ask if he or she wears glasses. This method of doing the ROS, however, requires a high level of competence. An additional problem is that the patient may believe that you are asking your question (e.g., "Are you having any headaches?") because of something that you see during the physical examination. This may create anxiety and distort the patient's response. Thus, it is important to preface your examination, or at least your questions, with a comment that you will be asking routine questions

---

CLINICAL KEY 6–1

A Functional Allocation of Time in an Initial History

- Introduction—1 minute
- Understanding the patient's life, habits, and interests—5 minutes
- Definition of chief complaint and present illness—15 minutes
- Definition of other active medical problems—5 minutes
- Major past medical and family history—8 minutes
- Review of systems (ROS)—3 minutes

for the sake of completeness rather than questions specifically related to the patient's illness or physical findings.

Some clinicians approach the ROS with standardized questionnaires that the patient fills out before the interview. (The Appendix presents several questionnaires useful for specific aspects of the history.) The use of such instruments, however, does not replace the ROS section of the interview but merely changes its character. Instead of asking directly about symptoms, the clinician reviews the questionnaire and asks for more detail regarding positive responses. The clinician also must determine whether the patient has understood the written words well enough to answer the questions accurately. A questionnaire is perfectly acceptable, but it is useful for the learner to conduct a complete ROS without the benefit of such instruments. Then, after you have developed a comfortable style, you might create a personalized questionnaire for future use.

You must also check out **pertinent negatives;** that is, symptoms a patient has not reported that would support one of your diagnostic hypotheses if it were present. If a patient presents with cough, for instance, a pertinent negative might be a lack of shortness of breath.

Several guidelines are useful in learning about and conducting a good ROS:

- It is not necessary to ask detailed questions about every symptom related to every organ system. **You can expand the net of your inquiry by first emphasizing symptoms related to the patient's principal complaint and by starting with general as opposed to specific yes/no questions.** For example, you can ask, "Are you having any trouble with your vision?" rather than "Is your vision decreasing?" or "Do you see double?" In other words, ask the patient about general difficulties with each system, then focus in on details of existing symptoms, and finally check out pertinent negatives.
- The ROS should be abbreviated or eliminated in emergency situations; it also can be completed at a later date if the patient is too tired or too sick to respond to a tedious inquiry at present.
- Anyone, even someone in perfect health, is likely to have some positive responses on a complete ROS. With each positive response, you should obtain enough detail to indicate whether the symptom is significant or trivial. As a general rule, significance relates to severity and duration: the more severe and the more chronic the symptom, the more likely it is to be important.
- The use of ambiguous terms such as indigestion, bowel trouble, or fatigue is adequate for initial screening. Then, if there is a positive response, the symptom must be defined more precisely.
- The ROS section of the history should be at the end of the interview so that you have had time to "size up" the patient and ascertain how to assess his or her responses (e.g., denial on the one hand or obsession with the trivial on the other).

CLINICAL KEY 6–2

The Style of Questions in the ROS

"I'd like next to ask some general questions about your health to make sure I haven't missed anything. I'd like you to think especially about things that may have bothered you recently (or in the past year since your last checkup). Okay?"

"Have you had any headaches or problems with your head and neck?"

"How about with your vision and your eyes?"

"What about your ears, nose, or throat? Any allergy or hay fever symptoms?"

"Any problems with your skin? Lumps or bumps or moles that concern you?"

And so on....

Clinical Key 6–2 presents the style of questions in the ROS that demonstrates these principles.

A Sample Review of Systems

The following sample transcript is neither comprehensive nor ideal, but simply a reasonable example conducted by a medical house officer. As you read through this interview (in which there are some good and some not-so-good features), think about how you might have phrased these questions, whether you feel important information is missing, and whether you feel any questions are excessively detailed:

I'm going to ask you a bunch of questions I ask everybody. They are very general questions and some of them have short answers. Do you find that you get fevers often?

No.

How about chills? Have you had any chills recently?

Yes, but I just took that as being, you know my hormones for my hysterectomy. That's what I took it as being.

Okay. Do you get night sweats?

Yes.

Do you soak through all your bed clothing?

No.

How much do you weigh now?

202.

How much did you weigh a year ago?

About 180–190.

What is the most you have ever weighed?

This.

You certainly aren't losing weight right now. Is that right?

Right.

Do you get headaches?

Sometimes. Maybe I'd say once a month. Maybe once every other month.

Do you have problems with your vision?

No.

Do you ever have double vision?

No.

Ever see spots in front of your eyes?

No.

How about blurry vision?

No.

Have you ever passed out?

No.

Blacked out?

No.

Do you often feel lightheaded?

No.

Do you hear ringing in your ears?

No.

Do you get a pain in your throat?

No.

Sore throats often?

No.

Does your neck hurt?

No.

Have you noticed any lumps or bumps anywhere in your body?

No.

Do your joints ache?

Yes.

Which ones?

Here.

Okay, you are pointing to your left knee and your back. How about other joints in your body?

No.

Do your muscles ache?

I just thought that it was my muscles in my leg.

Okay, fine. Do you get short of breath when you exercise?

I haven't exercised.

How about just walking around town?

No.

Can you climb stairs without becoming short of breath?

Yes.

Do you get pain in your chest?

No.

Have you ever gotten pain in your chest while you were exercising?

No.

Have you ever felt your heart fluttering or racing very quickly?

I don't think so.

Do your ankles swell on you?

No.

Are you able to lie flat in bed without becoming short of breath?

Yes.

Do you ever wake up in the middle of the night short of breath?

No.

Do you have to cough often?

No.

Ever cough up blood?

No.

Have you noticed any change in bowel habits, your bowel functions?

Yes.

How have they changed?

I don't pass my bowels as often as I did before I had surgery.

How often do you pass your bowels now?

Maybe twice a week.

Is the stool shaped as it was before or is it different? Is it thicker or thinner?

Thicker. Yeah, because a lot of times I have to chew some Feenamints to make it go myself.

Do you have diarrhea intermixed with this at all?

No.

Have you noticed any tarry black stools?

No.

How about blood in your stools or on your stools?

No.

Have you had any belly pain?

Yeah.

Where does your belly hurt you?

Right where I had my incision. Sometimes like only when I laugh.

It hurts you along the incision?

Uh-huh.

How about somewhere else in your belly?

Right here.

Okay, you are pointing to your right groin area.

It's just like—mostly like when I see something real funny and just like when I laugh. There is not any pain, it's just there. I just get a pain when I start laughing.

Have you noticed if you are very thirsty often? Do you find yourself drinking a lot of fluids?

Sometimes.

Do you think that you get cold more easily than some of your friends? Do you find that you put on heavy clothing when other people are not wearing jackets and things?

No.

Does the heat bother you more than you think it bothers other people?

No.

What is your energy level like?

So-so. It's moderate.

Do you become fatigued easily?

Sometimes.

How's your appetite?

Great.

What are the good and not-so-good features of this ROS? Among its good features are its completeness (almost every organ system is covered) and the way in which it is introduced. Also, the interviewer asks one question at a time and gives the patient sufficient opportunity to respond. However, there are also some problems. For example, the physician introduces a little medical jargon with the terms "night sweats" and "change in bowel habits," although many patients understand these terms. The more striking problem (and one common to the ROS) is the variation between lack of detail for some symptoms and overly elaborate detail for others. For example, the patient's complaints of headache, joint pains, and thirst are not further characterized; the clinician seems to have dismissed these symptoms as unimportant without additional inquiry. On the other hand, there appear to be too many specific questions on vision and on cough and various types of shortness of breath; one question, such as "Do you have any trouble breathing?" would do.

The trick is to achieve balance. Because the interviewer is asking questions presumably unrelated to the main problem, the ROS serves as a screening device. The questions are not hypothesis-driven, and the probability that a positive response indicates significant pathology is low.[2] Another way of putting this is that **the positive predictability (how often a certain symptom or symptom complex actually signifies a certain disease) of ROS responses is less than the positive predictability of spontaneous statements that arise in the course of the patient's elaboration of the present illness.**

The Positive ROS

Some patients give a very literal interpretation to the questions in the ROS, answering "yes" to almost every question. When this happens the task seems to be interminably tedious, and the interviewer fears that the history will never end. Sometimes, in addition to being positive, the answers are also given in great detail about relatively trivial matters. For example, although you may want to know if the patient wears glasses, you may have little interest in the fine details of how the patient's refractive error has changed in the past 5 years or what the patient feels about his or her optometrist. A difficult ROS might begin this way:

> Now I'd like to ask you a series of questions just to make sure we haven't missed anything important, okay?
>
> *Fine.*
>
> I'll start with your head, and we'll work our way down. Do you get headaches?
>
> *Oh, I'm used to terrific headaches all through my life, and one doctor said it was high blood pressure, though I didn't know it at the time.*

We seem to be off to a bad start as we do not expect or desire a severe, chronic problem to surface for the first time in the ROS; now, instead of zipping down the list of questions, the interviewer has to stop and ask for details about the headaches. When this happens, usually one of two things is going on: either the clinician has failed to inquire in an empathic way about other active problems and significant past medical history, or the patient has simply overinterpreted the question.

The best way to deal with this situation is to prevent it by asking about other active problems and significant past medical problems soon after the questions concerning the present illness. Not only does this maneuver uncover such problems early in the interview but it also facilitates seeing connections between these problems and the present illness. If this technique fails or if you forget to use it, you might try one of a number of other approaches:

- Bring the patient back to the present with a reminder that the focus is on currently distressing symptoms.

- Make the questions very general—"Have you ever had any stomach or bowel trouble?"—and ask for further details only when the response to the initial screening is positive.
- Encourage filtering out of unnecessary details by reminding the patient of time limitations, or by asking him or her to pick out the most important symptoms.
- Undertake much of the ROS while performing the physical examination.

TRANSITION TO THE PHYSICAL EXAMINATION

Medical interviewing, unlike other forms of the helper–client interaction, usually also involves a physical examination. The history and physical examination are different parts of the same process; if we focus on data gathering, it is difficult to pinpoint exactly where the history ends and the physical examination begins, or vice versa. For example, from the first moment the patient walks into your office or you walk into the hospital room, you begin to make observations about the physical condition of the patient. You observe skin color, affect, behavior, clothing, and mental status. The entire mental status examination, although part of the interview in that it involves no touching, is more properly considered as part of the systematic physical examination (see Chap. 9). On the other side of the coin, as you are doing the physical examination, you continue to interact with your patient, hoping to obtain not only physical information but also personal and symptom information.

It is difficult, at first, to go from talking to touching. Early in your clinical training, it is especially difficult to unglue yourself from your chair and approach the patient. In the hospital, paying attention to the patient's comfort, such as offering some water or changing the window blinds, may be appropriate. Ordinarily, when in the clinic or in your office, you will be interviewing a patient who is fully clothed. Although having a patient disrobe and put on an examination gown prior to the interview is often conducive to good office functioning, it is rarely conducive to patient comfort. It undermines respect for the person. Thus, the patient should be fully clothed, and you will be faced with telling him or her to get undressed when you are ready to start the examination. Clinical Key 6–3 presents how to be direct and clear about what is going to happen and why.

Here is how one clinician begins an examination of a new patient. Note the explicit directions as well as the ROS-type question asked at the beginning of the examination:

> Do you have any questions before we do your exam?
>
> *No.*
>
> Okay. Why don't you climb up here, and just sit there, just step around, and come around there. Okay. I am going to cover you and you can just sit there. I'm going to check your thyroid and your lungs and your heart, and examine your breasts. Have you had any thyroid trouble?
>
> *No.*

CLINICAL KEY 6–3

Making the Transition to the Physical Examination

- First, give the patient an opportunity for the last word. For example, "I think that's about it for now. Is there anything else we haven't covered or that you'd like to tell me before I examine you?"
- Second, tell the patient clearly what the game plan is. For example, "Next I'm going to do your physical examination, and then after that, we can sit down and talk about your problems and what tests you might need."
- Third, be very specific about what clothing the patient should remove, where to sit or lie, and in what position. For example, "I'm going to step out of the room for a moment now. Please get undressed down to your underpants and put on this gown. Put it on with the opening toward the back. And then sit on the end of the table up here."
- Let the patient know your focus is still on him: "I'll review your file while you're getting undressed and then I'll be back."

It is best for you to leave the room, or to pull a curtain across the room if one is available, while your patient gets undressed. In the hospital, of course, this is usually not a problem, but, even there, patients may want to use the bathroom or remove a dressing gown or robe. In office practice, when you are doing only part of a physical examination, it may be appropriate for the patient to remove only his or her shirt or unbutton several buttons. For specific parts of the examination, ask the patient to disrobe that area or, alternatively, say, "I'm going to untie (or unbutton or remove)...." If a female patient has large breasts, ask her for assistance in moving the breast for you to listen to the heart. This approach allows the patient to feel more like a participant and less like a victim.

CONVERSATION DURING THE PHYSICAL EXAMINATION

Although maintaining a conversation during the physical examination allows you to continue to gather data, it may serve other essential functions as well. You can use your communication skills to put the patient at ease, encourage the patient to feel like an active participant in his or her own care, and diminish the perception of a difference in power between the clinician and the patient, which becomes more marked during the physical examination. Here is how one patient describes these feelings:

Whether it be horizontal, or in some awkward placement on one's back or stomach, with legs splayed or cramped, or even in front of a desk, the patient is placed in a series of passive, dependent, and often humiliating positions. These are positions where embarrassment and anger are at war with the desire to take in what the doctor is saying. In this battle learning is clearly the loser.[3]

Use conversation to show the patient that you remember the complaint about abdominal pain while you are doing the abdominal examination, or use "small talk" to distract the patient so the patient's muscles will relax, making the abdominal or pelvic examination easier for the patient and more accurate as well. Keep talking to reassure the patient, and explain what you are doing. As a beginner you may find it difficult to converse while you also are concentrating on the sequence of things to do and the techniques for doing them. It is not difficult, however, to make such observations as:

- "I'm going to look into your ears now."
- "I'm feeling for your thyroid gland. Can you swallow now? I know it's difficult to swallow like that when someone asks you. Good."
- "I'm going to do a rectal exam now to check your prostate gland. It will make you feel like you are going to have a bowel movement, but don't worry, you won't."

It is also easy for you, and reassuring for the patient, to indicate that parts of your examination are normal. It is usually not particularly helpful to comment on every little thing you do, but if you know the patient is concerned about a particular system, it would be helpful to note your findings about that system right away. For the patient who comes in with chest pain, a comment that the heart and lungs sound normal can be quite reassuring for the patient (who need not be bothered at this point with the information that the heart may sound normal even when there is heart disease). Here is an example of how a clinician spoke to a patient during the parts of the physical examination that involved listening to the lungs and heart and palpating the breasts and abdomen. Notice the inclusion of a few ROS-type questions, education about breast self-examination, and attention to the patient's comfort ("Tell me if I hit any sore places.") as parts of the body are examined:

> Okay, I am just going to loosen this [unties gown in back]. How long have you been smoking?
>
> *About 3 years....*
>
> And you want to quit.
>
> *Well, yeah, I've been thinking about it.*
>
> Take a deep breath. Okay, out, good, and again.... Good. Now I am going to ask you to slip your arms all the way out and I am going to listen to your heart.... Okay. Sounds good. Now I'm going to check your breasts. I want you to put your hands up like this [demonstrates] and I'm just going to look at them first to see if there are any bumps....

Uh mm.

Okay, have you ever tried examining your breasts?

No, not really.

We recommend that everyone do it once a month; the best time is right after your period has stopped. Do your breasts get sore before your period?

Yes.

Okay, well, that is why it is best to wait until after your period starts when usually the lumpiness goes away and they're not tender to touch.... I am going to ask you to just hold this up ... and I want you to put your arms up over your head. What you do when you are checking is to do exactly what I'm doing.... Go all around the outside of your breasts like this ... up here is breast tissue and also up here ... so you are going to go in kind of a circle like this ... then spiral in until you get every part including under the nipple. Okay? Now I'd like you to lie down and we'll check your breasts again.... We always check them in two positions.... And I am going to check your heart.... Do you have any indigestion or trouble with your bowels? Now tell me if I hit any sore places.

The pelvic examination is a particularly personal and anxiety-producing experience. You should explain clearly what you are about to do and what the patient is likely to feel. Ask the patient if she has had a pelvic examination before. Whether she has or not, it is very reassuring to say something like "I'm going to pretend that this is your first pelvic examination and explain everything that I'm doing." The less experience the patient has had, either with pelvic examinations or with you, the more reassurance she will need. You should first touch the patient's inner thigh and then firmly but gently conduct the examination. You should describe the anatomy to the patient as you are doing the examination. As you become more experienced, you will be able to help her relax her muscles through your calm tone of voice, your gentle palpation, and your instructions about deep, slow breathing.

Here is how one clinician introduced a patient (who had requested a diaphragm for birth control) to her first pelvic examination. Everything is described with a relaxing, almost hypnotic, tone of voice; gestures are slow and deliberate (no sudden moves); and the clinician continuously looks at the patient's face to gauge her reactions:

The next thing I am going to do is a pelvic exam. These are all the things I am going to use, but I am not going to use all of them on you. Okay. These are the slides on which the Pap test is done, and these are the little brushes that I use to do the Pap test. See how soft they are? and this also, which I will roll around the cervix just like that [demonstrating], see, it is not sharp.... We usually do a culture for infection at the same time....

A culture?

Yes, and that is to check for infection. This instrument is cold, and that is really the worst thing about it. It is called a speculum and this is inserted very gently into the vagina and then opened very gently like that [demonstrating] so that I can see your cervix and see that it is normal. Okay? [Patient nods.]

What I will ask you to do is to put your feet into these things, which are called stirrups, these metal things, that's good, and now I want you to pull yourself all the way down to the end of the table like that, and practically feel yourself like your bottom is coming off the end of the table. Okay? That's fine. I am going to put this pillow under your head right there, okay, and I am going to shine a light on you so that I can see what I am doing and as I do things I will tell you what I am doing. Okay? Are you more or less comfortable?

I guess so.

All right, it is not very comfortable, that is true. Okay. Now what I am going to do is to look at the outside of you first. If you can just kind of relax, that's good. Now what I am doing is checking the labia, or lips. Good. Now you are going to feel my finger at the edge of the vagina, feeling where your cervix is. Do you know what your cervix is?

No.

Okay, that is the opening to your womb or uterus. Okay, I am just kind of locating it first, and that is just my finger again. Okay, now you're going to feel the cold metal which I tried to warm up a little bit, but usually it's still cold. Is that okay?

Mm hmm.

Now I insert it just until I can see your cervix so that I can do the Pap test. Okay, now I can see your cervix very clearly now....

Is that where I put the diaphragm?

Exactly, that is exactly where to put the diaphragm. Okay, now I am just using that soft brush to do the Pap test, okay?

Mm hmm.

And now I'm going to use one of those scrapers and sometimes you feel that scraping feeling, but usually what you feel is the pressure of the speculum being in place there.... Now I am just spraying those glass slides that I just took and that preserves them so they can be checked later. And now I am taking the speculum out. Are you still with me?

Yeah.

Now I am going to just check back inside your vagina, okay, and where my fingers are is where you put the diaphragm. Now I am going to ask you that when you go home you practice feeling where your cervix is. I am touching it right now. On you, it is a little bit off to your left side,

> okay, and it feels like the tip of your nose when you touch it. Okay.
> When I put one hand over here, between the two hands I can feel
> where your uterus is.... And I am touching it right now and it feels
> normal. Now I am checking on each side for your ovaries....
>
> *Can you feel all that?*
>
> Yes, I can feel all that, especially in someone like you, because you are
> very relaxed and I can feel everything. Okay, the next thing I am going
> to do is check your rectum and that will make you feel as though you
> have to have a bowel movement, right, that is just my finger in your
> rectum. That's kind of an uncomfortable feeling. It feels completely
> normal.

Notice how the clinician keeps talking, but frequently checks back with the patient, and is educating the patient all the while about her body and about the normality of the findings. Indeed, the proof that the technique is effective is in the patient's pleasure and wonderment ("Can you feel all that?") at the ability of a pelvic examination to tell so much and her ability to completely relax her muscles.

Your continued interview with the patient during the physical examination provides clarification and reassurance, and increases your efficiency. The new information aspect will gradually develop as you become more comfortable with the procedures of physical examination, so that concentration on the actual techniques can sink into the background and you are able to concentrate more thoroughly on your immediate observations. Until you are experienced, do not try to do the complete ROS during the physical examination. However, if you are looking at the eyes, for example, and this reminds you of an eye question you forgot to ask, go ahead and ask it. The physical examination is also a good time for "chit chat" with the patient, thereby finding out more about his or her life and lifestyle.

Finally, the physical examination itself has not only a diagnostic but also a therapeutic role. Simply touching the patient—the "laying on of hands"—may cause him or her to feel better and be reassured. Tactile communication opens up a channel of interpersonal response that can be very important in healing. In particular, specific attention to the painful areas of the body demonstrates that you have listened, understood, and are concerned about the patient's suffering.

ENDING THE INTERVIEW

When you have completed the physical examination, you reconvene the interview to terminate it. The goal of a good closure is no different from the goal of your entire interview and will be easier to attain if the patient understands from the outset the purpose of the interaction. The purpose will vary, depending on whether you are a medical student, resident, physician assistant, nurse practitioner, or attending physician with a long-term role in the patient's management. Overall, the patient should expect to feel understood and not be abused in any way. In history taking, this means that you have gotten the story straight and shown appropriate concern for his or her comfort, privacy, and modesty. The techniques of being accurate, empathic, respectful, and genuine apply to this part of the encounter as they do to all the other parts.

It is always a good idea to give the patient the opportunity to have the last word:

- "Anything else?"
- "Do you feel there is anything about what you have told me that I have not understood?"
- "Is there anything else you'd like to tell me or ask me?"

If you are a student, this may be the end of your contact with the patient. When you close the encounter, you should:

- Provide a summary of what the patient has told you.
- Be sure to let the patient have the last word or ask any additional questions.
- Give a pleasant thank you and goodbye.

If patients ask questions you cannot answer about their diseases or medical care, you should say something like "I am not able to answer that, but it is a good question to ask your doctor." This is a truthful answer whether you are unable to answer because you do not know, or because, although you do know, the question is more properly answered by the patient's physician.

When you have responsibility for a patient's care, however, the more typical closure implies a continuing **contract** between you and the patient; it acknowledges responsibility for solving problems and providing care. In this general context, ending a patient encounter, whether an initial evaluation or a short office visit, should include these actions on the part of the clinician:

- **Differential diagnosis or hypotheses.** What you share depends on the patient—how sick he or she is, how knowledgeable, and whether or not he or she has other sources of information. What you share also depends on the illness; some findings are pertinent to the illness, and others are incidental or trivial. Avoid discussing what is interesting to you but may be irrelevant to the patient.
- **Devise a problem list with priorities.** This is painstaking and difficult at first but becomes easier with experience. It is important to realize that the clinician's priorities often differ from those of the patient. Patients may be interested first in feeling better, second in their overall prognosis, and third in the specific diagnosis. Clinicians share these concerns but often (especially while in training) are more interested in making the diagnosis than in treating the symptoms. Treating the symptom is often not the same as treating the disease. Many trivial illnesses (e.g., simple upper respiratory tract infections) do not in themselves need specific medications but have symptoms that patients want treated. On the other hand, many significant

illnesses (e.g., hypertension) have no symptoms but, from the clinician's point of view, demand specific therapy.

- **Educate and negotiate.** The clinician should provide information so that the patient can make informed decisions about the illness and treatment. The clinician then answers questions and engages in negotiation to determine the optimal course of action consistent with the patient's beliefs and values (see Chap. 16).

- **Agree on a plan of action and clarify responsibilities.** Determine what will happen next and who will do what. The clinician may agree to order and interpret tests, talk with consultants, write prescriptions, provide information, or perform procedures. The patient may agree to take medication, modify diet, keep the follow-up appointment, or report further symptoms. Ideally, medical care is a partnership in which you negotiate an agreement or contract with the patient, but the character of that contract depends on the patient's illness (emergency care versus chronic antihypertensive therapy) and on the patient's acceptance of responsibility (see "Negotiation" in Chap. 16).

To conclude this chapter, we present an example of the closing minutes of an office visit with a patient who suffers from back pain:

> I don't find anything on my exam. I don't find anything that makes me think you have a pinched nerve. I think periodically you may be getting some nerve irritation and that's accounting for the pain that's shooting down your legs. What I think we should do, I want to check your x-rays that you had. I want to review those. I think you should get off of your feet at least for a day or two. Is that, are you able to do that?

> *Yeah.*

> You don't live by yourself?

> *No. I live with my daughter.*

> Okay, fine. I'm going to give you a couple of different medicines. I'll refill the Percocets, but I only want you to use that as needed. I'm going to give you another medicine called Motrin. Are you able to take aspirin?

> *Yes.*

> So, I'm going to give you Motrin, which is an anti-inflammatory medicine. I don't want you to expect any overnight relief from the Motrin, because it takes several days, sometimes up to a week. So I'm going to give you the Motrin, Percocet, and I'll give you a prescription for something called Pericolace, which is a very mild laxative and stool softener to make sure you don't get constipated. Do you have a heating pad at home?

> *Yeah, I have a moist heating pad.*

Wonderful. You can use that every hour if you like, but I don't want you using it for more than 20 minutes at a time. But you can use it up to 20 minutes out of every hour. All right? So, I want you to really cut down on your activity and then gradually increase your activity. But no prolonged sitting or standing, and no bending or heavy lifting. I want to see you next week, preferably on Friday.

What about my physical therapy?

I want to lay off that for now.

Now will you explain to me again what the Motrin is?

Motrin is an anti-inflammatory drug. It's an arthritic drug.

In other words, it's supposed to help the pain in the back?

A lot of the pain in back injuries is due to irritation of the tissues and this will quiet down that irritation of the tissues, that in conjunction with, first of all, the rest. I didn't feel too much muscle spasm in your back now.

Well, that has quieted down some. I had quite a bit in October. It sort of quit, but I still have the pain.

There's your prescriptions, here's the Percocet, only take that as needed for extra pain. The Motrin I want you to take one, four times per day: breakfast, lunch, dinner, bedtime, and you should take that continuously.... And remember, take it with meals or with something in your stomach, not on an empty stomach because it can irritate your stomach.... I want to see you next week, preferably on Friday, that will give us a full week. Okay? And we will see in a week, see how you are doing and, as I said, in the meantime, I'll review the x-rays. Okay? Anything else?

I wanted to mention to you. I had gone for a Pap smear and they said the Pap smear was normal, I mean I don't have cancer....

Notice how this physician shares the findings and clarifies the plan of action, including what he will do and what he expects the patient to do. Note, too, how the patient at the last minute brings up her concern about cancer possibly being the cause of her pain. The physician can now offer appropriate reassurance that the etiology of her pain is not cancer, and he will know that the patient's fear of cancer may reappear if the pain does not improve. It is not at all unusual for critical information like this to surface at the close of the interview when the patient feels comfortable and can see that he or she is being listened to. It is vital, therefore, that you demonstrate your open-ended attitude even as you close the encounter, as this clinician did with the remark "Okay? Anything else?"

SUMMARY ▪ THE ROS, PHYSICAL EXAMINATION, AND CLOSURE

The objectives of the ROS are to:
- Identify active problems not yet discussed
- Associate additional symptoms with current illness

The ROS may occur late in the interview, or parts of it may occur during the physical examination, when you chat with the patient to:
- Obtain more ROS-type information
- Learn more about the patient as a person
- Make the patient more comfortable.

After the examination, you close the clinical encounter by:
- Summarizing what you heard and what you found
- Devising a problem list and negotiating priorities
- Outlining a plan of action and responsibilities
- Continuing to educate the patient
- Giving the patient the last word

References

1. Platt FW, McMath JC. Clinical hypocompetence: The interview. *Ann Intern Med* 1979; 91:898–902.
2. Verdon ME, Siemens K. Yield of review of systems in a self administered questionnaire. *J Am Board Fam Pract* 1997; 10:20–27.
3. Eisenberg L, Kleinman A. Clinical social science. In: Eisenberg L, Kleinman A (Eds.). *The Relevance of Social Science to Medicine.* Dordrecht, Holland, D. Reidel, 1980.

Suggested Reading

Boland BJ, Wollan PC, Silverstein MD. Review of systems, physical examination, and routine tests for case finding in ambulatory patients. *Am J Med Sci* 1995; 309:194–200.

Coulehan JL, Schulberg HC, Block MR. The efficiency of depression questionnaires for case finding in primary medical care. *J Gen Intern Med* 1989; 4:461–467.

Cyr MG, Wartman SA. The effectiveness of routine screening questions in the detection of alcoholism. *JAMA* 1988; 259:51–54.

Johnson KB, Feldman MJ. Medical informatics and pediatrics. Decision-support systems. *Arch Pediatr Adolesc Med* 1995; 149:1371–1380.

Mitchell TL, Tornelli JL, Fisher TD, Blackwell TA, Moorman JR. Yield of the screening review of systems. A study on a general medical service. *J Gen Intern Med* 1992; 7:393–397.

Novack DH. Therapeutic aspects of the clinical encounter. *J Gen Intern Med* 1987; 2:346–355.

Older J. Teaching touch at medical school. *JAMA* 1984; 252:931–933.

Spitzer RL, William JB, Kroenke K, et al. Utility of a new procedure of diagnosing mental disorders in primary care: The PRIME-MD 1000 study. *JAMA* 1994; 272:1749–1756.

Wall EM. The predictive value of selected components of medical history taking. *J Am Board Fam Pract* 1997; 10:66–67.

Zimmerman M, Coryell W. The validity of a self-report questionnaire for diagnosing major depressive disorder. *Arch Gen Psychiatry* 1988; 45:738–740.

Zung WK. A self-rating depression scale. *Arch Gen Psychiatry* 1965; 12:63–70.

CHAPTER 7

I Shall Enumerate Them to You

● ● ● ● ●

THE CLINICAL NARRATIVE

*At least I have a grip of the essential facts of the case. **I shall enumerate them to you,** for nothing clears up a case so much as stating it to another person.*

Sherlock Holmes to Dr. Watson

in "Silver Blaze"

After you interview and examine your patient, you walk away, possibly with pages of cryptic notes. You may feel pretty clear about the story and already have a few inklings of differential diagnosis. The most important single part of your patient's workup is complete, but before progressing further, your next task is to put the story on paper, or "do the write-up." From the morass of the patient's symptoms and experiences, you have to choose what to include in the permanent clinical record. How do you do that? And how do you structure the story to make it most useful?

Because this text is limited to the skills of clinical interviewing, in this chapter we focus on how to conceptualize, format, and write down the clinical history. However, the patient record is, in fact, a literary genre with its own objectives and standards of practice. In this genre, a patient history does not normally stand by itself. Its proper format also includes physical and laboratory data, an assessment or formulation (e.g., what the clinician's hypotheses are), and a plan for diagnosis and/or therapy, not to mention subsequent entries like flow charts and progress notes. Consequently, to give a more complete picture of the clinical record, we also present some guidelines for the other, nonhistorical elements of your write-up.

This chapter consists of four sections. In the first, we consider some basic concepts about recording the written history and the purposes of a clinical record. Whose story is it, the clinician's or the patient's? The second section presents a basic outline for constructing the written history and physical examination. Next we comment on some of the advantages and disadvantages of the problem-oriented method of clinical record keeping. Finally, we consider the formal case presentation and other forms of oral communication among health care professionals.

TURNING THE HISTORY INTO THE WRITE-UP: THE CLINICAL NARRATIVE

Just the Facts?

Recording the history is not a question of "just the facts, ma'am." It is the end product, if you will, of a long process of selection, interpretation, and editing. What you write on paper is a result of at least four levels of selection and interpretation:

- The first level is the **patient's experience** or raw data; that is, the "facts" as they actually happened and what it was like for the patient to feel the throbbing headache or experience the room spinning around.
- The second level is the patient's **conceptualization of the experience;** that is, how the patient organized the facts to construct a story that lends meaning and coherence to the experience. This conceptualization draws on the patient's values and beliefs. He or she began to weave this story even before seeking medical help, but your questions and selective attention help create the current version.
- A third level is the **clinical tale,** the story you generate by means of the clinical interview. Because you speak a medical language and live in a medical culture, you may reconstruct the patient's story with additional characters (e.g., groupings of symptoms) or a somewhat different plot development.
- Finally, you select some of this story for the **write-up.** To do this, you apply certain canons of literary form. There are rules and guidelines appropriate to the write-up just as there are rules and guidelines appropriate to other literary genres like the short story or the nonfiction essay.

When we call the final product the "clinical history," it is easy to forget the interpretive and selective process that went into producing it. You are not simply a passive secretary or scribe. It is both inefficient and impossible to repeat everything the patient says. In this respect, it is useful to use the metaphor "interpreting a text" to describe diagnosis and problem solving in the clinician–patient interaction. What seems at first glance to be "just the facts" is actually an interpretation of the facts. You are trying to understand the meaning of the patient's story much as a literary critic tries to understand a text. The quality of your interpretation depends on your skill and experience, as well as on the text's underlying readability. The context in which you see a patient or read a sentence can be a major determinant in your interpretation. No single interpretation of a book or of a patient's illness is final; there should be continuous re-evaluation. In clinical practice, as in literary criticism, a "true" interpretation is validated through open discourse among peers and consultants.

Recording Personal Information

Because we tend to believe that what is written in the chart is *prima facie* true, and because the medical record has so many functions, the record can become a powerful source of misinformation. Errors, such as mistakes in observation or clinical judgment, tend to be perpetuated because so much emphasis is placed on the written word. A wrong diagnosis or a judgmental remark, once written, is difficult to eradicate. Keep this issue in mind, particularly when recording personal data about the patient.

What personal data should be recorded? Here are some guidelines that attempt to steer between the Scylla of biochemical approaches to the patient and the Charybdis of disrespect or sentimentality:

- Be cautious about recording the patient's attitude, lifestyle, expectations, and/or health belief system. Although it is always useful to have relevant knowledge of this sort about the patient, it is not always important to write it explicitly. Unless a patient's dramatic or dependent style is out of the ordinary range, privacy and efficiency dictate silence. If you need to communicate a patient's style or idiosyncratic beliefs to others because they play a significant role in patient care, then the information should be written in a descriptive, as opposed to a judgmental, way.
- Delete certain personal information from the written record, such as explicit description of sexual habits, problematic relationships, or criminal records, even though it may seem important. Imagining the chart being read by the patient is a useful criterion for what is appropriate to write.
- Include the patient's own words whenever possible, not just in the chief complaint. For example, recording that the patient describes the headache as "a deep pain like someone is twisting a screwdriver

inside my brain" tells a lot about the patient and is less judgmental than writing "patient describes the headache in a bizarre fashion," or "patient is histrionic."

- Minimize distortion by avoiding language that "pathologizes." In clinical practice we often use words that turn people, experiences, or feelings into "pathologies"; the plain language of human experience does not seem medical enough for us. We like to use "depressed" rather than "sad," and rarely do we describe patients as "discouraged" or "courageous." To make the record more personally descriptive, avoid words like *apathy, anxiety, denial, depression,* and *manipulative.* Try instead to use words like *determined, discouraged, hopeful, optimistic, brave, fearful, sad,* or *hopeless.* Likewise, beware of saying that the patient *refuses, declines,* or *has failed* the measures you prescribe.
- Use behavioral or functional descriptions to convey personal information. By simply describing how the patient spends his or her day, what his or her hobbies are, or what he or she does on weekends, you can sketch important features of the person without getting too personal. Such statements fit well into the medical record; the operative principle is to be descriptive, not judgmental.

FUNCTIONS OF THE CLINICAL RECORD

Memory Aid

Originally the medical record served only as a stimulus to jog a clinician's memory. Many physicians, for example, kept brief notes on index cards. The complete "text" was not on the card but in the clinician's mind. Although today we use more extensive records, we still remember details about our patients' lives and experiences that we do not write down.

Communication

The medical record serves to communicate with other health professionals. In the modern hospital or clinic setting, health care is a multidisciplinary team activity; for example, as many as 50 or more people may have legitimate access to an inpatient chart. Most of them will want to communicate their findings and their treatments to other members of the team. This communicative function leads to certain conventions regarding which observations are important to record and the form in which they ought to be recorded.

Quality Assessment and Research

A senior clinician evaluates his or her students and residents, at least in part, on the basis of the patient record they write. Hospital quality assurance and utilization review committees monitor the performance of physicians and other health professionals by reviewing their charts. The clinical record also serves as a data source. Retrospective chart reviews serve as one of the basic building blocks for clinical research.

Administrative and Legal Matters

Health care insurers use the chart to verify diagnosis and to establish that claimed services were actually provided. Quality control and cost-containment strategies involve reviewing charts and ascertaining "quality" at least in part on the basis of recorded data. Finally, the clinical record is legally discoverable and can be used as evidence in court.

FORMAT OF THE CLINICAL RECORD

Table 7–1 presents the elements usually included in a clinical write-up. Although there is broad consensus on these major features, detailed conventions about the way they are put together vary from hospital to hospital, clinic to clinic, and practice to practice. Some institutions use structured forms, at least for the more "objective" parts of the write-up, such as problem lists and physical examination; some use paperless computerized records; and others rely on old-fashioned handwritten notes. The following discussion is a generic one into which most institution-specific formats should fit.

TABLE 7–1

ELEMENTS OF CLINICAL CASE DESCRIPTION
Subjective
History
▪ Identifying data.
▪ Chief complaint: Use the patient's own words.
▪ History of the present illness: Organize the story.
▪ Other active problems: Outline what else is going on.
▪ Past medical history: Note hospitalizations, surgery, allergies, important illnesses.
▪ Family history: Use a genogram or table.
▪ Patient profile: Sketch with care.
▪ Review of systems: Record significant positives and negatives.
Objective
Physical examination
Laboratory data
Integrative
Assessment: The problem list
Plan

Identifying Data and Chief Complaint

The write-up begins with a succinct statement that identifies the patient and tells why he or she is seeking medical help. Often the patient's chief complaint, stated in the patient's own words in quotation marks, is the most effective descriptive statement to use. For example:

- Mr. Steven Maringo is a 47-year-old construction worker who came in because "I've had a sore throat for a month and it won't go away."
- Ms. Alice York is a 41-year-old chemist at Alcoa, with a history of "ulcers," who came in now because "I've had a burning pain under my ribs all week."
- Beth Salisbury is a 10-year-old fourth grader who came in because "my ear hurts" since yesterday.
- Mr. Fred Jones is a 32-year-old computer programmer referred by Dr. A. Zinger for evaluation of a persistent "washed out feeling" and lower extremity weakness.

When a patient has been referred, as in the last example, it is important to record that fact. Some patients may not have a chief "complaint" as such because they are coming in for a routine checkup or a driver's license examination. Whatever the reason, it is recorded in the patient's own words.

Other particularly relevant data may also be included in the introductory statement. For example, "Mr. Fred Jones is a 32-year-old, unmarried, African–American computer programmer who works at Ibex Industries." However, one should not try to pack this sentence with too many identifying features. Is the fact that Jones is unmarried or African–American relevant to his persistent "washed out feeling"? Maybe, but a thousand other features might be relevant as well. Although it is best to strive for simplicity here, many institutions have their own conventions about how to begin the write-up. Some, for example, might insist that you identify all patients by race and occupation, in addition to age and sex, no matter what their medical problems are.

Present Illness

The Present Illness section should reflect your interpretation and organization of the patient's story. Although the diagnoses may be in doubt, you should have a good grasp of the patient's problem(s), and organize the present illness description accordingly. The description should be succinct, with emphasis on:

- Time course
- Symptom characteristics
- Functional deficits

Use the patient's own words and voice when possible, but remember that *you* are the author here. Just because the patient rambles or has 13 different complaints doesn't mean that you should ramble as well. Your organization and choice of material should reflect *your* thinking about how the symptoms fit together, not the patient's.

For example, consider the transcription of an opening statement presented in Chapter 3 (p. 42). The written Present Illness section might begin thus:

> Mrs. P has been feeling "tired" and "worn out" even when she gets as much as 11 hours' sleep. Her sleep is interrupted by "hot flashes," although these are less frequent than they were previously.

The writer may choose to put the patient's concerns about nervousness and loss of libido under the Other Active Problems section (to follow), or may include them in the Present Illness, if he or she considers them aspects of the same problem (a depressive disorder, for example).

You will frequently encounter patients who have had multiple hospital admissions and specialty consultations, and who have records an inch thick. It is tempting to construct the present history of such a patient from old chart data, with little input from the patient. For example:

> Mrs. Ely was first found to have carcinoma of the breast in May 1995, after which she underwent a left simple mastectomy, followed by a course of local irradiation. In June 1999 she was noted to have bone mets in T4 and L1... [list series of medical interventions]... and today [in February 2001] is admitted to be evaluated for further chemotherapy.

This is not a history of an illness; it is a chronicle of medical events. Does the patient currently have symptoms? Why is chemotherapy being considered at this time, rather than last year or next month? The patient's voice is absent. Medical records can provide supplemental information that sheds light on the current problem, but it is never appropriate to construct a narrative based on data from old records and call it "present illness."

Other Active Medical Problems

It is useful to consider the Other Active Medical Problems section a separate section, although sometimes it may be integrated with the Present Illness section. Patients often have complex and chronic medical problems. A given episode of illness may well be an exacerbation of a chronic problem, or interact with another ongoing disease. Because of this, it is important to select continuing problems from the Past Medical History and to provide details about their current status. In the preceding example, if Mrs. Ely was admitted for symptoms of pneumonia, her history of breast cancer and chemotherapy would certainly be relevant, and would be recorded thoroughly in this part of the text.

Past Medical History

The Past Medical History section begins the more standardized or routine part of the write-up. By definition, it includes only those problems not directly (or obviously) relevant to the illness at hand. The format, as described in Chapter 4, should be as follows:

- Serious illnesses, from childhood to the present, including hospitalizations
- Surgical procedures
- Accidents and injuries
- Pregnancies, deliveries, and complications
- Allergies, including type and known allergens
- Current medications, including over-the-counter drugs, with dosages and schedule (these may also be listed under Other Active Problems)
- Health maintenance data, including immunizations and screening tests

Family History

The family history is best presented in a genogram that shows relationships in a diagrammatic form (Fig. 7–1). Squares represent males; circles, females. A diagonal line or "x" indicates that the person has died. Diseases may be indicated above or below the symbols. Alternatively, the family history can be presented in tabular form. This method is more efficient if the patient does not have much medical information about his or her family. Relationships can be indicated by abbreviations such as MGM for maternal grandmother, PGF for paternal grandfather, and so forth. Such a family history might look like this:

MGM (d. age 60s), unknown cause
MGF (d. age 70), heart attack
PGF (92), arthritis, forgetful

Social History and Patient Profile

The object of the **patient profile** is to give a picture of the patient as a functioning person and to record medically related or health-related behavior. The harried clinician should avoid making the person invisible and recording only whether he or she smokes tobacco or drinks alcohol. On the other hand, the writer should also avoid becoming too discursive or personal. Some considerations about how much personal data to include are presented in the next section. Approach writing the Patient Profile with a standard outline in mind, similar to the outline used during your interview, even though, in a given case, you need not necessarily write something for each item:

- Brief biography (e.g., place of birth, education, military service, and years in this locality)
- Current marital, family, and home situation
- Occupation and occupational history, including toxic exposures and stresses
- Lifestyle (e.g., religious affiliation, spirituality, personal interests, hobbies, travel, and exercise)
- Diet and nutrition

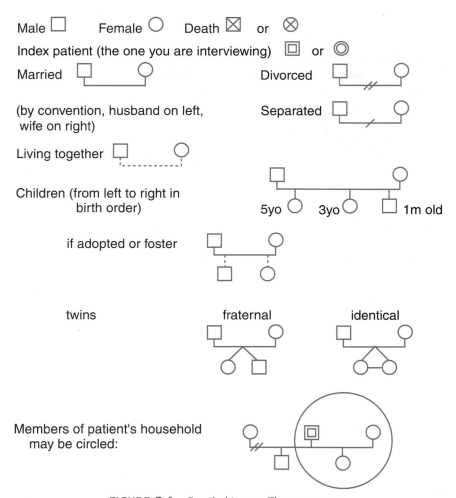

Male □   Female ○   Death ⊠ or ⊗

Index patient (the one you are interviewing) ▣ or ◎

Married   Divorced

(by convention, husband on left,   Separated
 wife on right)

Living together

Children (from left to right in
         birth order)   5yo 3yo 1m old

         if adopted or foster

         twins   fraternal   identical

Members of patient's household
    may be circled:

FIGURE 7-1   Family history: The genogram.

- Personal habits (e.g., use of tobacco, alcohol, and "recreational" drugs)
- A typical day's activities (this may be placed under Present Illness when a change in functional status is an important descriptor of the illness)
- Relevant feelings and beliefs (e.g., work satisfaction, perceived stresses, understanding of the illness, and attitudes toward health care)

Review of Systems

Data obtained in the Review of Systems (ROS) section of the interview may be incorporated into the written Present Illness, if relevant to the current problem(s); placed in a structured system-by-system ROS section; or simply left unwritten. Beginners should include a fairly comprehensive ROS to develop the discipline of considering each system in turn. More experienced clinicians will usually write a few positive findings and pertinent negative findings. They will then indicate that the rest of the ROS was "unremarkable" or "negative."

Physical Examination

Although there are many local variations, the overall format is standard. You begin with a statement about the patient's general appearance and continue with vital signs (respiration rate, blood pressure, pulse rate, and temperature) and the results of the examination of skin, head, eyes, ears, nose, throat, neck, lymphatic system, chest, back, breasts, heart, abdomen, rectum, genitourinary system, extremities, musculoskeletal system, nervous system, and, finally, mental status. Although you generally collect mental status data by talking rather than touching, they are recorded as part of the physical examination.

Laboratory Work

Results of diagnostic studies may be included as part of the initial write-up if they are routine or are available shortly after your interview and physical examination. In such cases, the results are part of the database on which your assessment and plan are based. There is no standard method of recording laboratory or x-ray findings. Perhaps the most efficient and efficacious way is to use appropriate flow sheets and not place these data in the midst of written text. Nevertheless, it can be useful to have a snapshot of basic studies (complete blood count and differential, urinalysis, serum chemistries, chest x-ray, or electrocardiogram) in the database to help buttress your initial assessment. Each institution has its own recommended set of routine laboratory work for new patients, or for patients admitted to the hospital. However, in recent years the emphasis has been on selecting diagnostic studies, rather than on ordering "routine" studies.

Assessment and Plan

A good way of organizing your assessment and plan is to use principles derived from the problem-oriented medical record system, which we will now address.

PROBLEM-ORIENTED RECORDS

Many health care institutions and clinical offices employ some version of the problem-oriented medical record (POMR). There are numerous variations of the POMR system, but we emphasize these basic elements that contribute to patient-centered care:

- **Database.** Each record should include a database that consists of the written clinical history, physical examination, and basic laboratory data. The narrative in the database should reflect the human story, rather than being merely a compilation of symptoms and diagnoses.
- **Problem list.** Each record should include a list that enumerates the patient's identified health problems, including currently active problems and those that have resolved. This list ought to be updated regularly. The problems may include expressed concerns of the patient, as well as observations and interpretations made by the clinician. Thus, a problem might be any of the following: a symptom or diagnosis; a physical sign or laboratory finding; or a personal, social, existential, financial, or functional difficulty. As further information develops over time, the initial problems may be clarified, condensed, divided, or resolved, and others may be added.
- **Structured entries.** Usually a structured format is used to write about each problem initially and in subsequent hospital or office notes. This format includes four sections:
  - ⇒ **S**ubjective, recounting symptoms and personal data
  - ⇒ **O**bjective, dealing with physical signs and laboratory data
  - ⇒ **A**ssessment, expressing the clinician's analysis of the problem
  - ⇒ **P**lan, stating the measures to be taken

  The acronym **SOAP note** or **SOAP format** acknowledges these four structural elements in each entry. This scheme presents a structured opportunity to assess subjective data and use them regularly in writing progress notes. The term "person-oriented data" is perhaps more appropriate here than is the term "subjective."
- **Flow charts.** The record may include preprinted flow charts and other devices to jog the clinician's memory, organize and display complex data, and enhance patient care.

PRESENTING THE PATIENT

The written case record may serve as the Federal Reserve Bank, but the oral case presentation is the day-to-day currency of clinical practice. Trainees and clinicians communicate rapidly and effectively about patient care by sharing well-organized vignettes that "capture" the patient and his or her clinical problem. As a student you may first encounter case presentation on rounds in the hospital, where the intern or resident gives a succinct summary of the case, ending with a differential diagnosis and plan of action. Less experienced trainees are generally expected to give longer, more "complete" case presentations, often lasting for several minutes, whereas more experienced trainees give capsule summaries lasting only a minute or two. As you become more familiar with case presentation, you will notice that some presenters come across as assured and energetic; at the end of their presentations, you can actually *visualize* the patient and understand the problem. But some presenters come across as tentative and disorganized; their patients remain elusive. Not infrequently, disorganized presenters will attribute much of the problem to their patients. "The story isn't clear," they'll say, "because the patient is a poor historian."

Oral case presentation is a clinical skill in its own right. In the next section we briefly outline the major features of case presentation and present some guidelines.

Guidelines for Effective Case Presentation

Know Your Patient

To present a patient effectively, you have to understand the story and have some idea of how the clinical evidence fits together. Clearly, if you have taken a good history, performed an examination, thought the case through and completed a written workup, you should be able to meet this threshold criterion. We can't emphasize enough how important it is to have a thorough grasp of the story before condensing for oral presentation. If you have questions about the primary data, go back to the patient. If you have questions about how items fit together, discuss them with one of your colleagues or supervisors.

Know Your Listener

What is the purpose of your presentation? What do you hope to accomplish? It makes a big difference whether you are presenting your patient on rounds in the context of general medical care, or to a specialty consultant, such as a cardiologist or a social worker. Bear your listener's expertise and interest in mind.

Understand the Power and Limitations of the Spoken Word

Readers can linger as long as they wish over a text, but listeners have to comprehend what you are saying as you say it. Clarity and organization are high priorities. The other side of the coin is your opportunity to engage listeners and direct their attention by telling a good story.

Sell the Story

To capture the power of the word, your style of presentation is crucial. You need to "sell" your patient and the narrative you've constructed. When you are giving a case presentation, you should seize the opportunity to bring the clinical data together in an effective and convincing way. At the end of your presentation, your listeners should have a vivid picture rather than a series of disconnected data points.

Format of the Case Presentation

1. **Opening Statement.** Begin with an opening statement much like the opening of your written report. This statement should provide a quick look at the patient as a person while, if possible, introducing the chief complaint in the patient's own words. You should not try to fully characterize patients and put them into pigeonholes, but rather to give a glimpse of living, breathing persons. For example, consider the following opening statements:

   "Mr. B is a 69-year-old retired salesman with diabetes, hypertension, coronary artery disease, and high cholesterol, who developed severe chest pain while he was driving his car to the mall this morning."

   "Mrs. R is a 47-year-old school teacher from Bayshore who presents with 3 days of increasing chest pain and productive cough."

2. **The Illness Narrative.** Present the history of the present illness and other active problems in a concise way. Remember that you are telling a story, not reciting a medical textbook or describing a random occurrence. You are also "selling" the story. Don't be afraid to be enthusiastic.

   The more structured sections of the history—past medical history, ROS, family history—can usually be handled by presenting only positives and relevant negatives. It is perfectly appropriate for a formal oral presentation to contain a statement such as the following:

   "Past medical history includes gall-bladder surgery in 1969 and chronic open angle glaucoma diagnosed some time in the 1980s. As far as the patient knows there is no pertinent family history. The review of systems was essentially negative."

3. **Patient Profile.** You would be surprised at how a patient can "come alive" by presenting a few human details. Yes, you do want to indicate whether the patient smokes, drinks, or uses recreational drugs. But it is easy enough to say, in addition, that he is a married steam-fitter who lives with his wife and has two grown children; or is an attorney who lives alone and plays semiprofessional baseball. These items may give your patient a human face while adding only a few seconds to your presentation.

4. **Physical Examination and Laboratory Data.** Your presentation will also include a targeted statement of physical findings and relevant laboratory data. Beginners may be asked to provide more completeness in this area (i.e., long lists of negatives).

COMMUNICATION AMONG PROFESSIONALS

The complexity and size of the health care team has increased enormously from the old days when the only players included the patient, the doctor, a nurse, and possibly a single consultant. Good health care now requires a team effort, whether it is for an inpatient, who has many consultations and services in a short period of time, or an outpatient, whose ongoing care may involve the cooperation of many health care providers. We often use the term "collaborative care" to describe the contemporary model. In collaborative care, one clinician, generally the primary care doctor, serves as a coordinator and integrator of the patient's total care. Other specialists collaborate both with the patient (in providing their specific services) and with the primary clinician (in making their contribution to the whole picture). The problem is that collaborative care often is *not* collaborative because clinicians fail to communicate promptly, appropriately, or completely.

Requesting Consultation

As professionals we are expected to communicate effectively with colleagues, consultants, and team members. Here are some pointers:

- Be specific about your reason for consultation. Remember that technical consultants (such as radiologists) need to know the nature of the problem and something about the patient as well. Thus, you should provide a short patient vignette when you request a procedure. For example, rather than simply scrawling "mammogram" across a requisition form, you might write, "Ms. B is a 49-year-old woman with fibrocystic breast disease who is very anxious about a tender new mass she discovered last month in the inferior lateral quadrant of her left breast."
- Make the request in an appropriate manner and level of urgency. In some cases you will simply send a request to the consultant's office; in urgent cases you will speak directly with the consultant, describing the situation and requesting an immediate evaluation.
- Make yourself accessible to the consultant to provide additional information or answer questions.
- Make sure the patient (or the patient's family) is aware of the consultation, understands its purpose, and has consented. This is normally not a problem with outpatients, who make their own appointments with consultants.
- Provide follow-up to your consultant.

Providing Consultation

- Clarify what the questions are and focus your patient evaluation on answering those questions.
- Respond to the patient and to the consulter promptly and flexibly. In addition to a written note, it is often appropriate to phone the primary clinician with your observations and impressions.
- Keep the primary clinician informed about progress or developments, if you continue to follow the patient.

SUMMARY ▪ THE CLINICAL NARRATIVE

In this chapter we present guidelines for translating your interview experience (and notes) into a written case write-up and an oral case presentation. The write-up and other parts of the medical record serve as memory aids, methods of communication, data for quality assessment and research, and administrative or legal documents. A typical format for the case description is outlined in Table 7–1.

We also discuss a number of additional points about clinical narratives and medical records:

- The present illness is a narrative of the patient's experience; it should read like a story.
- The problem-based medical record system includes several useful concepts that enhance patient care:
  - the initial database
  - a broad human perspective, rather than a narrow disease perspective
  - problem lists
  - respect for subjective data
  - flow sheets
- When recording personal information, be careful to respect the patient's privacy as much as possible.
- Use language that describes, but doesn't pathologize.

Oral case presentation serves as the basis for day-to-day communication among health professionals about patient care. Formal presentations should be concise, well organized, and designed to convey a clear picture of the patient's story, your findings, and a summary of your thinking about the case. Consultation and other forms of communication among professionals should be focused on improving patient care through efficiency and coordination.

Suggested Reading

Donnelly WJ. Righting the medical record. Transforming chronicle into story. *JAMA* 1988; 260:823–825.

Hawkins AH. *Reconstructing Illness. Studies in Pathography.* West Lafayette, IN, Purdue University, 1993.

Hunter KM. Doctors' Stories. *The Narrative Structure of Medical Knowledge.* Princeton, NJ, Princeton University, 1991.

Weed LL. *Medical Records, Medical Education, and Patient Care.* Cleveland, OH, Case Western Reserve University, 1970.

PART TWO

BASIC SKILLS IN PRACTICE: SPECIAL PATIENTS AND SETTINGS

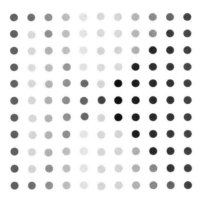

CHAPTER 8

Headed in the Right Direction

● ● ● ● ●

PEDIATRIC AND ADOLESCENT INTERVIEWING

Stuart rose from the ditch, climbed into his car, and started up the road that led toward the north. The sun was just coming up over the hills on his right. As he peered ahead into the great land that stretched before him, the way seemed long. But the sky was bright, and he somehow felt he was **headed in the right direction.**

E. B. White, *Stuart Little*

Why devote a separate chapter to pediatric interviewing? Are the medical histories of children and adolescents so different from those of adults? In the following pages, we take the perspective that children and adolescents are not merely "miniature adults." Not only is the style of a pediatric interview different from the style of an interview with an adult, but the style of the pediatric interview also varies dynamically from one developmental stage of childhood to the next.

CHILDREN VERSUS GROWN-UPS: SIMILARITIES AND DIFFERENCES

There are, of course, many similarities between pediatric and adult medical interviews. For example, the basic organization of a clinical history is the same for patients of all ages: chief complaint, history of present illness, past medical history, family history, patient profile, and review of systems. Similarly, skills and values that facilitate good adult interactions, such as empathy, respect, and confidentiality, are equally important in pediatrics.

The two most important differences between the adult and pediatric interview are the individuals who participate in the conversation and the topics emphasized at different stages of development. Parents or other family members often must provide information. This need is obvious in the case of a young child, but potential problems arise in gathering information, and the precise point at which a child has the skill to contribute his or her own story is not always easy to determine. With regard to topics, the prenatal history, for example, is vitally important in the case of a neonate but less so in the case of an adolescent. And the achievement of developmental milestones, which is critical to the routine assessment of a 6-month-old infant, is of minimal significance in the evaluation of a "straight As" second grader who presents with a sore throat.

SETTING THE STAGE FOR EFFECTIVE COMMUNICATION

A private and comfortable environment is essential to the pediatric interview. If the patient is in a hospital room with several beds and the neighbor's television is playing, visitors are chatting, and medical personnel are performing procedures, then families will feel uncomfortable talking about even mundane historical items, much less giving thoughtful observations of behavior or potentially embarrassing details. Before starting, suggest that the television and radio be turned off and, if possible, roommates be taken elsewhere by their parents or by staff members. Otherwise, draw curtains around the child's bed to provide at least the illusion of privacy. Similarly, you should see that an infant is comfortable and quiet (usually in a loved one's lap) before expecting the parents to be relaxed enough to provide you with detailed information. In the case of a preschool child, offering the patient a toy to play with may well improve the efficiency of an interview. At the beginning of an interview with a newborn's parents, spend a few moments admiring the baby; try to charm a 2-year-old toddler before interviewing the mother; ask a school-age child about a favorite television show or after-school activity before starting the interview. With children it is often easier to establish rapport *indirectly* by admiring a toy or a pair of new shoes rather than greeting the child too enthusiastically. Then, spend a few moments talking to the parent or guardian to give the child time to size you up (while you size up the child out of the corner of your eye). Here's how one clinician did it with a 4-year-old child:

[Entering quietly and looking first at the child's mother]: Hi there. So how's he doing?

[Mother]: *He seems fine. He did really well with the medicine. [Mother is sitting on the exam table and the child is walking around the room.]*

[Child]: *I want you to look at mommy's ears.*

That's a good idea. Would you like to help me?

[Child]: *...Okay.*

You can hold my stethoscope [handing it to child] while I get the light [reaching for otoscope]. [Looking in mother's ears] These look good. What about your friend Winnie the Pooh—can I look in his ears next? [Child hands stuffed toy bear to clinician.] They look good, too. Do you want to see? Now I can look in your ears, they look excellent. Very good. You did a very good job.

Notice how the clinician gives this child time to size up the situation, and provides an opportunity for the child to become familiar with potentially scary maneuvers. Sometimes the exam room becomes a three-ring circus when parents bring more than one child. In these situations, do the best you can to maintain your focus and use the opportunity to observe how the parent or guardian sets boundaries and expectations for the children.

Make no assumptions about the relationship of the caretaking adults to the child patient. The parents of an infant may not necessarily bear the same married name. Thus, the term "his father" rather than "your husband" or "the baby's mother" rather than "your wife" might be more appropriate until the parental relationship is better understood. Similarly, an infant and his or her parent may not carry the same surname. A brief glance at the registration form might reveal that the infant's name is Doe, while the mother's and father's name is Smith. Because you need to understand the relationship for the benefit of the child, it is best to ask, simply and nonjudgmentally, "I notice that your name is Smith and William's name is Doe. Can you explain the relationship to me?"

Finally, tailor your vocabulary to the level of understanding of the family members with whom you are speaking, although discernment of their verbal and clinical sophistication is subject to bias and may at times be difficult. Consider this aspect, too, in speaking with the child, who will understand more than you may expect if only you use appropriate words. For example, you could say to a parent, "Tell me about this rash." But you can say to a child, "Do you have any spots?"

TALKING WITH PATIENTS OF DIFFERENT AGES

The style and content of a medical interview, as well as its participants, vary enormously with the child's age. The questions you ask new parents about their baby will be very different from those you ask a teenager. The content of the medical history changes with age, just as the style and dynamics change. Topics that are obviously important in the prenatal visit or in the newborn interview become distinctly less important as the child matures and, indeed, may not be mentioned at all in the medical conversation with an adolescent. For convenience, we distinguish four types of pediatric interview: the prenatal visit, the visit with the infant or toddler, the visit with the school-age child, and, finally, the visit with the adolescent.

The Prenatal Visit

Ideally, the clinician responsible for the medical care of a newborn should meet with prospective parents before the birth. The **prenatal visit** allows the caregiver to obtain important medical information and establishes a partnership of mutual trust and respect. The diminished role of extended, multigenerational families means that in many cases the emotional and educational support for new parents may come from a clinician, rather than from family members. A brief, informal meeting initiates such a support system and dispels myths and preconceptions that the potential parents might have. The information you acquire during this prenatal visit includes a detailed family history, the parents' knowledge about child care, and their plans for feeding the baby (breast versus bottle) and for circumcision (yes or no). Practical issues like the schedule for well-child office visits, clinical fees, and telephone access also can be presented at this time.

During your meeting with prospective parents, obtain information about the family history: familial disease, previous histories of birth defects, and perinatal deaths. The purpose of this family history is twofold:

- To alert you to possible genetic disease in the infant
- To reassure or inform parents concerned about implications for their child of certain familial illnesses or tendencies

Listen especially for details of miscarriages and neonatal or childhood illness or death. The parents' health and their past medical history should be outlined in some detail, especially with respect to disease states that might endanger the life or health of the fetus during pregnancy. Pay attention to the physical, social, and emotional environment into which the child will be born. Parents' discussion of their plans for feeding the baby and their knowledge of child care inform your educational efforts.

This prenatal interaction also provides an opportunity to lay the groundwork for anticipatory guidance, that critical educational aspect of caring for children. For example, take the opportunity to discuss issues such as:

- The parents' perceptions of changes that will occur in their lives with the newborn's arrival
- Identification of support persons for the mother and father when the infant goes home
- The parents' knowledge of safety for the infant at home and in the automobile

- How the parents view preparation of siblings for the new addition to their family

The Infant and Toddler

During infancy and the preschool years, the child is the focus of the interview but usually not a participant. Although the patient may add little to the actual conversation, the interview is usually conducted while the infant or toddler is present. This small but important person serves as a catalyst to aid parents' recall of historical details. Also, parents are likely to be more comfortable if they are with their sick child, and certainly the child will be more comfortable with the parents. And when the child sees you interacting with the mother or father, the child is more likely to develop a (very tentative) feeling of trust.

A child who is fussy or in pain will only distract both you and the parents, however. The situation can be remedied with a pacifier or bottle for the infant or a familiar toy for the toddler. It is useful to carry around a colorful item or two to interest your preschool patients. Sometimes inexperienced clinicians either ignore the patient completely (to the consternation of parents) or try to become instant "buddies" with the child, forgetting that by 1 year of age most children are quite wary or even frightened of strangers. Moreover, illness may make the toddler irritable, and the clinical setting may be terrifying. A good compromise is to begin the encounter with a simple, friendly greeting, followed by the enthusiastic but brief examination of one of the child's own toys.

The medical history includes information about the perinatal period:
- Complications and problems during the pregnancy and labor (e.g., "Did you have any problems during your pregnancy or with your labor and delivery?")
- Problems during the first days of life (e.g., "Did Zac have any problems when he was born?")

If it has not already been obtained, you should take a careful family history as well. Ask about the child's crying, sleeping, and bowel and bladder function. Ascertain the child's immunization status, including reactions to the immunizations. Carefully review developmental stages, focusing on different milestones depending on the age of the child, and try to get a sense of the child's temperament (e.g., regular versus irregular habits, mellow versus intense reactions).

Here's how one clinician does a quick developmental screen on a 6-month-old:

> So. It's good to see you. You look as if motherhood is agreeing with you but I know it's hard work. How's Jacob doing?
>
> *[Parent]: He's doing really well. He's easier than Elizabeth was. He's very predictable, although sometimes in the middle of the night he wants to play.*

> He looks like a playful character and he clearly loves his mommy, and I can see he's not too sure about me. What's he doing for you?
>
> *[Parent]: Well he's rolling over both ways and if I sit him up he can stay there. Everything goes in his mouth.*
>
> That all sounds very normal. Have you ever seen him pass something from one hand to his other hand?

Notice how the clinician provides the parent with support and positive feedback and progresses from open-ended to more specific questions, building opportunities for anticipatory guidance even during this information-gathering phase of the encounter. Avoid leading questions (e.g., "Doesn't he sit up yet?"), which create needless anxiety (if he's *not* sitting up yet) and inhibit true answers and sharing of concerns. Sometimes a developmental history can be accomplished with a single question when there is an older normal sibling: "Tell me how Jacob has been for you compared to Elizabeth."

Nutrition questions are also important in your clinical history. A few screening questions often suffice:

- "How many ounces of formula (or, for older children, milk) does your baby take each day?" For breast-fed babies, "How many times does the baby nurse in 24 hours?" and "What's the longest he or she goes between feedings?"
- For older infants and toddlers, "Are there any foods your child refuses to eat?"
- "Does your child get much in the way of sweets and fast food?"

Because anticipatory guidance plays an important role in every interaction in this age group, try to obtain enough information to anticipate later discussions of accident prevention, feeding, toilet training, teething, and acquisition of normal speech patterns. The content of the interview varies with the reason for the visit: well-child care, an office visit for illness, a very sick child in the hospital, or a child about to have a surgical procedure. The child's demeanor and the parents' level of anxiety and ability to provide precise information about the child's illness will vary. Parents may be very focused on whether they have cared for their child correctly or have done anything to provoke or worsen an illness. Convey that the parent is a good parent. Parents may see their skills as parents being challenged and may answer questions "ideally"; at the same time they want to share their fears and worries. Sometimes, especially early in the interview, you may be unable to provide such reassurance and may need to say:

> I understand your concern about whether you should have given Molly that cold medicine, but I'd like to leave that aside for the moment and get back to how she's been acting over the last few days. When did you first notice that she wasn't her usual self?

Once you have established the history, you will be able to reassure the parents that they have not hurt their child or, alternatively, to educate them in the proper care of a sick child.

The symptoms of pediatric illness, particularly in the preverbal child, are often nonspecific and tell us more about how sick the child is than about precisely what the illness is. A 15-month-old cannot tell us that his or her left ear hurts; rather, he or she will cry, be irritable, have a fever, and possibly have a loss of appetite or even vomiting and diarrhea. If we are lucky, the child may tug at the affected ear, but many children with healthy ears do that as well. We have to rely on our physical examination to make the diagnosis of left otitis media. But if the child is exceedingly irritable, refuses to play, and refuses liquids, we may need additional diagnostic studies to rule out more serious illness such as meningitis. Table 8–1 lists the key information required in the infant and toddler interview.

TABLE 8–1

CONTENT OF INFANT AND TODDLER INTERVIEW	
Reason for Visit	**Topics Discussed**
Well-child visit	Parental concerns
	Prenatal and birth history
	Developmental milestones achieved
	Dates of prior immunizations. Is child current?
	Eruption of teeth
	Habits: sleeping, crying, and bowel and bladder function
	Intercurrent illness and other illnesses
	Nutrition history
	Cultural and family practices (feeding, taping umbilical hernias, keeping face covered to prevent colic, and so on)
Sick visit or admission to hospital	All of the topics discussed in a well-child visit
	History of Present Illness (see Chap. 3) with special emphasis on time of onset, initial symptoms, and subsequent symptoms
	Difficulty feeding—too slow, not at all, refusal of liquids, refusal of solids, or preference for water or juice as opposed to milk or formula
	State of hydration. When was the last wet diaper and how wet?
	Does the infant or child seem himself or herself?
	As playful, alert, and pleasant as usual? Acting sick?
	Temperature taken at home? (Rectal? Axillary?)
	Medications (including over-the-counter medications) already given and their dosages?
	What concerns the parents most? What do they think is causing the illness?
	History of recent similar illnesses in patient or family?

The School-Age Child

When a child reaches the age of 5 or 6 years, the interactive balance in the interview begins to change. Children are then more able to contribute substantially to the collection of data, but their reports are usually broad and sometimes difficult to interpret. Thus, you must turn to parents to provide accuracy and precision, while always trying to confirm the data with the small patient insofar as is possible. An enormous maturational range is found in elementary school–age children. You can expect to find behaviors ranging from shy, sullen, and silent to that of the garrulous child who cannot be stopped! Thus, as a sensitive interviewer, you must take your cues from observing the patient before deciding whether and how much to involve the child in actual history taking.

In general, the school-age child is a healthy child. Well-child visits emphasize historical information concerning immunizations, development, and nutrition, and the psychosocial aspects of a child's environment. Knowledge of the child's school performance and friends is necessary for the global understanding of a school-aged child's well-being. Anticipatory guidance at this age emphasizes accident prevention, both in the home and at school, and good nutrition. Special aspects of the content of the interview of the school-age child are indicated in Table 8–2.

TABLE 8–2

CONTENT OF SCHOOL–AGE CHILD INTERVIEW	
Reason for Visit	**Topics Discussed**
Well-child visit	Parental concerns
	School progress, school readiness, relationships with peers
	Developmental milestones achieved? At what age?
	Habits (eating, sleeping, continence)
	Age-appropriate play?
	Similarities to and differences from peers
	Significant past and birth history
	Illnesses since last visit
	Nutrition
	Dates of prior immunizations
Sick visit or admission to hospital	All of the topics discussed in a well-child visit
	History of Present Illness (see Chap. 3) with special emphasis on parent's observations
	Child's descriptions of symptoms
	Medications (including over-the-counter medication) already tried
	Similar illnesses in household or peer group

The Adolescent Patient

Your interactions with teenagers are potentially the most complicated and difficult of any interviews you will conduct. Because the adolescent person is frequently ambivalent or confused by his or her own feelings and resists talking about them, you will notice a lot of silence during these interviews. Yes/no and other types of closed-ended questions will yield extremely brief answers that leave you struggling to come up with more questions. Moreover, during the adolescent years, patients take an increasingly active role in their own health care, while their parents move progressively into the background. This is a change that many mothers and fathers, as well as their teenage children, find difficult.

You may initiate the interview with an unfamiliar teenager with a direct, unaffected introduction:

> Hi, I'm Dr. Smith and I'm glad to meet you. Tell me what made you decide to come to see me or [as is often the case] why your parents made you come in.

Sit down and meet the teenager at his or her level with some eye contact that allows for natural breaks. Remember that initially you are a stranger and must establish a basis for trust. Many clinicians try to become instant friends with teenagers, succeeding only in confusing or antagonizing them. It is important to be the person you are (see "Genuineness" in Chap. 2): if you're not "cool," don't try to be. It is appropriate to talk with adolescents alone for part of the interview, if not for the whole interaction. Most parents are cooperative and will leave the room without difficulty when you explain:

> You know how important it is for you to feel that you have a private and confidential relationship with your doctor? Most of my young patients feel the same way. So I'm going to ask you to leave while I talk with Jamie. Is there anything you'd like to tell me before you go?

When speaking with an adolescent, establish that your conversation is confidential. Whether the information is potentially embarrassing or not, build trust by assuring the patient:

> I always want to make it clear to all my patients that what they tell me is private. I will not repeat anything you say unless you give me permission to do so or I'm worried about you and we need to tell a responsible adult, like if you get very sick or something. But you know, your Mom cares about you and may have some concerns about what we do today. If she asks me anything, in order to protect your privacy, I'm going to tell her that she needs to ask you. So you might want to think about what you'd like to tell her, and we can talk about that some more at the end of our visit.

This kind of statement not only nourishes the adolescent's desire for autonomy but also acknowledges the parent or guardian's rightful interest in the child who has not yet achieved full adult status. It also implies that parents and their children should talk about important things, even those that are difficult, such as sexuality.

The sexual history is a critical (but particularly difficult) topic for adolescents, which must be covered when there are genitourinary or gynecologic symptoms and also to help prevent and screen for sexually transmitted disease and pregnancy. As with patients in any other age group, you should use clear language that the patient understands and proceed from less intimate questions ("Tell me about your family and friends." "Do you have any special friends?" "How about boyfriends or girlfriends?") to more intimate questions ("Do your friends go on dates?" "How do they feel about having sex?" "How do you feel?" "Are you sexually active now?"). If you are uncomfortable with these issues, it is okay to say so. Useful approaches include:

- "I'm uncomfortable talking about this but as your health care provider I need to find out if you're at risk for HIV and other illnesses."
- "Do you have any questions about your body? About sex? About how not to get pregnant? Have you thought about birth control?"
- "Are your friends (or the kids at school) having sex? How about you?"
- "Some kids your age get pretty serious about relationships and start having sex. How about you?"

Patients should be given time to respond and allowed to answer in their own way with your assurance that the information is confidential. Teenage males should be queried about their risk of getting someone pregnant, just as teenage females should be asked about their risk of pregnancy.

One problem, of course, is making sure that when you use a term such as "sexually active," you are sure the patient understands what you mean. Young teenagers vary widely in their sexual knowledge and experience; among 14-year-old girls, you will find those who have already been pregnant and others who will look wide-eyed and disbelieving that you could even think of asking such questions. For this reason, questions about their peer group as well as questions that do not imply any right answer or particular level of experience are useful. For example:

Some girls your age who are late with their period will worry that they may have gotten pregnant. Have you had any worries like that?

No, because I know I can't be.

You can't be. Tell me more.

Well, I didn't have sex. I don't even go with boys; none of my friends do.

Sometimes the conversation takes a different turn:

Some girls your age who are late with their period will worry that they may have gotten pregnant. Have you had any worries like that?

Well, I thought about it.

Tell me more.

Well, I don't really think I can be.

Did he touch you or did he put his penis near you or inside you?

Notice the need to be simple and precise in your language so that you can be sure that you are obtaining accurate information.

Important information to obtain from the teenager centers around the teenager's interaction with his or her environment and social world. In a sense, the patient profile or social history is *the* history in the adolescent. Tactfully posed questions dealing with drugs and alcohol, safety, sexuality, contraception, and sexually transmitted diseases are an important part of a medical history in this age group. But even the most tactful interviewer often has difficulty breaking through the outward reserve that many adolescents show. If this is the case, posing sensitive questions in the past tense is sometimes helpful. For example, rather than asking, "Do you smoke cigarettes?" you might ask, "Were you smoking cigarettes 6 months ago?" This avoids direct confrontation. Here is another example of how you might "open up" a silent and possibly angry adolescent interview:

I'm sorry that your father dragged you in here against your will. I know if I were in your shoes I'd be pretty angry. But since we have this time together, do you think we could talk about some of the things that have been going on in your life? None of this is any of my business unless it's okay with you for me to get to know you better. I'd like to hear more about how you've been feeling.

Other important issues to discover during the interview are:
- School performance
- The presence or absence of close friends
- Behavioral difficulties both at home and at school
- Stress and stressors, and symptoms such as anxiety or depression

Ideally, you should obtain most of this information directly from the adolescent rather than from a parent or guardian. Topics important to review during the visit with the adolescent patient are listed in Table 8–3.

SUMMARY ■ Techniques for Interviewing the Young Patient

Even the toddler can provide important data in the history, and many older children do not require intermediaries to transmit their stories.

To make the most of your interactions with pediatric patients:
- Approach the young child indirectly by first admiring a toy or item of clothing.

TABLE 8–3

CONTENT OF ADOLESCENT INTERVIEW	
Reason for Visit	**Topics Discussed**
Well visit	Parental concerns and confidentiality in the clinician–patient relationship
	School progress and peer relationships
	Habits (eating, sleeping, physical activity)
	Smoking, alcohol and drug use
	Sexuality and sexual activity
	Past history (illnesses, medications, allergies)
	Interval history (any illness or symptoms since last visit)
	Immunizations (and related childhood diseases)
	Lay the groundwork for anticipatory guidance:
	Diet and exercise
	Injury prevention (bicycle, motor vehicle, firearms)
	Smoking, alcohol and drug use
	Sexuality, contraception, unintended pregnancies, STDs
	Stress, depression, hopelessness
Sick visit	Reason for coming (parents' view, adolescent's view)
	History of Present Illness and related Review of Systems
	Boundaries of confidentiality (what parent needs to know when adolescent is sick)
	Possible relationship of sexual activity and substance use to current symptoms
	An abbreviated review of well-visit topics if the sick visit is also a first visit to the office

STDs = sexually transmitted diseases

- Understand the parent or guardian's view of the illness to lay the groundwork for assuring them that they did not cause it.
- As children get older, involve them more and more in the interview, choosing words they understand.
- Help families understand common problems and developmental milestones, laying the groundwork for anticipatory guidance.

To make the most of your interactions with adolescents:

- Establish the confidential nature of your relationship, as well as its limits and boundaries.
- Avoid yes/no type questions that tend to produce brief responses ending, ultimately, in silence.
- Address topics such as drug and alcohol use, sexuality, and safety.

Suggested Reading

Bennett HJ. Using humor in the office setting: A pediatric perspective. *J Fam Pract* 1996; 42:462–464.

Johnson KB, Feldman MJ. Medical informatics and pediatrics. Decision-support systems. *Arch Pediatr Adolesc Med* 1995; 149:1371–1380.

Steiner BD, Gest KL. Do adolescents want to hear preventive medicine counseling messages in outpatient settings? *J Fam Pract* 1996; 43:375–381.

CHAPTER 9

A Different Silhouette

● ● ● ● ●

INTERVIEWING THE GERIATRIC PATIENT

*A human being sheds its leaves like a tree. Sickness prunes it down; and it **no longer offers the same silhouette** to the eyes which loved it, to the people to whom it afforded shade and comfort.*

Edmond and Jules deGoncourt, *Journal*, July 22, 1862

In this chapter, we consider some of the special sensitivities and skills required for effective interviewing of older or geriatric patients. Who are these "older" patients? Consider this opening exchange between a physician and a woman in the office for follow-up of hypertension and chronic diarrhea:

So how are you?
Okay, I guess. I guess it's just old age.
What about old age?

When does old age begin? This patient was 88 years old; but what if she had been only 78, 68, or 58? Although you should have special concerns if a 58-year-old patient complains of "old age," you will find it difficult to have any hard and fast rules about when an "older person" has become "old." (One older patient with a sense of humor describes old age as that time of life when the word "doctor" becomes a verb!) The 68-year-old chief executive with

143

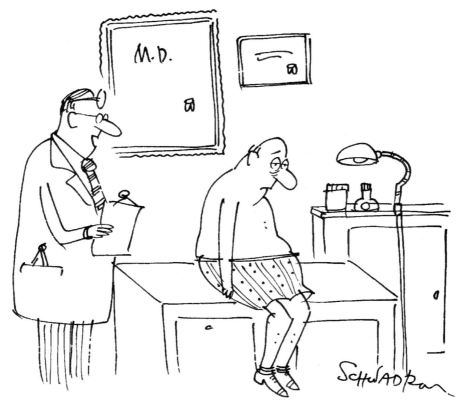

"Mr. Haroldson, I'm taking you off trying to stay young."

neither health problems nor plans to retire is certainly not the same kind of older person as the 68-year-old retired mill worker with oxygen-dependent chronic lung disease and recent memory loss. The former would find questions about his ability to perform routine activities of daily living insulting if not bizarre; the latter would find such questions very relevant to his overall management. So the approach to older persons is individualized and geared to the patient's stage of life without making rigid classifications based on chronologic age.

We now explore special aspects of history taking in this group, including the style and content of the interview, mental status testing, and the problem of the "third party" and confidentiality in caring for elderly patients.

THE STYLE OF THE INTERVIEW

The short vignette just presented illustrates the way in which many elderly patients attribute their symptoms to normal aging and may require open-ended prompting ("What do you mean by 'old age?'") to discuss symptoms that could indicate a specific disease process as opposed to senescence. Patients may attribute nocturia or joint pains, for example, to aging, even though these symptoms may, in fact, indicate specific diseases, such as congestive heart failure or rheumatoid arthritis. Moreover, vague symptoms may have special implications in the elderly, as in the case of a 90-year-old man with pneumonia who experiences loss of appetite and feelings of malaise rather than a more typical presentation with fever and cough. Likewise, chronic symptoms must be distinguished from acute or unstable symptoms. For example, the sudden onset of urinary incontinence requires a different approach than does a report of incontinence of many years' duration. You also will notice that the pace of the interview is often slower and that the elderly infuse their medical stories with a lifetime of experience that demands our respect. These are just some of the stylistic changes that you will note as you interview the geriatric patient.

Consider this example of a 77-year-old woman with end-stage renal disease:

> So, hi, it's nice to see you back. How've you been feeling since you left the hospital?
>
> *Well, each day is a little better and with that new fluid pill I'm not gaining any weight. But I'm very tired, more tired than I used to be. You know, my husband—he's 95 years old—just got out of the hospital, too. I'm taking care of him and I'm taking care of myself. But it's in the Lord's hands and I have a family in my church. They bring food, they help out. I used to be the choir director.*

Notice how the clinician gives the patient time to respond, in the process learning much about not only the patient's illness but also how she's managing with it. It is clear, too, (from what she volunteers in her response) that this patient's cognitive skills are intact.

THE CONTENT OF THE INTERVIEW

In addition to changes in style, the geriatric history emphasizes somewhat different content areas as well. For example, remote events, such as childhood history, are usually not relevant and may be obtained with a minimum amount of detail, with questions like "Any unusual illnesses when you were a child?" The family history is also less important because most familial diseases will have expressed themselves by the time a person reaches old age. Family history takes on a different twist because you are now looking not only at the preceding generation but at the patient's children and grandchildren as well. For example, an older woman whose daughter has breast cancer may herself be at increased risk of the disease and may not know that, in fact, it was breast cancer that took the life of her mother 40 years earlier. Moreover, elderly persons may worry about the health of their children and grandchildren, and your interest in their families provides an opportunity to explore those concerns.

Perhaps the most striking difference in the history of elderly patients is the need to assess their functional status in terms of everyday activities and their abilities to do those things necessary to sustain and enjoy life. The social history (or patient profile—see Chap. 5) includes most basic activities of daily living, including the ability to eat (chew and swallow), sleep, bathe, dress, walk or move about unaided, and maintain continence. (What *can* the person do? What *does* the person do?) The ability to cook and to perform simple household chores also must be assessed. Several useful rating scales are available for measuring functional status or activities of daily living[1]; the high points are described in Clinical Key 9–1.

Details about diet include consideration of specific nutrients such as calcium (needed to prevent osteoporosis) and fiber (which may help prevent constipation and treat diverticular disease or hemorrhoids). You should also assess sexual feelings and function, but this must be done sensitively and in

---

CLINICAL KEY 9–1

Special Aspects of the History in the Elderly Patient

Topic	Sample Questions
Normal sleep-wake cycle	"Are you able to sleep when you want to sleep and not sleep when you don't want to?"
Continence of bowel and bladder	"Can you manage by yourself in the bathroom? Can you get there in time?
Dietary habits	Who helps you with the shopping and cooking? Let's go through what you eat on a typical day so I can see whether you're getting everything you need."
Mobility	"Do you have any trouble getting around? Going up or down stairs? Have you had any falls?"
Medications	"Let's go through all the pills you brought with you. Tell me how you take each one."
Alcohol use	"Tell me how much alcohol you drink on a typical day. What about other days?"
Support system	"Do you have family or friends or neighbors you can call when you need help?"
Vision/hearing	"Are you able to see what you want to see? Hear what you want to hear?"
Memory	"Have you been having any problems with your memory?"
Depression	"How have your spirits been?"
Sexuality	"Have you had any change in your interest in sex?"

context. Frail, sick, or widowed elderly patients may find questions like "Are you sexually active?" or "Are you having any sexual problems?" surprising, if not downright inappropriate. It is better to give the patient plenty of room to answer, based on his or her own situation. For example, "As people get older they sometimes find that their marriage changes. How has it been for you?" and then "Has anything changed in your sexual relationship?" Change in sexual function also may be related to specific illness, rather than to age per se. For example, "I can see that you're having problems with the circulation in your legs. Sometimes when men have this problem, they also notice problems getting an erection. Have you noticed anything like that?"

Another content area of special importance in elderly persons is the detailed review of all medications—over-the-counter as well as prescription drugs. This is best accomplished by asking patients to bring all their pill containers with them, even the containers of drugs they no longer take. Questions about alcohol intake should not be neglected, but the CAGE questions (see Clinical Key 5–3 on p. 81), though useful, are not as sensitive in the elderly. Adding questions about the frequency and quantity of alcohol consumed increases one's ability to detect abuse or dependence in this age group. Finally, immunization status, including diphtheria–tetanus, influenza, and pneumococcal vaccines, and any adverse reactions to these immunizations, is an important part of the geriatric history that often is given insufficient attention.

MENTAL STATUS ASSESSMENT

The Informal Assessment

The interviewer must facilitate a technically competent interview with patients who may be frail, hard of hearing, visually impaired, or suffering from memory loss. You always quickly and inconspicuously assess cognitive function in the opening moments of the interview, usually without a formal mental status examination. The purpose of this informal assessment is to determine whether the patient is competent to give his or her own history and what assistance might be needed to help ensure accuracy and precision of medical data. How is this informal assessment accomplished? First, certain clues about mental status arise even before the examination, as you observe the interaction between patient and family members or caretakers:

- Does the patient himself or herself call to make an appointment or to report symptoms?
- Does he or she arrive in the office alone, having driven a car, or taken a bus or taxi?
- Does the patient forget an appointment even when reminded with a postcard or phone call?

Patients who cannot remember having made appointments also may be unable to remember medications or to recall and precisely report symptoms that they experience.

Next, as you enter the examining room or the patient's hospital room, pay careful attention to the patient's level of alertness (awake or drowsy). The patient sedated with a narcotic to alleviate renal colic may not be able to tell you very much (other than that he or she is feeling better now) until the medication wears off. Is the patient alert enough to focus attention on you and follow you from one question or statement to the next? Problems with alertness are common in hospitals and are probably under-recognized. You should also note the patient's general appearance and behavior. Does he or she appear socially appropriate? Is the patient clean and quiet, or disheveled and agitated? Is the patient physically active or slow and retarded? As you begin the interview, you next assess the patient's verbal output or speech. Is it relevant or irrelevant? Rambling or reticent? Repetitious or almost mute? Coherent or incoherent? These characteristics, in turn, tell you a great deal about the patient's thought process and content. Is the pattern of thought logical or tangential? Is the patient preoccupied with thoughts of death? Does he or she have an obvious delusional system?

Here is an example of the opening moments of a follow-up visit with a 76-year-old woman who was brought in by her family because of weight loss and abdominal pain:

You said you've been feeling sad.

Yeah, my mother died before the baby was born, and I just started talking to the women about it and all of a sudden I said I couldn't. It's just sad. Well, I raised a boy, his name was Andy, and he stayed in Europe and he couldn't get out there and he was about 10 years or something like that. And then my sister, you know, wanted to come back and I went to look for the money we were trying to collect for. So I went up and—you know how it is—and on a Sunday I went over there and the baby was born.

How would you describe this patient's thought process? Although her statement does seem vaguely related to the issue of sadness, it is difficult to follow the thread of this story, and it is certainly not a response to the question. We would describe it as rambling, tangential, and probably incoherent. It is typical of this patient, who could not really remember how she had been feeling. This is dementia, not psychosis.

In observing the patient, you will also certainly notice mood and affect. Is the patient flat or sad? Anxious or inappropriately merry? Cooperative or combative? Although orientation to time, place, and person may be obvious in the opening moments of your interview as you engage in social "chit chat" with your patient, be aware that many mildly and even moderately demented older persons retain excellent social skills that belie their cognitive deficit. We are reminded of two elderly women, both 93 years of age, who came to the office one day for back-to-back appointments. The nursing and reception staff commented, "Aren't they doing well!" But in reality, one was doing well and the other was not. Each exhibited the social amenities of saying hello, observing how much she liked her clinician, and commenting on the weather. One then went on to give a detailed account of her arthritic symptoms over the past month. The other, despite enthusiastically greeting her doctor, whom she had seen many times before, replied as follows:

> *It's so very nice to see you. You're such a grand person.*
>
> Why, thank you. It's nice to see you, too. Do you remember who I am?
>
> *Well, you look very familiar. What's your name again?*

The patient's ability to remember becomes readily apparent as the history proceeds and you try to gather precise information about symptoms. The elderly gentleman who repeats items in his history at different parts of a brief interview may not remember that he has already told you these details. The patient who says she has been feeling fine despite her family's concern about her repeated complaints of chest pain may not remember these episodes of pain. Indeed, sometimes you encounter obvious factual contradictions, such as a patient with surgical scars on her abdomen who states that she has never had surgery.

In the following encounter with an elderly, demented patient, the patient simply cannot remember his recent symptoms; rather, he is only aware of how he feels at present:

> Do you know who I am?
>
> *Well, I don't know, no.*
>
> I'm Dr. Smith.
>
> *Oh.*
>
> I'm glad to see you today. How have you been feeling?
>
> *Oh, I don't know, just all poured out.*
>
> Weak, are you weak?
>
> *I imagine to a certain extent, but it seems just that nothing just seems to be right.*
>
> [Taking pulse] Your pulse feels good today.
>
> *I'm glad there's something good about me.*
>
> Do you feel there's not much good about you?
>
> *Oh well, I guess I'm just average.*
>
> How's your heart been treating you?
>
> *Oh, it never did bother me.*
>
> How are you sleeping at night?
>
> *No trouble at all.*
>
> How's your appetite?
>
> *Always with me.*

In such situations, we ordinarily dismiss the possibility of a useful interview with the patient and seek information elsewhere. In this example, the clinician spoke with the demented patient's wife, who stated that his appetite was poor, he was having a lot of trouble sleeping, and he was frequently short of breath. Be aware, however, that dementia may be mild and variable; you need to listen carefully for inappropriate responses or evidence of confusion. It is useful early in the interview to detect these problems, which will otherwise lead to faulty data collection. Only then are you ready to proceed with eliciting the chief complaint and history of the present illness.

Formal Mental Status Testing

As summarized in the preceding paragraphs, much of the information required for formal mental status testing is readily obtainable during a careful medical interview. Usually, these observations are sufficient to assess your patient's reliability and to rule out a significant organic mental problem such as delirium or dementia. Sometimes, however, it is important to perform a more complete mental status evaluation that includes specific descriptions of the following:

- Appearance and behavior
- Attention and alertness
- Speech and language
- Mood and affect
- Memory and orientation
- Thought process and content
- Judgment and insight
- Abstract thinking, knowledge, and calculation

One semiquantitative tool that is often useful in this respect is the Mini-Mental Status Exam.[2] Although this widely used questionnaire does not cover all the attributes of a complete mental status examination, it does give a relatively rapid numerical score that estimates cognitive function. In the hospital, the Mini-Mental Status Exam can be used to follow patients with fluctuating mental status by administering it at various times, such as in the morning and evening. In the outpatient setting, it can be used to evaluate and follow patients who have problems with cognitive function over the course of months or years.

The Folstein Mini-Mental Status Exam is shown in Table 9–1. Low scores or scores that change over time suggest neuropsychiatric or neurologic disorders such as delirium, dementia, or the so-called pseudodementia of severe depression. False-positive results may occur in patients who cannot concentrate because of extreme anxiety or thought disorder. In highly intelligent patients, the test may not be very sensitive and false-negative results may occur. Such problems should be noted during the test; when in doubt, more complete cognitive testing (which is beyond the scope of this chapter) should be done.

Clinicians are often reluctant to do mental status testing and find it awkward to incorporate these tests into their interview format. Indeed, the data

TABLE 9–1

THE FOLSTEIN MINI-MENTAL STATUS EXAM

	Score	Maximum Score

Orientation

| What is the (year) _____ (season) _____ (month) _____ (date) _____ (day) _____? | ( ) | 5 |
| Where are we (state) _____ (county) _____ (town) _____ (hosp.) _____ (floor) _____? | ( ) | 5 |

Registration

| I am going to name three objects and I want you to repeat them after me. (Interviewer, give one point for each correct answer. Repeat the objects until the patient can name them all—six trials maximum.) Number of trials ( ). | ( ) | 3 |

Attention and Calculation

| I am going to ask you to do some subtraction. Think of the number 7. I want you to subtract 7 from 100. Now subtract 7 from that and keep on going. 100, _____, _____, _____, _____, _____. Stop. Alternative: Spell "world" backwards. | ( ) | 5 |

Recall

| Please name the three objects that I had you repeat after me just a short while ago. (Interviewer, give one point for each correct answer.) | ( ) | 3 |

Language

Please name these for me. (Show patient a watch and a pencil.)	( )	2
Now, please repeat the following: "no ifs, ands, or buts."	( )	1
Now I am going to ask you to do something for me. "Take a paper in your right hand, fold it in half, and put in on the floor."	( )	3
Now I want you to read this and do what it says. (Interviewer, hand the patient a card that says "Close your eyes.")	( )	1
Now, please write a sentence for me on this blank piece of paper. (Interviewer, give the patient a blank piece of paper and ask him or her to write a sentence for you. Do not dictate a sentence; it must be written spontaneously. It must contain a subject and verb and be sensible. Correct grammar and punctuation are not necessary.)	( )	1

Visual-Motor Integrity

Please copy this design. (Interviewer, on a clean piece of paper, draws intersecting pentagons, each side about 1 inch, and ask him or her to copy it exactly as it is. All 10 angles must be present and 2 must intersect to score 1 point.)	( )	1
TOTAL SCORE	( )	30
INTERVIEWER: Assesses patient's level of consciousness along continuum.		

| Alert | Drowsy | Stupor | Coma |

SOURCE: From Folstein MF, Folstein SE, McHugh PR. Mini-mental state: A practical method for grading the cognitive state of patients for the clinician. *J Psychiatr Res* 1975; 12:189–198, with permission of Pergamon Press PLC.

obtained are not really part of the medical history as such, but, more correctly, are part of the objective database, akin to the physical examination. Patients also may find specific questions about memory or cognition stressful. To ease these tensions, it is best to introduce mental status testing after the history part of your interaction, either just before or just after your physical examination. By this time, you will already have developed a relationship with your patient as well as an understanding of what some of his or her problems are. Such knowledge gives you a way to introduce this part of your evaluation in a straightforward and natural way. For example:

> I've noticed that as we've been talking there are some things you have trouble remembering. Would it be all right if I test your memory?
>
> *How do you do that?*
>
> Well, I will ask you questions, some of which will seem silly to you and easy, and others may be hard for you. Would that be okay?

or

> Do you ever forget to take your medication?
>
> *No, I never do.*
>
> How do you remember?
>
> *That's the first thing I do every day. But sometimes my memory is not so good. Sometimes I forget things I'm going to say.*
>
> Is that a new problem for you?
>
> *No, it has been for some time. I guess at 88, what can you expect?*
>
> At 88 I think you're doing fine. Would it be okay for me to test your memory so we can get an idea of how much of a problem it is?

During the examination, patients will be more relaxed if you provide support and encouragement, especially when they struggle with finding the correct answers. For example:

> Please name this for me. [Interviewer shows a patient a pencil.]
>
> *Well, it's something for something to say in, I don't know.*
>
> Would you know how to use it?
>
> *No, I don't think so. I couldn't even write my name anymore.*
>
> You couldn't write your name anymore? Do you know what you could use this for?
>
> *I have no idea.*
>
> Okay, well it's a pencil.
>
> *A pencil.*
>
> You can write with it, you just do like this and you can write with it. I see that you wrote your name pretty well here.

Notice in this case how the physician provides information and positive reinforcement to the patient (an 82-year-old man with multi-infarct dementia) who, in fact, made a connection with the object ("I couldn't even write my name anymore") but was unable to actually name it or to describe its use.

THE THIRD PARTY

No discussion of interviewing elderly patients would be complete without mentioning the issue of autonomy and the role of concerned family members or caretakers. Difficulties arise when the patient and "concerned others" disagree on the extent of disability caused by dementia or other illness, or when the patient and family disagree about the value of some proposed plan of treatment. In the case of a failing or frail octogenarian with mild dementia, it is often difficult to evaluate competence for medical decision making or to assess the legitimate interests of family or caretakers. Within the interview, we may hear different histories: The family of an 80-year-old woman reports that she leaves the stove untended and soils herself, but the patient denies these problems. Family members may want to see the clinician in private, out of the patient's earshot, and then forbid the clinician to discuss their concerns with the patient. Or a daughter brings her mother to the office pretty much against the patient's will. How do you respect the concerns of family members and at the same time nurture the patient's autonomy?

The preceding sentence contains two words that summarize the last paragraph (and indeed this entire section on interviewing elderly patients): respect and autonomy. First, you should approach your elderly patient with the same respect and concern that you have for any other patient. Your contract as a clinician includes honesty, privacy, and confidentiality, as discussed fully in Chapter 11. Consequently, while being sensitive to the family's concerns about what "grandma" should or should not be told about her condition, it is important for you to emphasize her right to know and the fact that most elderly patients respond well to being fully apprised of their situation.

Moreover, you should be sensitive to the patient's feelings about privacy, and minimize the involvement of a third party in the interview if the patient so wishes. Respect for other family members demands that you make them aware at the outset of your clinician–patient contract: you will not collude with them to withhold information or to "help" the patient against his or her competent wishes. Second, insofar as it is possible, nourish the patient's autonomy. Some elderly patients have deficits that render them temporarily or permanently incompetent to make medical decisions. But even if your patient is judged incompetent, you continue to have an obligation to respect his or her interests. Sometimes you may disagree with family members about just what the patient's best interest is. For example, optimal medical treatment of an elderly, mildly demented man with heart disease might require a low-salt, cholesterol-lowering diet. This diet may eliminate most of the foods that he has enjoyed eating all his life. The patient's daughter might insist on sticking to "the letter of the law," cooking him only bland food that he doesn't like. Perhaps she believes this is in "Dad's best interest." "He doesn't know what's good for him," she tells you. Doesn't he? It might be far more beneficial to the patient as a person at age 80 to enjoy life and enjoy eating than to have a small reduction in his cholesterol level. In this case, the clinician's obligation (nourishing autonomy) might be to counsel the daughter to provide a more enjoyable—though perhaps less medically "correct"—diet for her father.

SUMMARY ▪ TECHNIQUES FOR INTERVIEWING THE ELDERLY PATIENT

To make the most of your interactions with geriatric patients:
- Try to get the patient's own story rather than going through an intermediary, however well-meaning.
- Adapt your interview style to a slower pace.
- Assess mental status through both informal observation and formal testing.
- Assess problems with activities of daily living.
- Do a detailed review of all medications, including over-the-counter medications.
- Respect the patient's life experience and nourish his or her autonomy.

With the ability to adapt your interview in both content and style to different age groups, you have begun the process of building on your basic skills and applying them to different situations and different types of patients.

References

1. Duke University Center for the Study of Aging and Human Development. *Multidimensional Functional Assessment: The OARS Methodology,* 2nd Ed. Durham, NC, Duke University, 1978.
2. Folstein MF, Folstein SE, McHugh PR. Mini-mental state: A practical method for grading the cognitive state of patients for the clinician. *J Psychiatr Res* 1975; 12:189–198.

Suggested Reading

Adams WL, Barry KL, Fleming MF. Screening for problem drinking in older primary care patients. *JAMA* 1996; 276:1964–1967.
Bowie P, Branton T, Holmes J. Should the mini-mental state examination be used to monitor dementia treatment? *Lancet* 1999; 354:1527–1528.
DeVore PA. Computerized geriatric assessment for geriatric care management. *Aging* 1995; 7:194–196.

CHAPTER 10

For the Moment At Least I Actually Became Them

● ● ● ● ●

CULTURAL COMPETENCE IN THE INTERVIEW

... for the moment at least I actually became them;
whoever they should be, so that when I detached myself
from them at the end of a half-hour of intense concentra-
tion over some illness which was affecting them, it was as
though I was awakening from a sleep.

William Carlos Williams, *The Autobiography*

Cultural competence in the interview is the ability to understand, accept, appreciate, and work with individuals of cultures other than one's own. In this context we use the word "culture" very broadly to include ethnicity, race, sexual orientation, and gender. Thus, to be culturally competent also means to avoid stereotyping, prejudice, class-ism, homophobia, and sexism in your everyday interactions with patients.

Culture drives the patient's values and beliefs regarding health and illness, and expectations regarding therapy. By "values" we mean the patient's fundamental moral and existential commitments and, in particular, how those commitments manifest themselves in the patient's attitudes and behavior. "Beliefs" means both general and specific understandings about what causes illness, how it develops, what you can do about it, and what will happen if you don't. Values and beliefs inform expectations. The first section of this chapter deals briefly with the ways that values and beliefs affect patients' decision making and behavior regarding illness. The next section considers the skills of cross-cultural interviewing, including situations in which the patient speaks little or no English and a translator is required. In the remainder of the chapter, we discuss cultural stereotypes and the various elements that contribute to personal health beliefs, and present a framework for eliciting the patient's interpretation of the illness.

THE PATIENT'S VALUES AND YOUR OWN

Values lie at the core of any clinician–patient encounter. The patient values life and health, as does the clinician. The patient presumably also values the clinician's help, and we expect the clinician to respect (value) the patient. Although these implicit commitments are important, today's cultural diversity requires us to explore patient values more explicitly because values may differ. A clear example arises in caring for dying patients: one person may consider life so sacred that it should be preserved at all costs, whereas another places greater value on quality of life. Advance directives are designed to reflect such commitments and the health care decisions that derive from them (see "Advance Directives" in Chap. 13). Similarly, in the care of the chronically ill, you will find that some patients place a very high premium on personal independence and self-determination, but other patients are more oriented toward family relationships and interdependence.

Religion and culture make substantial contributions to the development and maintenance of human values. Specific religious values sometimes significantly affect medical treatment, such as "sanctity of life" in decisions about withholding or withdrawing life-sustaining therapy, or "purity" in decisions by Jehovah's Witnesses not to accept blood transfusions. In other cases, cultural values play a major role in decision making. Native Americans, for example, value a process of group decision making by the family that appears to conflict with the concept of personal autonomy.

As clinicians, we need to be aware of our own values. We tend to assume that our medical explanations for illness phenomena and medically indicated forms of treatment represent "reality" rather than beliefs, and are self-evident. Our beliefs reflect the high value we place on attempting to control the world (and our lives) by using science, and the tendency to devalue ambiguity and unscientific explanations. Some clinicians are more tolerant than others of patients with alternative values. One of the first steps toward respecting and trying to understand patients who disagree with us is a commitment to personal reflection and self-awareness.

INTERVIEWING PATIENTS OF A DIFFERENT CULTURE AND LANGUAGE

It is perhaps easiest for clinicians to understand the importance of health beliefs when patients clearly have a different ethnic or cultural background from their own. In our culturally diverse society, it is now common for Anglo clinicians to encounter Hispanic patients; Indian clinicians, Vietnamese patients; Russian clinicians, Haitian patients; and vice versa. Language is only the most obvious barrier to communication in these situations. Even when the patient or clinician speaks the other's language, it may be difficult for them to express deeply held beliefs or complex medical explanations in a nonnative tongue. Moreover, the clinician's understanding of the patient's personal world (e.g., dietary habits, family constellation, and health-related behaviors) may be compromised by cultural ignorance or insensitivity.

Cultural Sensitivity

The fact that patients appear in your clinical office does not necessarily imply that they share your belief system regarding the etiology and treatment of illness. Table 10–1 presents some examples of cultural beliefs about the causes of disease or illness. In many parts of the world, the concept of bodily imbalance is the basis for a traditional understanding of ill health. For example, some Hispanic cultures subscribe to a folk physiology that requires a balance between "hot" and "cold" humors for optimal health. One becomes sick when an imbalance occurs. Moreover, certain diseases are characterized as cold (i.e., having a preponderance of cold humors) and others as hot. Medicines and other treatments are categorized similarly. To restore the appropriate balance, one must treat a cold illness with a hot medicine, and vice versa. The unsuspecting non-Hispanic clinician who is unaware of these distinctions and who prescribes hot for hot will likely encounter resistance and perhaps noncompliance. Similar notions of illness as imbalance, or disharmony, occur in Chinese (yin/yang), Indian, and Native-American cultures. In each case, conventional

TABLE 10–1

EXAMPLES OF BELIEFS ABOUT DISEASE ETIOLOGY

• Upset in the body's balance or harmony
  • Yin/yang (Eastern Asia)
  • Hot/cold (Central America)
  • Body, mind, spirit [Ayurvedic] (India)
• Soul loss (Native-American)
• Spirit possession (Ethiopia)
• The Evil Eye (Mediterranean, Middle East)
• Challenge or punishment from God (Christian Fundamentalist)

medical treatment may either be consistent or inconsistent with culturally rec-ommended therapy. The Western clinician must understand the patient's be-lief system well enough to recommend a treatment plan that will be synergis-tic with those beliefs.

Differences of culture also may lead to other miscues and misunder-standings (see Table 10–2). For instance, American phrases or idioms may be taken literally by persons who have learned English as a second language: a Korean patient understood a question about preoperative anxiety ("Are you getting cold feet?") as an inquiry about the temperature of his feet. Health care professionals also use medical jargon and "plain" language differently from their patients. One striking example (not as prevalent as it once was) derives from the "high blood–low blood" folk physiology in African-American and rural white populations in the American South. In these cultures, people equate hypertension (high blood pressure) with "high blood," which they in-terpret as excessive blood thickness or volume. This condition is believed to cause strokes because excess blood backs up in the brain. The same people use the term "low blood" for anemia, which they believe puts a strain on the person's heart. Thus, "high blood" and "low blood" are considered to be op-posing blood conditions when, in fact, they involve two completely different organ systems. It is difficult for patients who use these words in this way to ac-cept the idea that they can have high blood pressure ("high blood") and ane-mia ("low blood") at the same time.

Another example is the almost universal use of "negative" in medicine as a good finding:

> You don't have to worry, Mrs. Nguyen, your tests were negative.
>
> *Oh my God, I knew it... I knew this was coming. What will I do? This is what I was afraid would happen.*

This Vietnamese–American patient has understood the word "negative" (quite reasonably) to mean a bad outcome. Thus, the doctor has inadvertently confirmed her fears.

Other language miscommunications involve words or expressions that seem neutral to the clinician, but are inflammatory or disrespectful from the

TABLE 10–2

CULTURAL MISCUES AND MISUNDERSTANDINGS
• Idioms ("To tell you the truth, I think she is getting cold feet.")
• Same language, different meaning (Is positive good? Is negative bad?)
• Inflammatory word or comments (racist, sexist)
• The polite "yes" ("Yes, doctor" may mean "No.")
• Eye contact (In some cultures "open" eye contact may be embarrassing or even threatening.)
• Touching (Touching may be therapeutic in itself, or a barely tolerated necessity.)

patient's perspective. Consider the contemporary American woman's feelings of disrespect (based on sexism) when a clinician refers to her as a "girl," or the African-American man's outrage (based on racism) when a white American refers to him as a "boy." The use of a patient's first name may have a similar negative effect. Although middle-class American society revels in the informality of quickly placing relationships on a first-name basis, in many other cultures such a practice is considered extremely disrespectful, especially when the speaker is addressing a significantly older person.

Nonverbal behaviors also may lead to cross-cultural misunderstandings, as when the clinician uses direct eye contact (a "good" skill you learn in school), then discovers that he has insulted his Native-American patient or embarrassed his Asian patient. Likewise, touching, which in secular American culture is considered a positive (perhaps even essential) aspect of a clinician–patient encounter, may be problematic in some cross-cultural situations, especially when the clinician and patient are of different sexes.

Guidelines for Cross-cultural Interviewing

In many cross-cultural encounters, the patient does not speak English, or speaks English poorly, and the clinician needs a translator to assist in the interview (see "Challenges to Understanding Exactly," in Chap. 2). Clinical translation services should be widely available, reliable, and of high quality. Translators ideally should have received training in clinical translation, because, besides having competence in both languages, they need to be familiar with health care concepts and situations, and they must be knowledgeable about the cultural issues raised in this chapter. They also should exhibit good communication skills. Often, however, such a person is unavailable, and other clinical staff members, family members, or friends must serve as the translator. Clinical Key 10–1 presents some guidelines to keep in mind when interviewing a patient through a translator.

If at all possible, avoid using a close friend or family member of the patient as a translator. Such a person may not be able to provide accurate (and thorough) translation for several reasons:

- Lack of sufficient fluency in English
- Lack of clinical knowledge and experience
- Hesitancy to ask probing personal or intimate questions
- Hesitancy of the patient to reveal personal or intimate information in this person's presence

Sometimes, however, there is no alternative but to speak through a family member. This situation may not cause a problem for simple, nonthreatening communication about straightforward matters, but in more complex situations, the clinician should do everything possible to arrange for a professional interpreter.

Commonly, however, your patient will have some command of English and will be able to provide the basic clinical information. Nonetheless,

CLINICAL KEY 10–1

Guidelines for Cross-cultural Interviewing

If interviewing through a translator

- Use trained clinical translators, if possible, rather than family members or "pick-up" office or hospital staff members.
- Speak directly to the patient, not to the interpreter.
- Avoid technical jargon, rather than relying on the translator to transform your jargon into everyday language.
- If you suspect a problem with translation, change the wording and revisit the issue. Be sure the translator knows what you want.
- Determine the patient's reading ability in his or her own language before using written materials for patient education.

When the patient speaks English

- Determine the patient's level of fluency in English and arrange for a translator, if needed.
- Ask how the patient prefers to be addressed.
- Assure the patient of confidentiality. Rumors, jealousy, privacy, and reputation are crucial issues in close-knit traditional communities.
- Employ a speech rate, tone, and style that promotes understanding and shows respect for the patient.
- Consider alternatives to direct questions. Patients from traditional cultures may respond better to a more conversational approach.
- Check frequently to determine patient understanding and acceptance.
- Understand your own cultural values and biases and accept those of others.
- Develop a basic understanding of the cultural values, health beliefs, and illness behaviors of the particular ethnic or religious groups you serve.

See also *Multicultural Information and Resources,* Boston, MA, Children's Hospital, 1997.

language may prove to be a barrier to discussing more sophisticated or complex topics, or to talking about personal matters. Sometimes it is unclear whether language itself is the barrier, or whether the barrier is cultural practices that prohibit airing certain topics or revealing certain information. Clinical Key 10–1 also includes a series of guidelines regarding cross-cultural interviewing in English. If it appears that the patient would be more comfortable conversing in his or her own language, it may be helpful to use an interpreter even though the patient is ostensibly competent in English. Table 10–3 gives some examples of English terms that may pose problems in translation to the equivalent medically relevant concepts in other languages.

TABLE 10–3

FREQUENTLY MISTRANSLATED MEDICAL TERMS	
Term	**How to Avoid Misunderstanding**
Allergy	Often a question about allergies is interpreted as meaning, "Does the medicine make you sick?" To distinguish side effects or ineffectiveness from true allergy, ask about specific allergic manifestations (e.g., "Does it cause a rash?").
Anxiety, nervousness	Use a variety of terms referring to both physical and psychological manifestations to elicit a history of anxiety. Ask about fears, racing heartbeat, sweating, and so on.
Blood tests	"Taking some blood" may be frightening and difficult to understand. Be explicit about the amount (expressed in teaspoons, rather than "tubes") and the purpose of the tests.
Dizziness	Distinguishing lightheadedness from vertigo can be challenging in translation. Make sure that the interpreter (or patient) understands the distinction between "unsteadiness" or "drunkenness" and the sensation that the room is spinning.
Fever	In cultures that divide illnesses into "hot" and "cold," the word "fever" may be used to refer to any hot disease, even in the absence of measured variation in body temperature.
Sensation of "pins and needles"	The literal translation of this term would be meaningless in languages other than English. Many Mexicans use the term "hormingas" (ants) crawling on the skin. This example illustrates the importance of avoiding idioms or metaphors when translating to a different language (or culture), or making sure that the interpreter understands the English idiom.

Adapted from Rothschild SK. Cross-cultural issues in primary care medicine. *Dis Mon* 1998; 44:293–319, at p. 312.

HEALTH BELIEFS IN THE INTERVIEW

A Multiplicity of Cultures

Cultural values and beliefs are not the only factors that influence how persons understand health and illness or conceptualize health care. Religious, gender-based, socioeconomic, educational, environmental, familial, and personal factors also play roles. Thus, although cultural generalizations provide us with useful information, they should not be used to **stereotype** the attitudes or behavior of individual patients. Consider the following global statement: "In Hispanic cultures people believe that they have little or no control over natural forces in the world." Such a statement might be helpful to clinicians insofar as it provides a context for understanding expressions of fatalism among Hispanic patients. But such a generalization is harmful if it is used to stereotype an individual and to justify not educating and engaging him in his own health care, for instance. Likewise, the statement that women in traditional Arab cultures are expected to express their pain loudly may be true from an anthropological perspective. It also may help us understand a patient's behavior. But a clinician who uses this generalization to discount or minimize an Arab patient's expression of pain is engaging in cultural stereotyping.

Sometimes using the concept of "culture" helps us to understand the common experience of groups of people who may not at first blush appear to constitute cultures. Take, for example, the culture of deafness.[1] The deaf community has its own language, traditions, and rules of social contact. The life experience of deaf people may foster negative attitudes toward health care professionals who focus on deafness solely as a disability, rather than as an alternate (and extremely rich) way of being in the world. The term "hearing impaired," which may have clinical usefulness, in no way captures the self-image of persons born into the deaf world. In taking care of a deaf person, the culturally competent clinician must be sensitive to cross-cultural aspects of the encounter. Here are a few examples:

- Deaf persons rely on touch and vision rather than on sound to get another's attention. Touching that is considered appropriate in deaf culture might seem aggressive or uncomfortable in the hearing community. Likewise, exaggerated hand waving or stomping of feet (to produce vibration) to attract attention is acceptable behavior.[1]
- Because deaf persons value face-to-face encounter (which is essential for signing), leave-taking is often an extended process, rather than an abrupt "goodbye."
- American Sign Language (ASL) is the native language of deaf Americans; spoken English is their second language. Thus, miscommunication is likely to occur, especially with sensitive or complex topics, even when the patient reads lips well or the communication is in writing. It is often desirable to enlist an ASL–English translator.

Likewise, we might view the medically underserved population as a separate, identifiable culture, even though underserved communities in the United States may include individuals from many different racial and ethnic identities. These communities are generally characterized by low socioeconomic status, multiple social problems, poor access to needed services, and skepticism or distrust of the health care system. One benefit of conceptualizing the underserved as an identifiable culture is that, by doing so, one establishes a context for understanding how difficult it is for some patients to think and act like "we" do regarding the benefits of health care, or the beneficence of health care institutions. Clinical Key 10–2 summarizes skills that assist you in reaching across the cultural divide to make a therapeutic connection with patients from underserved and disadvantaged communities. Before being able to enlist the patient's cooperation, to explain the situation effectively, or to empower the patient to improve his or her health, you must first establish "contact" through empathy. To understand the patient, you must listen carefully to both cognitive (health beliefs) and affective (anger, powerlessness, etc.) aspects of the communication and respond with understanding and a commitment to serve.

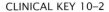

CLINICAL KEY 10–2

Elements in Interviewing Patients from Underserved Populations

EMPATHIZING with the patient's concerns, frustrations, failures, and successes
- Listen to the patient's expressions of frustration, failure, and anger.
- Elicit a detailed patient profile, including health concerns and beliefs.
- Express solidarity and a commitment to serve.

ENLISTING the patient's interest and cooperation
- Frame the medical problem in a language and a belief system that the patient understands.
- Recognize and validate the patient's priorities.
- Inform the patient of the problem's importance and the value of addressing it.

EXPLAINING the rationale of treatment and the process relevant to care
- Avoid medical jargon and statistical explanations.
- Be specific; give explicit, concrete instructions.
- Provide low-literacy instructional materials in the patient's native language.

EMPOWERING the patient to partner with the clinician
- Give positive feedback regarding the patient's successes.
- Elicit the patient's concerns about cooperation with the treatment program.
- Seek the patient's explicit personal commitment to participate.

SOURCE: Adapted in part from Rothschild SK. Cross-cultural issues in primary care medicine. *Dis Mon* 1998; 44:293–319, at p. 334.

Personal Health Beliefs

Like most people, health care professionals often look upon culture as a characteristic of people who look or speak differently from themselves. We may readily acknowledge that illness-related beliefs make a difference when treating people of other cultures, but we ignore the wide spectrum of beliefs and healing practices presented by ordinary people in our own society regardless of age, cultural background, or education. We have a cultural blind spot—our own beliefs seem so obviously true that we don't realize that they are culturally determined.

Although culture may provide the context for personal beliefs, such beliefs develop from a variety of sources: childhood experience, formal education, interactions with family and friends, television, newspapers, the World Wide Web, and so forth. One's conceptualization of illness, threshold for seeking professional assistance, and expectation for cure are based on one's personal belief system. Most people do not share the same blind faith in medical science that health professionals often have. As clinicians, we look to physiology, microbiology, and probability for answers. When you are seriously sick, however, it is difficult to believe that your illness is a random event or a matter of probability. If 22% of persons exposed to a certain virus become clinically ill and, of these, 14% develop jaundice, you ask, "Why me? Why was I one of the small percentage who got sick and came down with jaundice? What does my illness signify?"

One type of personal meaning derives from the patient's underlying value system and personality. If a patient views her illness as a justified punishment from God for putting her mother into a nursing home, she may continue to experience symptoms and dysfunction even after the pneumonia has cleared up. If another patient attributes his heart attack to personal weakness in the face of business pressure (e.g., "I just don't have what it takes"), he may well deny its seriousness and resist treatment. Another type of personal meaning has to do with concepts of how illness happens; patients may believe, for instance, that high blood pressure is caused by stress, a cold is caused by sitting in a draft, and cancer is caused by high-voltage power lines.

Eliciting Health Beliefs

Clinical Key 10–3 presents a framework for eliciting patients' beliefs regarding health and illness. This cultural status exam constitutes a kind of screening test to ascertain whether the patient's beliefs and expectations will conflict with medical explanations or treatment and interfere with the clinician–patient relationship. Such beliefs might prevent you from effectively influencing the patient's behavior unless you utilize them (or, at least, consider them) in your therapeutic plan.

The questions at the descriptive level simply recap the complete characterization of symptoms that we discussed in Chapter 3 (p. 48). It is important to discover precisely what your patient identifies as the major problem for which he or she is seeking help. The ostensible reason for coming, or chief complaint, may not, in fact, be the actual reason for coming, or may be only a part of it. Sometimes you must probe further to get the whole story and to put it together coherently. The questions at the conceptual level address the patient's understanding of the cause, appropriate treatment, and probable outcome of the illness, as well as the premises and logic that he or she uses as the basis of those concepts. Patients who are aware that they have beliefs that conflict with medical orthodoxy may not initially feel comfortable explaining them, thinking that you will dismiss them or become angry. Thus, it is necessary to set the stage by developing an empathic connection so that the patient will trust you.

The questions at the personal level deal with the idiosyncratic personal meaning of symptoms. Here again, mutual respect and trust must be present

CLINICAL KEY 10–3

Cultural Status Exam: The Patient's Interpretation of Illness

Interpretive Level	Examples
Descriptive	How would you describe the problem that has brought you to me?
	What are the main difficulties this problem (sickness, illness, disease, or misfortune) has caused for you?
Conceptual	What does the illness do to you? How does it work?
	Why do you think it started when it did?
	What kind of treatment do you think you need?
	What are the results you hope for? What will happen if you don't get treatment?
	Apart from me, who else can help you get better? How can they help?
Personal	Why did you (in particular) get sick?
	What is most frightening about your sickness?

Adapted in part from Kleinman A, Eisenberg L, Good B. Culture, illness and care: Clinical lessons from anthropological and cross-cultural research. *Ann Intern Med* 1978; 88:251.

before patients will express their deepest fears or venture their most closely held beliefs (e.g., that the illness is a punishment for past sins).

Fragmentation of Beliefs: Info-Fragments

In today's world, beliefs about illness are often fragmented and contradictory, many of them falling into the category of simple misinformation. People are constantly exposed to health-related "info-fragments" from television, radio, magazines, newspapers, and the Internet. From these, a person may garner a variety of "facts" and opinions, many of which will be inconsistent with others. For instance, a patient may learn in one article that, to be healthy, he or she should eat a low-fat diet. Another article will stridently argue for a low-carbohydrate diet. An item from the Internet will cite scientific studies that "prove" the efficacy of a low-protein diet. But how can a diet be low in all three major foodstuffs? This inconsistency may be obvious to someone who understands physiology and nutrition, but to many patients these beliefs about diet are not necessarily inconsistent. They have all three info-fragments floating in their head, and they apply each of them in different situations. This condition makes it difficult to have good nutrition and contributes to anxiety about diet.

Consider some additional info-fragments related to health care:

- Cancer is caused by electromagnetic radiation from power lines.
- Fish oil prevents heart disease.
- Vitamin C cures the common cold.
- Stimulating the immune system can cure cancer.
- Wearing a copper bracelet can ameliorate arthritis.

To many people the world is awash with new and exciting medical "discoveries" every day. Consider this segment from a routine follow-up visit by a 65-year-old woman to her primary care provider:

> *Green tea. Is it bad? I won't take it if you say not to [holding out a paper to her physician with information about green tea on it]. I take selenium and magnesium and lots of vitamins, but I really have to lose weight. So what do you think?*

And what do you want to take this for?

> *I'm fat. They say this works, or should I go to Weight Watchers? I don't know.*

There's....

> *... no magic, I know, I know. What's the matter with me? I just have a healthy appetite. I don't snack, I don't like candy, but I do like to eat. Look at what else I found [produces a handout on tomatoes and lycopenes in prostate health] and its not written by a cuckoo. How I got this is, a man called in to this doctor who was presenting a report on TV. And said that his PSA was 30 and he had had biopsies, which were okay and how to bring his PSA down. And this doctor recommended this. So I'm making my husband take it. [Her husband's PSA is 6 and the biopsies are negative, but she is very worried he has prostate cancer.]*

Well, I'm not sure what to say about your husband. But as far as the green tea goes, it won't hurt you. On the other hand, I think you've learned something from the fen-phen experience. I know you were very frightened when all that came out about the side effects. You can lose the weight but the trick is keeping it off, you're gonna have to eat less. The way fen-phen took the weight off was that you ate less while you were on it. Green tea or anything else for that matter is no different.

> *I do want to lose the weight. I promise that when I come back from Florida I will have lost the weight.*

Twenty pounds can make a big difference to your health.

The patient first asks about green tea as a weight-loss modality and shows the clinician the source of this info-fragment (a handout from a natural food store). She also indicates that she takes "selenium, magnesium, and lots of vitamins," presumably as a result of other info-fragments about healthy lifestyle or weight loss. At the same time, she acknowledges knowing about a different method of losing weight—Weight Watchers. She has obviously heard her physician's explanations in the past ("There's no magic"), but she cannot bear to abandon the shimmering allure of info-fragments. In fact, she tosses out another one, the use of tomatoes and lycopenes to promote prostate health, while assuring the physician that the blurb from the Internet wasn't written by a "cuckoo," the implication being "so it must be true." The clinician acknowledges the info-fragments without surprise or anger. While indicating a lack of specific knowledge about them, she refocuses the conversation on the basics of nutrition and physiology—to weigh less you have to eat less. She also refers to the patient's anxiety-producing experience with fen-phen, gently bringing home once again the fact that "there's no magic."

Sometimes health care professionals contribute to misinformation. Consider the following excerpt from a conversation between a physician and a patient seeking medical care because of epigastric pain and "heartburn":

> *I take shots for allergies and I take two aspirins every day for my blood pressure.... I don't eat any sugar, any salt.*
>
> Two aspirins for....
>
> *Every morning.*
>
> For what, why do you take that?
>
> *Trying, trying to thin out my blood to keep my pressure down, I try to keep it around 100.*
>
> I see.

Later in the same interview the patient comes back to the issue of aspirin and blood pressure in this way:

> *But I always take two aspirins, I've taken two aspirins for years.*
>
> Where did you get into that habit?
>
> *Ah, when I was in the military in '78 and '79.*
>
> Um humm.
>
> *A German doctor told me that, ah, if you take two aspirins with milk in the morning, he says, it lowers your blood pressure and thins things out.*
>
> Um humm.
>
> *And I've always ... my blood pressure is always like 100, 110, it's real low.*

If you accept this person's basic premise, he has a perfectly logical belief regarding aspirin and blood pressure. He assumes that high blood pressure is caused by "thick" blood. If so, and if aspirin thins the blood, it is reasonable to take aspirin to prevent hypertension. This particular belief is likely to be simply a piece of misinformation. (It is, however, somewhat similar to the cultural "high blood–low blood" beliefs described earlier.) The clinician could easily remedy this misinformation by explaining that blood pressure and blood coagulation involve two entirely different systems. In this case such an explanation would be particularly important if, in fact, the patient has gastritis or peptic ulcer, which may have been caused by the aspirin, or if he subsequently develops hypertension and needs medications to lower his blood pressure.

SUMMARY ■ CULTURALLY SENSITIVE INTERVIEWING

In this chapter we address the patient's pre-existing values, beliefs, and expectations regarding illness and health care as they relate to the medical interview. Clinicians who practice in cross-cultural settings are usually aware that many patients hold traditional health beliefs. However, as clinicians we must also learn to recognize that "culture" is not simply an attribute of people who appear to be different from us. The dominant American culture fashions our own beliefs and many of our patients' beliefs about illness. The human experience of illness is never free of values or meaning.

- Language is the vehicle of culture. High-quality health care requires effective professional translating services when the patient does not speak English. In many cases, translation also improves the quality of communication even when the patient is generally competent in English.
- Cultural competence does not stereotype. Cultural values and beliefs are not the only factors that influence how persons understand health and illness, or conceptualize health care. Religious, gender-based, socioeconomic, educational, environmental, familial, and personal factors also play roles.
- The concept of culture helps us to understand patients from many different types of community, such as the deaf community and the medically underserved.
- In eliciting a patient's interpretation of his or her illness, use questions that address the descriptive, conceptual, and personal aspects of these beliefs. Knowledge of these factors is essential for you to understand the effects of serious or chronic illnesses, as well as to promote optimal therapy.
- Many beliefs about illness and therapy are fragmented and contradictory, rather than being tightly integrated into a coherent system. To optimize patient care, you must identify and address these info-fragments.

References

1. Barnett S. Clinical and cultural issues in caring for deaf people. *Fam Med* 1999; 31:17–22.

Suggested Reading

Carrillo JE, Green AR, Betancourt JR. Cross-cultural primary care: A patient-based approach. *Ann Intern Med* 1999; 130:829–834.

Cooper-Patrick L, Gallo JJ, Gonzales JJ, Vu HT, Powe NR, Nelson C, Ford DE. Race, gender, and partnership in the patient-physician relationship. *JAMA* 1999; 282:583–589.

Flores G. Culture and the patient-physician relationship: Achieving cultural competency in health care. *J Pediatr* 2000; 136:14–23.

Galanti GA. *Caring for Patients from Different Cultures. Case Studies from American Hospitals.* Philadelphia, University of Pennsylvania Press, 1997.

Kleinman A, Eisenberg L, Good B. Culture, illness and care: Clinical lessons from anthropological and cross-cultural research. *Ann Intern Med* 1978; 88:251.

Like RC, Steiner RP, Rubel AJ. Recommended core curriculum guidelines on culturally sensitive and competent health care. *Fam Med* 1996; 28:291–297.

Morris DB. *Illness and Culture in the Postmodern Age.* Berkeley, University of California Press, 1998.

Multicultural Information and Resources, Boston, MA, Children's Hospital, 1997.

Rhian FL et al. Educating medical students for work in culturally diverse societies. *JAMA;* 1999; 282:1–11.

Shapiro J, Lenahan P. Family medicine in a culturally diverse world: A solution-oriented approach to common cross-cultural problems in medical encounters. *Fam Med* 1996; 28: 249–255.

CHAPTER 11

The Real Satisfaction

● ● ● ● ●

COMMUNICATING WITH THE PATIENT IN THE OFFICE SETTING

It's the humdrum, day-in, day-out, everyday work that is **the real satisfaction** *of the practice of medicine; the million and a half patients a man has seen on his daily visits over a forty-year period of weekdays and Sundays that make up his life. I have never had a money practice; it would have been impossible for me.*

William Carlos Williams, *The Autobiography*

Most medical care takes place in the clinician's office, rather than in a hospital. Yet students have traditionally learned how to interview by doing "histories and physicals" on inpatients. In the past, the range of patients and illnesses seen in the hospital was reasonably broad. A person might spend 2 weeks as an inpatient after an uncomplicated heart attack, or a week receiving intravenous antibiotics for pneumonia, so it was convenient for students to spend an hour or more doing a complete history and physical. Recovering patients often welcomed the student's company and attention. Today, however, hospitalized patients are generally very ill and not representative of the spectrum of clinical practice.

Although we call it "the real satisfaction," interviewing in the office setting presents particular problems. Normally, the clinician does not have an hour or more to spend with each patient, nor do patients necessarily expect to spend their day sitting in a clinician's office; thus, efficiency and thoroughness may seem to be in conflict. But because of its longitudinal nature, ambulatory care practice presents many opportunities to use interviewing skills to enhance patient care and develop effective relationships. The first section of this chapter introduces various ways of gaining efficiency and focus to improve communication in the clinical office setting. Subsequent sections consider special issues: managed care, the interview as a tool in preventive medicine, and the crucial role that confidentiality and truthfulness play in everyday clinician–patient interactions.

GAINING EFFICIENCY AND FOCUS

Although hospitalized patients today are sicker and have shorter stays than in the past, interviewing them is, in some ways, straightforward. Usually only one principal problem has caused the hospitalization (chest pain, for example, or rectal bleeding), even though chronic disorders (such as diabetes or hypertension) will affect the patient's care. Thus, what we call a "linear" approach to the patient's history makes sense: a complete exploration of the chief complaint and history of the present illness, followed in order by other active problems, past medical history, and so forth. We can start at A and proceed to Z. And we may have adequate time to do so.

Outpatient practice can be more complex and unpredictable. One patient may come in with a simple acute problem such as a sore throat; another may come for follow-up of a chronic disorder such as arthritis or hypothyroidism; a third may arrive with vague symptoms like malaise or fatigue. Often, a patient we believe has come in for a follow-up visit surprises us with a new complaint or asks, "What was my last cholesterol level, and why haven't I had it checked recently?" It is not unusual for a patient to present acute, chronic, and preventive issues in a single 15- or 20-minute visit. And your other patients are waiting. What to do?

Clinical Key 11–1 presents a short list of skills for achieving efficiency and focus. In the following sections, we address each of these issues in turn and illustrate how good interviewing skills may convert sources of frustration into opportunities for better patient care.[2]

Solicit the Patient's Agenda

Sometimes a desire for efficiency tempts us to abandon an open-ended interviewing style in favor of more focused questioning. We think that if we ask just the right questions or follow an algorithm, we will save time. If the patient has chest pain, we will stick to chest pain questions; if he has an upset stomach, we will concentrate only on gastrointestinal (GI) questions, and so forth.

CLINICAL KEY 11–1

How to Achieve Efficiency and Focus in the Office Setting

- Solicit the patient's agenda.
- Negotiate priorities.
- Orient the patient to the flow of the encounter.
- Maximize patient understanding.

Another temptation is to cut off the patient before he or she finishes the opening statement, or perhaps even the chief complaint. It might be difficult to imagine a medical history without a chief complaint, but consider the following examples:

EXAMPLE 1

Hello. You're here because of back pain?

Yes, I have lower back pain. And....

How long have you had it?

EXAMPLE 2

Hi, how have you been? Let's see, I had you come back today to see how your depression is doing.

That part's okay. But....

How many pills are you up to now?

EXAMPLE 3

How's it going?

Not too well, lot of discomfort here [puts his hand on back] down the arch and here under the arm and, ah, here, and this here....

How about the pacemaker clinic, were you there this morning?

Notice that the clinician, not the patient, has stated the chief complaint in these examples. The clinician has closed the inquiry to other problems or symptoms by indicating what topics may be discussed. In the third example, the clinician completely ignores the patient's obvious back discomfort because he thinks of him as a cardiac patient. Marvel and colleagues[1] found in their study of practicing family physicians that the average time a patient was allowed to speak before being interrupted was only 23 seconds! Patients who are initially cut off are likely to be dissatisfied and try again and again to return to *their* concern, or they may simply give up and not have their problems addressed. How often the heart patient fails to have his arthritis evaluated because aching joints are not on the clinician's agenda!

Paradoxically, *you save time by remaining quiet and allowing patients to have their say.* Open-ended questions allow you to generate hypotheses quickly without relying on the patient's hypotheses about his condition. Although questions such as, "How's your diabetes?" or "How's your chest pain?" may sometimes be useful, they should be delayed until later in the interview.

Here are examples of better ways to initiate the encounter:

EXAMPLE 1

Hi, Mrs. Jones, I'm Dr. Walker. Nice to meet you.

Same here.

What brings you here today?

I'm having a problem with my back. It's still bothering me. And for the past 10 years, I've had a chronic problem with phlebitis in the legs, and I have some problem with my feet swelling at times and therefore circulation in both legs. But right now I'm having a devastating problem with my lower back. It's been going on ever since about the 20th of October. And I would like to see if I could get into a diet program.

A diet program?

Uh huh.

First, why don't you tell me about your back.

EXAMPLE 2

What brings you here today?

Well, for several weeks now I've had these lumps on my head; they're really itchy. My neck hurts, too. I think it's from when I had that accident, you know, it keeps acting up. Since I am here, I might as well have it checked.

Okay. Have you had any other medical problems recently?

EXAMPLE 3

Tell me why you came today.

Well, I haven't had physicals on a regular basis. I'm feeling like I'm getting to a point where I ought to do that.

So you need a good physical.

Right.

You sure it's not a specific problem you noticed?

Not really.

Okay. But if you think of something while we're talking, don't hesitate to mention it. How has your health been?

These clinicians begin with open-ended questions that permit the patient to state a chief complaint and elaborate a bit on other concerns, so that the full range of patient concerns is on the table. In the third example, the clinician notices the patient's apparent hedge ("Not really," as opposed to "No, not at all") and reassures him that he is welcome to bring up symptoms as the interview progresses. In the second transcript, the clinician listens to the patient's full response, then encourages additional disclosure, "Have you had any other medical problems recently?" Marvel and coworkers[1] found that patients who were permitted to state all their concerns used only 6 seconds more on average than patients whose clinicians interrupted or redirected them. However, those who *were* interrupted more often brought up additional concerns later in the interview, thus prolonging the interaction. The extra 6 seconds you invest in listening to the patient's opening statement may be the most critical time of the interview, avoiding frustration and anger on the part of both clinician and patient and ensuring that the patient's "hidden" agenda does not remain hidden. **Do not interrupt!** This skill saves time.

In ambulatory care, the patient's needs dictate the character and completeness of your clinical history at any given time. One history might be a database on a healthy person seeking guidance about cardiac risk factors, another patient may have an acute illness that demands immediate attention, and others are returning for follow-up of chronic conditions that are influenced by medical, emotional, and social factors. Additionally, some chronically ill patients present with acute, perhaps unrelated, problems. Here is an example of a woman scheduled for a routine follow-up visit. She had developed a new symptom and some nonmedical concerns. The first-year family practice resident summarized the situation as follows *(we have annotated the text to indicate the different types of problems)*:

L.B. is a 50-year-old divorced woman whom I am seeing in follow-up for newly diagnosed diabetes mellitus and hypertension *[chronic diseases]*. She has been on glipizide and her concerns for this visit are that about 1 week ago she experienced a dramatic change in her visual acuity *[acute problem]*. She states that even with her glasses she is still unable to read as she had before. She can't see, her vision is blurry. She denies headaches or eye pain. She denies any other neurologic deficit. No numbness or tingling, no swelling of her extremities. Ms. B's other concern is that the Department of Labor states that if she has been ill, she is unable to collect unemployment benefits *[economic and social concern]*. She requests a note stating that she is medically cleared to continue seeking work and, therefore, eligible for unemployment benefits. Her other problem is that she can't sleep because of anxiety, both about her job and also because of her former husband, who keeps threatening her... *[emotional and social concern]*.

Given this complexity, you frequently cannot attend to all the issues in one visit. Fortunately, you do not have to. The complete database evolves and develops, changes and extends, over the course of your ongoing relationship with the patient.

Negotiate Priorities

What if the patient offers more complaints than you can handle in the time allotted? When the patient presents several concerns, you must establish priorities and set an agenda. What has to be attended to today? What can wait until next week or next month? What problem is of most concern to the patient? To the clinician? When there is disagreement between clinician and patient about these priorities, it is the clinician's responsibility to take the lead in negotiating a resolution of the conflict (see Chap. 16). Undisclosed agendas lead to missed diagnoses, not to mention angry patients (who feel that they did not get what they came for) and frustrated clinicians (who get telephone calls the same day from patients who have just left the office and now have "new" complaints).

After the patient's opening statement, the clinician should encourage the patient to "lay the cards on the table" by specifying all of today's concerns. This initial phase establishes the range of problems and their breadth, but not their depth. It may be likened to the overture of a musical score, in which each theme is briefly introduced but then set aside, to be developed more fully later. In music, certain conventions and the composer's artistry determine the order in which the themes or melodies may be developed. In clinical interviewing, the clinician and the patient decide how to proceed. When one problem is not clearly more urgent than another, the patient may be the one to decide how to use the limited time. But when there is an urgent problem that the patient does not recognize, or if the patient is not capable of making decisions, the clinician must play a more direct role in setting the agenda.

Orient the Patient to the Flow of the Encounter

When a patient has several nonurgent problems, a summary statement followed by a question and an explanation of your strategy may help:

> You've mentioned three concerns—your weight, this pain in your foot, and the premenstrual symptoms. Since our time is limited, which one would you like to focus on today [or first]?"

or

> I can see that you're really bothered by this itching in your feet [summary statement and interchangeable response]. But I noticed that your weight is up about 10 pounds and you seem a little short of breath. Since our time is limited, is it okay if we check out your heart and lungs first?

It is easy to overlook new problems when a patient is scheduled for what looks like a routine follow-up visit and you start the interview off with, "How's the diabetes doing?" as opposed to, "How have things been going lately?" The latter is totally unrestricted and may even invite nonmedical responses like, "My health is great, but my job is driving me crazy." "How has your health been?" or "How have your medical problems been doing?" are intermediate queries restricted to whatever concerns the patient perceives as health-related. "What can I do for you today?" is a good beginning; it is open-ended, yet indicates the desire to focus on "today."

Here is an example of how you might begin an interim history for a patient with a number of chronic health problems:

> Tell me why you came in today.
>
> *Just my regular visit. Dr. Smith said I had to come back for a checkup.*
>
> A checkup?
>
> *Yeah, he said I needed to have my blood sugar rechecked after he changed the medication.*
>
> Okay, fine. We can certainly take care of that. Anything else I should know about or that we should discuss before we get to that? Are you having any other problems?
>
> *Well, since my last visit I've noticed some trouble with my breathing.*

Notice how the interviewer makes sure nothing else is going on. The blood sugar may not be an immediate priority if the patient has developed shortness of breath, possibly suggesting congestive heart failure. This search for other active problems (OAP, see Chap. 4) is an essential part of every initial or follow-up outpatient interview. Unlike the initial interview of a hospitalized patient, where the discussion of OAP tends to occur after the complete development of the history of the present illness, in the ambulatory setting (particularly for those with chronic disease), the discussion of OAP occurs early. The search for OAP is essential in setting the agenda to make the most efficient use of your time with the patient and to prevent the "hand-on-the-doorknob" phenomenon.

We close this section with a 60-year-old woman who scheduled an appointment because she had been having chest pain. Notice the clinician's confusion as the patient states her chief complaint:

> How are you feeling today?
>
> *Oh, not too good. I still have that goofy headache.*
>
> You still have the headache?
>
> *And it's, I would say, one side, just sick. It's on the right side, and it starts here and it goes to the top of my head.*
>
> Have you ever had a headache like this before?
>
> *Oh, I've had headaches ever since 1965. I would take attacks and my blood pressure was very high and the doctor gave me medication.*
>
> I see. Is there anything different about this headache that you have right now compared to your other headaches that you've had?

> *Compared to the other headaches, this one is not quite as bad. But I've had it several days and it started about Sunday, and I'm worried about my blood pressure. Then I started having those chest pains.*

> And you've been having chest pains? Tell me about them [search for OAPs].

> *Well, they're right here. [Patient points to right pectoral area and then reaches around to her back.] It's right up in here and down around in there. Sharp. Like I went to pick up something off the dresser and it just grabbed me.*

> Okay. And you're also worried about your pressure? [OAP]

> *When I went to the store, I took it on the machine. It was a hundred and ninety something.*

> Okay. What would you say is the thing that's worrying you the most right now?

Notice that the clinician has established both the range of problems (at least three) and their urgency (none seems particularly urgent—the headaches are old and no worse, the chest pain is probably musculoskeletal, and the blood pressure taken in the office is 140/90). Given the limited time available, the clinician now turns the agenda over to the patient, who will dictate which concern to deal with during this encounter. (By the way, this is the patient we met in Chapter 5 who actually answered the last question by saying her main worry was "how to get those bills paid." So the agenda in this case was, indeed, completely hidden until the patient was permitted to decide how best to use the visit.)

Maximize Patient Understanding

Studies repeatedly show that medical treatment is "taken as directed" in only 50% or less of cases. Understanding is one of the most important factors in patient adherence to therapy. We prefer not to use the term "noncompliance" because it evokes the image of a passive, irresponsible patient behaving like a child; in fact, patients often have very good reasons not to follow instructions. Nonetheless, treatment is often compromised because the patient simply does not understand the nature and severity of the illness, the nature of the medication, the specific directions for taking it, or the expected outcome of treatment.

If clinicians attempt to explain these issues to their patients, why don't patients remember what they are told? Investigators have shown that personal characteristics, such as age and intelligence, generally do not play a major role in how much is remembered. Likewise, writing down the information, which on the surface would appear to be a fail-safe method, leads to better recall only if the patient is motivated to read the instructions and understands their importance.

Patients are more satisfied with their care and follow instructions better if they remember what the clinician tells them. Here is an example of the final part of a diagnostic interview in which, among other problems, the clinician appears to pay little attention to conveying understandable information:

> Okay, Mr. H., you've been having these problems for some time and I think they warrant further investigation. I'm not quite sure right now, some of your symptoms seem to be upper GI but some seem to be colonic as well. It could be an ulcer problem, it could be inflammatory bowel disease. I think the first thing to do is to schedule a flexible sigmoidoscopy and then we'll go on from there. I can do the flex sig in the office here later on this week. The nurse can give you an exact time and meanwhile we'll get you scheduled on the x-rays. You'll need a barium enema, probably air contrast, and then an upper GI series....
>
> *Is that test you mentioned, is that where you insert a tube in my rectum? I had one of those about 2 years ago, I could hardly stand it....*
>
> Well, it's not the most comfortable thing, but it is important, it's the only way you can get to the rectum, look at it, see the problem. It's not as bad as you think.
>
> *The main problem I'm having is this bloated feeling, and the indigestion. I didn't think it was so serious. Isn't there some medicine?*
>
> As you said, it's been bothering you for quite some time so I think we ought to get to the bottom of it. You can never be too careful. The problem with the GI tract is that, a lot of times, symptoms seem to blend together and it's hard to know what you're dealing with unless you look.
>
> *Do you think it might be something serious, I mean like an ulcer or something?...*
>
> Well, it could be an ulcer, but it's not typical. I think we'll just have to do the workup and see. In the meantime, I'm going to give you an antispasmodic drug to take, you can take it with every meal and at bedtime. I'll give you a prescription. We'll see what happens.

Let us focus first on the clinician's initial statement. How could he have presented the information to help understanding? First, he could have used words and phrases the patient was more likely to understand. He should not have used the terms "inflammatory bowel disease" and "flexible sigmoidoscopy" unless he intended to explain them, or at least check to determine whether the patient knows what they mean. Medical jargon can easily creep into conversations with patients, but it need not. You should be able to describe in plain language what you think is going on in the patient's body.

Second, the clinician in the example could have been specific about the problems being considered, the steps in the diagnostic plan, and the benefits and risks of his approach. Instead, he spoke in general terms like "further investigation" and "go on from there." What does that mean? Although he was uncertain about the precise diagnosis, he could have been more explicit about the options and, more importantly for the patient's peace of mind, the likely outcome: Will I get better? Is my condition serious? Is it likely that I'll need surgery? Eric Cassell coined the term "vague reference" to characterize this technique of tangential communication with patients, which often leads to increased, rather than decreased, anxiety about the problem because it encourages the patient to "imagine the worst."

Third, this clinician could have stated the most important information concisely at the beginning. Patients are more likely to remember the initial chunk of information than they are to remember data presented later. You should hook the patient's memory by giving a succinct statement that puts the problem in a frame of reference and leads to "Here's how we'll deal with it." The clinician might then employ another technique, repetition, to bring home the salient points in subsequent discussion.

Finally, at the end of the segment, the clinician could have asked how much the patient understood and given some feedback. Simply asking the patient to repeat what you have said and then giving feedback substantially increases patient satisfaction as well as accurate recall of information. The clinician also could have encouraged questions. These techniques for maximizing patient education also help avoid the "hand-on-the-doorknob" phenomenon.

Taking the example as a whole, we see that the clinician is attempting to share his uncertainty with the patient. The clinical situation is truly ambiguous and the clinician's statements convey that fact, but the *manner* in which he conveys the ambiguity is neither educational nor anxiety reducing. In fact, it creates new questions while leaving the old one ("Is it something serious?") unanswered. This clinician also avoids giving the patient any advice about the problem. Although the diagnosis is unclear, the clinician does have considerably more knowledge about what the symptoms mean and what might be done about them than the patient has. The clinician could have decreased some of the patient's uncertainty while mobilizing his efforts to address the problem constructively. For example, here is how the same clinician, on a better day, might share his findings and arrive at a plan with the patient:

> Well, Mr. H., you've had a difficult time with this problem, but I believe we'll be able to get to the bottom of it and find out what's wrong. We will have to do some additional tests, though, before we can say for sure. Your main symptoms, the cramps you get and the loose bowels, are most likely caused by a problem in your colon, one that we call irritable bowel syndrome. That means that there's a spasm in the muscles of your large bowel and that gives you the cramps and so on. But your other symptoms, that bloated feeling in the stomach and pain up there, they also suggest an acid problem, like ulcer or gastritis.
> *Are any of those serious?*

They're all medical problems that can be treated or cured. There's nothing to suggest that you have something really serious like cancer, for example. It could be an ulcer, but I think it's more likely that irritable bowel syndrome can explain all of your symptoms.

I really want to get to the bottom of this, I just can't take it any more. I just can't get my work done feeling like I do now.

It sounds as though these attacks have really gotten to you....

I'd say I'm almost paralyzed.

Okay, I understand. What I'd like to do is to schedule some tests today. One of them is a flexible sigmoidoscopy; that's a procedure in which I insert a flexible tube into your rectum. I can look through it and check the lining of your bowel, like for irritation or hemorrhoids. You'll come back to my office for that. The other two tests are x-rays, one of the large bowel and one of the stomach and small bowel.

Do you think it might be something serious, like an ulcer or something?

What are you thinking about? Possibly it could be an ulcer....

Well, ulcers can kill you, can't they?

It sounds like you heard something bad about ulcers.

My uncle bled to death from one. First they said it was an ulcer, then it didn't heal, he couldn't eat anything. Finally they found out it was cancer.

And you're worried that this could be cancer, even if the tests show something else?

I don't know. Like I say, I can't take it any more. My nerves are part of it, maybe.

Let's take this a step at a time. First, your symptoms and my examination do not show any suggestion of cancer; we have no reason to suspect it. As I said, it really sounds like either an acid problem or irritable bowel. That's the most likely. Let me explain that a little more....

This time the clinician has used several techniques that will enhance understanding and cooperation (Clinical Key 11–2). He also actively elicited the

---

CLINICAL KEY 11–2

How to Maximize Patient Understanding

- Use plain English, rather than medical jargon.
- Use concrete and specific language; avoid vague reference.
- State the important message first, then use repetition to reinforce it.
- Ask the patient to restate the message.
- Give corrective feedback.
- Provide opportunities for questions.

patient's beliefs ("It sounds like you heard something bad...") and considered them in his explanation. The patient is likely to be more satisfied than in our first example and to go home feeling less anxious.

SPECIFIC ISSUES IN MANAGED CARE SETTINGS

Managed care has become the norm, rather than the exception, in American clinical practice. Insurers now "manage" the services available to a given patient by offering comprehensive systems of care that range from preventive services and primary care through subspecialty and tertiary care. Managed care programs require each person to identify a participating primary care provider who coordinates the patient's total health care. Another desirable feature is an emphasis on prevention, including programs for health promotion and behavioral medicine (e.g., smoking cessation).

The more troublesome features of managed care arise not so much from the concept as from its current implementation. Because health insurance in the United States is overwhelmingly employer based, people often must change their insurance when they change jobs or when their employer signs a contract with a different insurer. These frequent changes often require patients to change their primary care provider. A second troublesome feature arises from the "dark side" of making the primary care provider integral to the system. Because many patients are accustomed to dealing with several different specialists, they may perceive the requirement to obtain referrals from a primary care provider as burdensome. Moreover, when generalists attempt to provide care that is more rational by limiting the fragmentation of services, thereby acting as the patient's advocate, some patients believe them to be acting as gatekeepers to prevent access to a desired service. This conflict in beliefs and expectations may fuel dissatisfaction among both patients and clinicians.

Although some clinicians and patients believe that these problems originated with managed care, in fact, they are general features of clinician–patient interactions and not limited to certain settings. Hence, we consider them as additional challenges in office practice.

"Coerced" Change

Consider this opening exchange between a patient and her new clinician at Magna Care, a managed care program:

> What can I do for you, Ms. B?
>
> *Well, they told me I had to come in and see you. What happened is, my health insurance changed and now I can't see my regular doctor anymore. I've been going to him for about 10 years now. He knows my whole history, everything....*

This clinician has a serious handicap: the patient seems upset that she can't see her "regular" doctor and has only come because "they" told her to. The patient's opening statement is not about her symptoms, but about her frustration and possible anger. The temptation here is for the clinician to ignore or minimize the patient's concerns and try to proceed immediately with the chief complaint. For example, he might say, "Okay, but tell me what your medical problem is," or "That's too bad, but we can get copies of the records... Now what is your problem today?" The second statement acknowledges the situation, but fails to consider the patient's feelings. It implies that the clinical record captures everything that's important in a clinician–patient relationship, that people are interchangeable.

How might this clinician respond in a more effective way? Consider the following two statements:

RESPONSE 1

[After a few seconds pause.] It sounds as if you had a good relationship with your doctor.

RESPONSE 2

It must be really frustrating when that happens. You probably just picked my name out of the book and you don't know what to expect.

In both cases the clinician gives an empathic, interchangeable response (see p. 27). The first response demonstrates an understanding of the cognitive content (previous relationship); the second focuses on the affective content (frustration). Either is appropriate in this situation, but the second response goes a bit further because it addresses an additional area of concern: the patient's uncertainty of what to expect from a new clinician. It gives the patient permission to verbalize her fears. For example, the conversation might continue:

Well, yes, I just had to go through the Magna Care list, so I tried you because it's pretty convenient to get to your office. My regular doctor was Dr. Samuels, just up the road in Port Jefferson. He's been treating me for years for my diabetes and arthritis.

Oh, I know Dr. Samuels. He's a very good internist. I understand why you hate to be forced to leave him. Well, I'll try to do a good job for you, too. And we can send for a copy of your records at Dr. Samuels' office.

This vignette of "coerced" change serves as an example of the general rules to begin listening at the beginning and to attempt to remove barriers to effective communication as soon as you identify them.

Dueling Agendas/ I Can Take Care of That

How can I help you, Mr. C?

They told me I had to see my PCP [primary care provider] to get these referrals. [Brings out a list.] I have an appointment next Tuesday with Dr. Nephron, who treats me for blood pressure, so I need that one today. And then my regular follow-ups with my allergist, my diabetes specialist—by the way, my sugar's high—and my cardiologist are due. So I thought I'd better get those referrals now, so I don't have to keep calling your office. And while I'm here, I was also wondering if you could recommend a good specialist for my stomach?

How would you feel if you were this patient's primary care provider? The patient is acting as if the clinician were a clerk or a gatekeeper, whose sole function is to handle the paperwork to enable him to see an array of specialists. This PCP—to use today's jargon—is bound to feel unappreciated and perhaps angry, and might be tempted to reply, "Wait a second, that's not how things work here. I'm the one who decides what referrals you need!" This would almost certainly lead to a needless confrontation. The problem, of course, is that the patient and clinician here have radically different agendas: the clinician sees herself as taking care of the patient and addressing his illness, the patient views her as an administrative cog.

Dueling agendas demand a direct approach. Unlike the coerced change example, it is unlikely that simple facilitative responses will encourage the patient to accept the generalist's care. The issue here is a radical misunderstanding of (or disagreement with) the role of the PCP. If the clinician tried a simple interchangeable response like, "Well, Mr. C., it sounds as if you have quite a few medical problems," the patient is likely to agree and indicate that that is precisely why he needs so many doctors. What is required here is a clear and relatively complete educational statement:

Well, Mr. C., it sounds as though you've needed quite a few specialists and certainly if you have an appointment with Dr. Nephron on Tuesday, I agree that we should arrange a referral for you. But today we're scheduled for a new patient visit—that means a complete checkup—so I think we should get started so I can understand your problems better. Did you have a primary care doctor before you joined Magna Care?

Not really. I used to go to Dr. Smith for colds and things, you know, maybe once a year, but he never did any testing, just wrote me a prescription for antibiotics or something.

OK, then, let me start by explaining how I view my role. I'd like to be your main doctor and coordinate all your medical care. And I'd like to get to know you better, so that maybe together we can work on improving your health. If we decide that you need to see a specialist, then he or she will report back to me and we can talk about it. Now I don't think we can start out with all these referrals ... first, I need to understand your health problems. So I suggest we start from what's bothering you right now, your stomach, and then we can talk about your sugar and your heart and so forth. How's that?

Well OK, but it's a long story....

This, of course, is not a miraculous resolution to dueling agendas: there will probably be continued tension over referrals, the need for additional education and, possibly, confrontation. Note, however, four aspects of this clinician's approach:

1. She immediately acknowledges the patient's most pressing request: the appointment with Dr. Nephron. Whether or not a nephrologist is required, the PCP minimizes the disruption to the patient's expectations by acceding to that referral. Presumably, she decided the referral would buy her some time to establish a relationship based on education and negotiation.

2. She immediately begins to establish the ground rules, including the fact that she views herself as the patient's major care provider. The message to Mr. C is clear, although not yet fully detailed.

3. She states her case without reference to Magna Care rules or expectations; good medical care should be justified on its own merits. If she had said, "You're in Magna Care now, so let me explain the restrictions they have on referrals to specialists...," she would, to some extent, be opting out of the therapeutic role by engaging in a game of "us versus them."

4. She is reasonable and friendly in her explanation. She speaks firmly, but she has not yielded to the understandable impulse to begin with, "What do you think this is, a supermarket where you can come in and pick out anything you want?"

Dueling agendas are often obvious in managed care arrangements, but this dynamic is important in all forms of clinical practice. We present additional examples in the section on "Papers, Forms, and Clearances" later in this chapter and consider the subject in more detail in Chapter 16.

COMMUNICATING ABOUT PREVENTION AND HEALTH PROMOTION

Many patients now expect health care professionals to address prevention and health maintenance, and actively seek out those who address these issues. Good clinician–patient communication is central to prevention and health promotion. The medical interview allows you to identify the patient's risk-related behaviors, personal preferences, and needed preventive services. Interviewing skills also facilitate health education, negotiation, and counseling regarding healthy lifestyles. In these ways the interview is a powerful tool for promoting better health. Table 11–1 outlines the components of a preventive health assessment, which normally should be embedded in the initial patient interview.

Immunizations and early detection (screening tests) are easy to neglect in ambulatory medicine because office visits are commonly short and highly focused. Clinicians may forget to build a database regarding a patient's immunization status and appropriate screening tests. Thus, it is important to include such questions as part of the past medical history during the initial interview and to make them a prominent part of a patient's annual checkup. Table 11–2 summarizes the results of an informative study on clinical interviewing and prevention,[3] which demonstrates that clinicians often fail to ask about prevention and health promotion. In this study, clinicians inquired about basic prevention issues less than half—or even less than one-quarter—of the time.

Begin your segment about prevention and screening tests with a brief introduction, such as "Now I'd like to ask a few questions about preventive care" or "I'd like to ask about things that keep you healthy." As part of the initial medical history, the patient profile (see Chap. 5) should also provide you with information about major cardiovascular and cancer risk factors. Other risk factors may be identified in the past medical history and family history. This information-gathering phase of the clinical interview sets the stage for later negotiation with patients (see Chap. 16) to alter their risks.

TABLE 11–1

PREVENTIVE HEALTH ASSESSMENT
• Introduction: "Now I'd like to ask you a few questions about keeping healthy." • Immunization status: "Can you recall anything about your immunizations?" 　• Basic immunizations 　• Boosters: "When was your last tetanus shot? Flu shot? Pneumonia shot?" • Screening: "Have you ever had your cholesterol checked?" 　• Age- and gender-specific screening tests: "When was your last Pap smear?" 　• Appropriate screening intervals 　• Screening behaviors (breast self-exam, testicular self-exam) • Family history: "Are you concerned about anything in your family that might put you at risk?" 　• Diseases and disorders predisposing to high risk: "Has anyone in your family had colon cancer? Breast cancer?" • Specific risk factors: "I'd like to ask you some questions about things that might put you at risk for certain diseases." 　• Behaviors: cigarette smoking, abuse of alcohol and other drugs 　• Exposures: occupational and environmental factors, multiple sexual partners, unprotected intercourse 　• Clinical findings: obesity, hypertension, diabetes • Lifestyle issues (see Chap. 5) 　• Nutrition: "Tell me about your diet." 　• Exercise: "Do you exercise regularly? Tell me what you do for exercise." 　• Stress management: "What do you do to prevent stress in your life? How do you cope with stress in your life?" 　• Health beliefs (see Chap. 10)

TABLE 11-2

LIKELIHOOD OF SELECTED HEALTH TOPICS BEING COVERED DURING A ROUTINE HISTORY (Percentage of Physicians Who Covered the Topic)	
76% to 100%	*26% to 50%*
Reason for visit	Immunizations
Specific concerns	Recreational drug use
Past illnesses	Breast self-examination
Current medications	Frequency of Pap smears
Occupation	Relationship with spouse or partner
Family history	History of depression
Tobacco use	Sexual activity
Alcohol use	*0% to 25%*
Menopause	History of STDs
Chest pain history	Sexual partners besides spouse
Mammogram history	Number of sexual partners
51% to 75%	Condom use
Prior hospitalization	Sexual partners with known HIV risk
Drug allergies	Injection drug use
Cholesterol check	History of transfusions
Last Pap smear	
Exercise history	

HIV = human immunodeficiency virus; STDs = sexually transmitted diseases
Adapted from Ramsey PG, Curtis JR, Paauw DS, Carline JD, Wenrich MD. History-taking and preventive medicine skills among primary care physicians: An assessment using standardized patients. *Am J Med* 1998; 104:152–158, at p. 156.

TRUTHFULNESS AND CONFIDENTIALITY

Maintaining Confidentiality

Confidentiality is an ancient concept in medicine. The Hippocratic Oath states, "What I may see or hear in the course of the treatment or even outside of the treatment in regard to the life of men, which on no account one must spread abroad, I will keep to myself holding such things shameful to be spoken about."[4] The American Medical Association's principles of ethics state that "a physician ... shall safeguard patient confidences within the constraints of the law." The ethical principle of respect for persons dictates a right to privacy that is violated if we make personal information available to others. Confidentiality is not only ethical but also useful, as it facilitates openness of communication and a trusting relationship between patient and caregiver, thereby enhancing therapeutic effectiveness.

Confidentiality does not simply mean keeping an occasional big secret, but rather indicates a daily pattern of respect for patients and their stories. Discussion of cases with one's friends, roommates, or spouse is generally inappropriate, even when the information in question is not strictly personal. Of course, some people do have a right to know. Health care is a collegial enterprise. Clinicians function as members of teams, so we often need to discuss patients with our peers, consultants, and other professionals. As a learner, one has a particular obligation to discuss patients with teachers. Even here, however, discretion is important. It is rarely justifiable to talk about patients on crowded elevators or in other public settings. In the hospital, presenting patients at the bedside is often a good teaching technique, but it may infringe on confidentiality if a roommate can hear the discussion of a patient's illness and personal life.

Another important way of maintaining confidentiality is to write only appropriate information in the patient's clinical record (see Chap. 7, p. 115). You should approach the record as a document that the patient has the right to review at any time and that others (e.g., office staff) will be seeing. Especially with regard to sensitive information, you should always ask yourself whether writing a particular item in the chart is important to your patient's care. Some examples of sensitive information include details of sexual practices, a criminal record, marital conflict, and financial difficulties. Mental illness, suicide attempts, and substance abuse must be recorded but should be handled sensitively. In some cases, it might be possible to write a brief "neutral" note to jog your memory, without expressing lurid details.

Confidentiality is challenged in small and not-so-small ways every day in practice. Consider this example of a 58-year-old woman who comes to you for follow-up of hypertension:

> So how have you been?
>
> *Well, I'm fine, it's my daughter I'm worried about. [Her 28-year-old daughter is also your patient.] I don't know if it's stress or she's just taken on too much or she's got something wrong with her. I know she's talked to you.*

Actually, the daughter has not talked to you. But do you say that you haven't seen her daughter for months? Even though the patient seems to assume that you have recently dealt with her daughter's problem ("and why aren't you doing anything about it?"), it is best to reply:

> Well, I know you appreciate that Jane's relationship with me is confidential.

Ideally, the patient agrees and says:

> *Of course, I know I can talk and you can listen and that you can't say anything. I know. I wouldn't want it any other way.*

If, on the other hand, she persists in asking about Jane's condition:

> *But you know how Jane is. She doesn't take care of herself. If you just let me know what her problem is, I'll make sure she follows your instructions.*

I can hear that you're really concerned about her. And I'm sure she doesn't want you to worry. So the best thing would be for you to sit down with her and explain how you feel.

Limits and Exceptions to Confidentiality

Confidentiality is a qualified duty, not an absolute one. Table 11–3 lists some standard exceptions to the rule of confidentiality. If a patient develops a seizure disorder, for example, the law may require that this fact be reported to the state motor vehicle licensing agency. This action might lead to the driver's license being suspended until the patient is medically stable for a specified period. Such laws are intended to prevent automobile accidents, but they may cause hardship for the individual whose license is suspended. Similarly, reporting suspected child abuse or domestic violence can cause a great deal of short-term family disruption and suffering, but the clinician who judges that abuse is probable must report it. The law supports the clinician because the state has a duty to protect the interests of vulnerable persons who cannot protect themselves.

It is becoming harder to maintain confidentiality. Tension is growing between the dictates of privacy and the demands of interested third parties. These problems result from:

- Health care arrangements in which the clinician is actually employed by a third party (e.g., health maintenance organization, managed care

TABLE 11–3

JUSTIFIED EXCEPTIONS TO CONFIDENTIALITY
Required by law*
Gunshot wounds
Specified communicable diseases
Child abuse or neglect
Dog bites
Licensing requirements (e.g., drivers, pilots)
Court subpoenas
Threats of harm to patient or others
Death threats
Suicidal tendencies
Communicable diseases

*These are examples; specific requirements differ by jurisdiction. Get to know the law in your state.

company, or corporate medical department) and may, therefore, have obligations other than those to patients.

- The use of broad, open-ended release forms to obtain patient care data to assess disability, insurability, and employability.
- Computerized medical information systems to which large numbers of people might have access.

These forces highlight the need to explain to patients that in some situations you may be obliged to share information. When such a situation arises, notify the patient and attempt to secure his or her permission. Failing that, be truthful about what is required and what you intend to do. If you diagnose a case of syphilis or tuberculosis, for example, explain that the law requires you to submit a report to the health department. While describing the public health reasons for this requirement, you are also giving the patient crucial information about communicability and its implications for his or her behavior. Here are examples:

- "You had a seizure and I'm not permitted to let you drive because you could hurt someone if you had a seizure while you were driving."
- "I'm required by law to let the county health department know so they can make sure that your contacts are identified and treated."

There are special problems and considerations regarding confidentiality in the care of adolescent patients, whose privacy ought to be respected even though they are legally minors (see Chap. 8), and geriatric patients, who may in some cases no longer have decision-making capacity (see Chap. 9).

Papers, Forms, and Clearances

Paperwork is the bane of modern clinical practice. Individuals have medical forms to be completed for jobs, school, insurance, public assistance, nursing homes, social programs, driver's licenses, and more. Likewise, health insurers require the proper paperwork to justify payment for medical or laboratory services, referrals to specialists, and so on. Truthfulness in everyday medical practice requires honesty in the way we handle these bureaucratic headaches, even though we are not inclined to devote our finest literary efforts to grinding out such administrative fodder.

Two issues frequently arise with regard to clearances and certifications in primary care. In one case, the patient asks that information be suppressed:

- "Don't put down that I'm a diabetic. After all, my diabetes is in good control. And it'll cost me plenty in extra insurance premiums."
- "Listen, that nervous breakdown was 3 years ago. It won't happen again. I'm all right now."

What should you do, given that telling the truth might well result in significant adverse consequences for your patient?

Because you must *be honest* in answering explicit questions on the form, explain to the patient beforehand what the medical record contains to avoid false expectations when giving consent for you to share medical information. For example:

- "It would be great if I could leave out your diabetes, but I have to be honest. Besides, how we are treating your diabetes is all over your records. If the company requests your chart, and sometimes they do, they'll see that you and I lied, which won't be much help to you."

However, you can take the time to *write additional explanatory material* if you believe that it will benefit the patient. You might indicate, for example, that the diabetes is in excellent control or that the episode of depression has completely resolved with no residual symptoms.

Finally, *don't volunteer information* unless you have reason to believe it is relevant. Often, a final item will be something like, "Are there any other significant medical problems or conditions?" There is no need here to detail the patient's medical history; simply put what might, in your clinical judgment, be significant to the insurance or job or program in question.

A different problem arises when patients ask you to make false or unsupported assertions about their illness or disability. The patient's insurance carrier or the state welfare department might ask if, in your opinion, the patient is "totally disabled." Perhaps you are unable to ascertain objective evidence of disability or the evidence is quite limited. In this case you should provide a truthful assessment based on your clinical observations. For example, "Yes, Mr. X does have diabetes, but there are only minor symptoms and no long-term sequelae." Or, "Yes, Mrs. Y does have degenerative joint disease but this, in my opinion, cannot explain her chronic pain." (Of course, chronic pain is in itself a severe disability, whether or not an objective cause can be identified.) Be truthful in your medical assessment; you should never make assessments of disability that are not warranted by your clinical judgment. Often you will be asked only to provide data, which another specialist clinician will interpret to determine disability status. You can, of course, decline to complete a form if you feel that your opinion is not in the patient's best interest.

SUMMARY ▪ COMMUNICATION IN THE OFFICE SETTING

Office practice can be a source of great professional satisfaction, but it also presents challenges to clinician–patient communication. New institutional and insurance arrangements exacerbate these interactive concerns and present new concerns. In this chapter we review skills that help you achieve efficiency and focus in the encounter, thereby enhancing your ability to help the patient and prevent dissatisfaction:

- Allow the patient time to state his or her concerns. It doesn't actually take any longer.
- Negotiate priorities. Then set the agenda.
- Explain the issues in plain language and check for understanding.

- If the patient has come to you because of a coerced change of clinicians, confront the issue directly. Empathize with the patient. Indicate a willingness to work together.
- If you and the patient have dueling agendas, confront the issue directly. Explain the options, while respecting the patient's experience and expectations.

Other issues pertinent to office interviewing include concerns about health promotion and prevention, confidentiality, and truthfulness in day-to-day clinical practice:

- The interview is important both diagnostically (establishing the patient's risk factors) and therapeutically (laying the groundwork for behavior change).
- Confidentiality is a primary value in medicine, but not an absolute one.
- Patient advocacy is an important part of primary care practice, but it must be based on truthfulness.

References

1. Marvel MK, Epstein RM, Flowers K, Beckman HK. Soliciting the patient's agenda. Have we improved? *JAMA* 1999; 281:283–287.
2. Ramsey PG, Curtis JR, Paauw DS, Carline JD, Wenrich MD. History-taking and preventive medicine skills among primary care physicians: An assessment using standardized patients. *Am J Med* 1998; 104:152–158.
3. Hippocrates, translated by Jones WHS. The Loeb Classical Library, Cambridge MA, Harvard University Press, 1923.

Suggested Reading

Gross DA, Zyzanski SJ, Borawski EA, Cebul RD, Stange KC. Patient satisfaction with time spent with their physician. *J Fam Pract* 1998; 47:133–137.

Levinson W, Stiles WB, Inui TS, Engle R. Physician frustration in communicating with patients. *Med Care* 1993; 31:285–295.

Realini T, Kalet A, Sparling J. Interruption in the medical interaction. *Arch Fam Med* 1995; 4:1028–1033.

Seelert KR, Hill RD, Rigdon MA, Schwenzfeler E. Measuring patient distress in primary care. *Fam Med* 1999; 31:483–487.

PART THREE

CHALLENGES IN INTERVIEWING

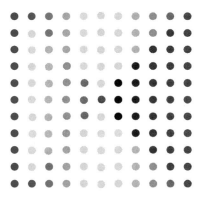

CHAPTER 12

Seal Up the
Mouth of
Outrage

· · · · ·

DIFFICULT
PATIENT–CLINICIAN
INTERACTIONS

Seal up the mouth of outrage *for a while*
Till we can clear these ambiguities
And know their spring, their head, their true descent....

William Shakespeare, *Romeo and Juliet*, Act V, Scene 3

In our interactive model of the medical interview, both the interviewer and patient play an active role in generating data that are as accurate and precise as possible. Sometimes interviewing is easy: the patient is alert, helpful, concise, and spontaneous; the problem is relatively straightforward; and there are no awkward topics, such as a sexual problem, or conflicted feelings. On other occasions the interviewer—and usually the patient also—becomes aware that the encounter is going poorly. We label particular patients or situations "difficult" when we make such an assessment—something is wrong, I'm stuck. The problems might arise from the patient, the clinician, the subject matter, or from extraneous events. We have already discussed (pp. 4–9) how

TABLE 12-1

DIFFICULT PATIENT-CLINICIAN INTERACTIONS	
Process problems (see Chap. 2)	*Interactive styles*
Technical impairments	Orderly, controlled
Organic impairments (delirium or dementia)	Dramatic
Language barrier	Long-suffering, masochistic
Style impairments (see Chap. 3)	Guarded, paranoid
Reticence	Superior
Rambling	*Somatization*
Vagueness	*Difficult feelings*
Topical problems (see Chaps. 5 and 6)	Anxiety
Sexual functioning	Anger
Positive review of systems	Depression
	Clinician's and patient's feelings about each other

SOURCE: Adapted in part from Kahana RJ, Bibring GL. Personality types in medical management. In: Zinberg NE (Ed.). *Psychiatry and Medical Practice in a General Hospital.* New York, International Universities Press, 1964, pp. 108–123.

observer bias and instrument precision affect the quality of any medical observation, whether it be a gallium scan, cardiac auscultation, or the clinical history. Any of these observations can be improved, but it takes attention, skill, and ingenuity to do so.

Table 12–1 presents a taxonomy of difficult patient–clinician interactions, including some problems involving process and topics that regularly arise during clinical interactions. Social and cultural issues are covered in our discussions of health beliefs (see Chap. 10), telling bad news (see Chap. 13), alternative medicine (see Chap. 14), and negotiation (see Chap. 16). In this chapter, we discuss interactive styles, somatization, and the difficult feelings of both patients and clinicians. These categories help us clarify and discuss aspects of the "difficult interview," although we rarely see these problems in pure form and often the differential diagnosis of problem interviews is complex.

INTERACTIVE STYLES

Occasionally the patient's interactive or personality style interferes with obtaining objective and precise data. Of course, everyone has a personality style, but under stress, such as that which accompanies illness, distinct coping behaviors may become exaggerated or even dysfunctional. Identifying your patient's style gives you important information about how he or she perceives the illness, filters or colors the historic data, and interacts with other people in other situations. Kahana and Bibring,[1] in a classic paper, presented observations on personality styles and suggested ways of coping with them during the interview to maximize the clinician's ability to obtain accurate data. The styles are:

- Dependent and demanding
- Orderly and controlled
- Dramatizing or manipulative
- Long-suffering or masochistic
- Guarded or paranoid
- Superior

Although rarely seen in "pure" form, these styles orient our discussion.

The Dependent, Demanding Style

These persons strive to impress the clinician with the urgent quality of their requests. They need special attention, massive reassurance, and constant advice. You may first identify them as optimistic, compliant, and "good" patients, because they often begin by making you feel that you are the only one who has ever cared about them or understood their problems. You soon find, however, that they expect a limitless amount of attention and care. Another term for this type of patient is "dependent clinger."[2] When their need for your constant attention is unmet, they become depressed or withdrawn, or blame you in a complaining or vengeful way. Trying to meet the dependent, demanding patient's every demand may drive you to exhaustion.

Dependent tendencies frequently (and temporarily) come to the fore in many acutely ill patients. You should address these needs with respectful, empathic, and generous care directed toward physical and emotional comfort. When this pattern becomes exaggerated or chronic, however, you must set limits. Clinical Key 12–1 presents a few guidelines for resolving some of the difficulties posed by patients with this interactive style.

The Orderly and Controlled Style

Some persons cope with their stress by attempting to gain as much knowledge as possible about their situation and to use this knowledge as a way of handling their anxiety. They are punctual for appointments, conscientious in taking medications, and preoccupied with the right and wrong ways of carrying out your instructions. Sickness threatens these patients with loss of control. They may present a list of carefully thought-out questions or a precise diary, detailing the frequency and severity of each symptom. They find the scientific approach congenial to their way of thinking and respond well to a professional, systematic sequence of history taking, physical diagnosis, laboratory studies, and therapy. These patients must be permitted to take charge of their own medical care and be given positive feedback about their efforts and abilities.

Because patients of this type are often on the same wavelength as the health professional, they may not appear to present a difficult situation. But their style suggests that, to minimize anxiety or anger and to optimize health care, you should consider the guidelines presented in Clinical Key 12–2. The following transcript is an example of a clinician talking with an orderly, controlled patient:

CLINICAL KEY 12–1

Interviewing the Dependent, Demanding Patient

- Suspect this problem when new patients make you feel that you are the only clinician who has ever understood them.
- Specify limits of your "contract" with the patient:
  - Provide written instructions.
  - Set follow-up appointments.
  - Set limits on phone calls.
  - Set limits on prescription refills.
- Avoid making promises that you cannot keep, such as solving nursing or insurance problems.
- Emphasize patient responsibility:
  - For understanding the nature and characteristics of health problems.
  - For behavior change and adherence to therapy.
  - For fulfilling his or her part of the therapeutic contract.
- Remind the patient that available time is limited, despite your interest and concern. Try a statement such as "You certainly have a lot of important problems, but since our time is so short, I'd like to get back to the reason you came into the hospital."
- Do not take credit for remission in the patient's symptoms, because you will likely be blamed for a relapse.

CLINICAL KEY 12–2

Interviewing the Controlled Patient

- Take an orderly and systematic approach to your clinical interview, providing frequent "road markers" (indicators of where you are and where you are going).
- Explain every symptom, disease, laboratory test, or procedure in detail.
- Don't leave any loose ends.
- Explain the purpose of each maneuver during the physical examination, especially if it appears unusual or prolonged:
  - Summarize frequently.
  - Take notes to indicate your interest and thoroughness.
  - Avoid mentioning any vague hypotheses, unusual aspects, or jumbled considerations you might have. Keep those to yourself.
- If you don't know, say so, and describe a plan for finding out.

How have you been?

I was trying to remember if I was supposed to call you. I think, I don't remember when I called last and now I couldn't remember if I was supposed to call you again or not.

Well, that's fine. I just was hoping that you hadn't tried and not gotten through or something like that. I understand you got new glasses. Has that helped?

I don't see the slightest difference.

You're not happy because you're having trouble seeing?

I'm not happy because I don't see as well as I would like to see. I can't see numbers well.

Does the eye doctor give you an explanation?

Well, he keeps talking. He talks to me, referring, speaking to me as "your cataract" and I said to him plainly, I said, "You referred to my cataract many times. You have never told me I have a cataract. Do I?" And he said everyone over 30 years old has a cataract. So that's....

So that's really not an answer. So you don't know whether it's the cataract, whether you have it in both eyes, or whether there's some other problem.

I don't know and I can't get a straight answer.

And later in the interview:

I wanted to tell you about that and I'm trying to think if there is anything else I should tell you. I don't remember anything. Of course, some of the problems are getting worse but I don't consider that something that wasn't expected. I assume that's what we should expect. Everything else is pretty much under control.

Notice how carefully this patient uses her words. When the clinician says, "You're having trouble seeing?" she corrects this wording with "I don't see as well as I would like to see." Similarly, she does not say, "There isn't anything else I should tell you"; she says instead, "I don't remember anything" (and this is interesting, because she is elderly and troubled about her recent memory). Notice her concern with doing the right thing, being compliant ("I was trying to remember if I was supposed to call you"). Consider the importance to her of thorough explanation, and how disquieted she is by the ophthalmologist's evasiveness ("I can't get a straight answer"). She accepts the fact that "some of the problems are getting worse," because "I don't consider that something that wasn't expected." Note how the clinician is able to clarify her concerns while avoiding explanations about a problem with which he is unfamiliar (i.e., her eye problem, for which she sees an ophthalmologist).

The Dramatic Style

This patient may charm you, fascinate you, frustrate you, and eventually make you angry. The pain is "the worst pain I have ever had ... it's with me all the time, day and night, nothing seems to help.... I haven't been able to sleep in weeks...." This person may have a need to be at stage center and may resent your interest in other duties and other patients. Such patients may look upon illness as a drama. At a deeper level, though, the patient may consider sickness a personal defect, a sign of being weak, unattractive, or unsuccessful. Sometimes, particularly when they make us uncomfortable, we describe such patients with judgmental terms, such as histrionic, hysterical, manipulative, or seductive.

Generally, clinicians should allow patients to tell their stories in their own words. We advocate that the interviewer provide direction, but do so without the high-control style that yields poor data and distant relationships. There are times, however, when the issue of control becomes more central to the interview process, and the dramatic patient's need for control may prevent you from obtaining the information you need. Sometimes the problem permeates the entire history. At other times, it may be limited to a particular facet. For example, a patient who abuses drugs may steer the discussion to a more neutral area every time you approach the question of substance abuse.

At times the patient's dramatic or manipulative style may lead to behavior usually not appropriate to a professional relationship, such as when he or she notices your new watch or hairstyle, compliments you on your good taste, or asks personal questions about your social relationships or sexual preference. Clinical Key 12–3 presents some guidelines for deflecting this type of behavior and getting beyond the dramatics into a more effective form of communication. Taking a thorough clinical history in a respectful atmosphere while demonstrating that you are in charge is the best way to build a solid relationship and to establish a treatment plan that will be acceptable to both you and the patient.

The Long-suffering, Masochistic Style

These patients are "help rejectors,"[2] who present a history of continual suffering from disease, disappointment, and other adversity. They see their lives as a never-ending story of bad luck. Often they disregard their own needs to help other people. Despite apparent humility, these patients may tend to be exhibitionistic about their fate. With regard to medical care, they may feel that no treatment will help them; when one symptom or illness disappears, another mysteriously takes its place.

The long-suffering patient will not "buy" reassurance and optimism. In the interview, you should avoid being overly optimistic or cheerful. You also should steer clear of easy answers like focusing on the patient's strengths or accomplishments (which might be a good strategy with another patient) or in-

CLINICAL KEY 12–3

Interviewing the Dramatic Patient

- Listen and observe as the patient talks. Ask yourself, "What does the patient gain by this behavior?"
- Remain calm, gentle, and firm.
- Feed back what you hear, using frequent summaries to regain or stay in control.
- Remain descriptive, not judgmental or evaluative; focus on the how, not the why. For example, "I've noticed that when I try to ask you about drug use you tend to change the subject," as opposed to "Why don't you answer my question?"
- If the patient asks you a personal or uncomfortable question, try reflecting back with a statement such as "Well, we're really not here to talk about my opinion.... I'm interested in hearing more about you. How did you handle that?"
- Identify the patient's strengths and feed them back, profiling the "healthy person within," as well as the patient who sits in front of you. For example, "I can see that you enjoy being an attractive woman and you enjoy being taken care of by a man. How do you meet those needs in your life?"

sensitive and patronizing remarks like "I'm sure you'll be feeling better in no time." These patients cannot be talked out of the severe nature of their suffering. Although they may not regard talking to a trainee as therapeutic, they may like the idea of being able to help you by permitting you to do a medical interview. Accept the patient's pessimism with a statement such as "It sounds as though you don't think there is much hope of getting better."

Consider the following interchange with an 82-year-old woman who is experiencing failing abilities and is trying to care for her severely demented 89-year-old spouse:

How have things been going for you?

Well, not much different. Same as usual. Same problems, same lack of solutions. I'm not saying that anyone would give me a different answer, but I still don't have to like it.

Yeah, you feel that you've gotten that answer to a lot of problems.

I feel that I've gotten that answer everywhere. Everything that I have problems with. Everything, that is, except Dr. Jackson, who wants to operate on my throat....

Which you don't want.

No. Pretty hopeless, isn't it.

Well, I think you're doing about as well as anyone could do.

> *Well, I don't know, maybe I am. Again I say it's not good enough, but I don't suppose there's any good enough in a situation like that.*

> How do you feel about the medication right now? Do you think it's helped your spirits at all?

> *I like to believe it does. I can't be real sure because I don't know how I'd be feeling without it, but I try to imagine it soothes me some.*

> Good.

> *I don't think it's doing me any harm.*

> Good. What about getting some extra help at home? Have you made any progress with that?

> *I don't know. The reason I have resisted is because I had a sister-in-law who could not live alone and she had an endless succession of people that I know stole from her and robbed her.*

> The best thing is to get either someone that you know well or a person who is recommended by someone you trust.

> *That's true, but I don't think that person exists.*

> I wish there were something I could do to help.

> *I don't expect you to have solutions. It's just how things are. Nothing can change.*

This kind of interchange is enough to make any clinician feel pretty hopeless as well. Note the patient's repeated return to the theme of no solutions. The most optimistic she gets (and it is not much) is "I like to believe" that the antidepressant she has been taking is helpful, at least "I don't think it's doing me any harm." The interviewer finally gives up making suggestions and begins to share the patient's pessimism: "I wish there were something I could do to help." The patient, in turn, paradoxically offers reassurance ("I don't expect you to have solutions").

The Guarded, Paranoid Style

Some patients are inclined to be suspicious of health care professionals and the medical care establishment. They may present a long list of slights from others and openly point out how the illness was mishandled; or they blame others for their illness. During stress, the patient may become even more anxious, guarded, suspicious, and quarrelsome. In turn, you may find yourself feeling constantly on guard, as if to avoid being "caught" in a competitive relationship.

These patients often express disgust about their previous interactions with health care professionals. Their clinicians not only failed them but also were insensitive and perhaps were in collusion with a system "rotten to the core." You may be presumed guilty by association. The patient may say with great exasperation, "All I want to know is if I've had a heart attack. Why doesn't my doctor tell me yes or no? Why is he keeping it from me?" It is rarely useful to unravel such a question, as you are unlikely to have the needed information and the patient may think that you are taking sides. A better strategy is to acknowledge and accept the patient's suspicions with a statement such as "It must be terribly frustrating, not knowing." Then try to proceed with the interview by reminding the patient that although you cannot help with that particular problem, "I am interested in hearing more about the symptoms that brought you here." Clinical Key 12–4 indicates some additional points to consider when interviewing the guarded patient.

The Superior Style

These patients are self-confident and may appear smug, vain, or even grandiose. They often come across as persons who feel they are entitled to the best of everything. They may demand the most senior clinician or the most well known specialist, and may be very condescending or arrogant toward trainees or younger professionals. They may attempt to control the clinician—sometimes by making many demands and sometimes by threatening litigation. Instead of having faith or trust in their clinicians, their relationships are characterized by entitlement. Often, such patients react to situations that occur in the office or hospital with anger and hostility—anger that can impinge upon you as caregiver. The suggestions presented later in this chapter for dealing with anger are also appropriate for this patient.

This style may reveal itself for the first time when the patient experiences unusual stress. Consider this example of a young actor who had never had difficulty interacting with his clinician until he developed a "cold or flu or something which normally I would just wait until it went away except I'm involved in a show right now." The dialogue continues:

CLINICAL KEY 12–4
Interviewing the Guarded Patient
- Remain friendly and courteous.
- Clearly explain your strategy for diagnosis and treatment.
- If you are a trainee or a consultant, pay particular attention to identifying your role and clarifying its limitations.
- When the patient makes a provocative statement, do not contradict, argue, or try to convince the patient otherwise.
- Openly acknowledge the patient's suspicious attitudes. Do not ignore them.
- Clarify your understanding of the patient's beliefs, while indicating that you do not necessarily agree with them.

> *And it's the leading role in a rather important production and we open*
> *this Thursday (clears throat) and I went into this cold.*
>
> You open this coming Thursday.
>
> *And I went into a cold; it feels like it's been in my system for about 2*
> *weeks, but then on about Thursday it started clearing up. Then because*
> *of an audition Friday morning I got like 6 hours of sleep. Friday I started*
> *to feel coldish, Saturday I felt terrible, yesterday I felt terrible, so I feel I*
> *just need some kind of prescription ... to be able to deal with it.*

So this patient who would "normally just wait" suddenly feels entitled to treatment for a problem that is self-limited and that has no definitive therapy. It is as though the patient is saying, "I know there is no cure for a cold, but since I'm the lead in an important production you must make an exception and cure me." This sounds paradoxical and illogical. In such a situation, one might respond:

> There's no cure for the common cold! Actors are no different from anyone else!
>
> *If you won't help me I'll find someone who will.*

But things will likely go better if you say:

> I can understand your concern, what with this production and all. As you know, there's no cure for the common cold. But why don't I take a look at you and maybe I can recommend something to get the symptoms under control so you'll feel in better form.
>
> *Okay. I sure hope there's something you can do.*

SOMATIZATION

The Nature of Somatization

Many patients have symptoms that are difficult to account for on the basis of "organic" disease. Some of these patients have syndromes that resolve over a relatively short period. Others have multiple and recurrent physical complaints that span many years, many clinicians, and many diagnostic workups, yet the story as a whole never seems to make pathophysiological sense. Sometimes the patient will tell you that "Doctors have never been able to find anything" or "They said it was all in my head." Others will bring you a series of medical diagnoses and treatments: gallbladder disease, uterine fibroids, osteoarthritis, degenerative disc disease, abdominal adhesions, and hypothyroidism. Although they ascribe their symptoms to these diagnosed disorders, these patients improve only partially and temporarily when treated and soon develop new ailments.

Such patients—often called "somatizers"—suffer real pain and often develop real disability, even though their problems resist ordinary disease categories. Somatization is a process whereby people experience and express emotional discomfort or psychosocial stress in the language of physical symptoms. As Nathaniel Hawthorne wrote, "A bodily disease, which we look upon as whole and entire within itself, may, after all, be but a symptom of some ailment in the spiritual part."

We consider somatization here for three reasons:

- Patients with functional somatic symptoms are frequently encountered in clinical practice, and they often consume large amounts of clinical time.
- Somatizing patients are often difficult to interview.
- The clinical interview and thorough review of the past medical history are critical to the diagnosis of somatoform disorders.

Table 12–2 presents a differential diagnosis of somatization as a psychiatric disorder. In the somatoform disorders (3b in Table 12–2), the process of somatization is a primary feature, and specific diagnostic criteria apply. A larger group of patients suffer functional somatic symptoms but do not meet the criteria of the *Diagnostic and Statistical Manual of Mental Disorders, Fourth Edition* (DSM-IV) for one of these conditions or for any other psychiatric disorder.

Somatizers use more medical services, require more sick leave and disability, and perceive themselves as less healthy than medically ill patients. Their interpersonal relationships, families, and ways of looking at the world are all affected by unending sickliness. Medical care itself provides a positive feedback loop that validates the patient's sickliness, creating new anxiety ("If no one can find out what it is, it must be something strange and terrible") and causing additional suffering.

TABLE 12–2

DIFFERENTIAL DIAGNOSIS OF SOMATIZATION

1. Occult physical disease
   a. Syndromes of unknown etiology (e.g., fibromyalgia, chronic fatigue syndrome)
   b. Diseases with subtle, multisystem manifestations (e.g., systemic lupus erythematosus, multiple sclerosis)
2. Secondary somatization
   a. Secondary to known chronic disease
   b. Secondary to other psychiatric disorders
      Adjustment reactions
      Alcohol or other substance abuse
      Panic and other anxiety disorders
3. Primary somatization
   a. Transient functional somatic symptoms
   b. Somatoform disorders
      Hypochondriasis
      Conversion reaction
      Psychogenic pain disorder
      Undifferentiated somatoform disorder
4. Factitious disease

Somatization in the Medical History

Three types of symptom generation may be considered manifestations of somatization within the clinical interview:

- **Patients may amplify symptoms** of acute or chronic organic disease, or may preferentially report somatic symptoms (while de-emphasizing emotional symptoms) of psychiatric conditions. One example of this process is "masked" depression, a condition that is often poorly diagnosed and treated by primary clinicians. Patients with masked depression may report a chief complaint of fatigue, for instance, and be unaware of their low mood. In such cases, the interview must be directed toward identifying those suppressed symptoms that complete the diagnostic pattern of depressive disorder. In most depressed primary care patients, the condition is not truly masked because they report their affective symptoms if asked directly. The problem is that their clinicians often do not ask.

- **Patients may report psychophysiological disturbances** (e.g., headaches, tachycardia, palpitations, or irregular bowel movements) mediated through autonomic or other known pathophysiological mechanisms. Many patients have these sorts of problems, and each can be diagnosed as a separate syndrome, such as irritable bowel syndrome, fibromyalgia, muscle contraction headache, and premenstrual syndrome. If you obtain a history of multiple, recurrent, or disabling syndromes of this type, give some attention to the process of somatization. Don't lose sight of the forest because you are carefully studying every tree.

- **Patients may experience actual conversion symptoms.** These symptoms serve a symbolic function in the patient's life, actually representing or replacing an emotion, rather than being nonspecific responses to conflict or life's stress. Consequently, conversion symptoms may not correspond to known physiological mechanisms or anatomical distributions. They often develop acutely (an important historical feature). The patient's description of a severe deficit (e.g., complete loss of feeling in the left leg or paralysis of the right arm) does not correspond at all with the physical signs. The patient is unaware of the symbolic meaning of these symptoms.

In clinical practice, you will commonly encounter amplified or psychophysiological complaints, either separately or in combination. True conversion symptoms are not rare but are infrequent. Virtually any symptom can be a manifestation of somatization; it need not be weird, complex, or inexplicable. In fact, when evaluating a patient for somatization, you should concentrate on the pattern, logic, and context of the symptom, rather than on trying to decide whether dizziness, for example, is more likely than dysuria to represent somatization. Look for "positive" features in the clinical history suggesting somatization, rather than taking the "negative" approach of ruling out every conceivable organic disease. Table 12–3 presents nine such positive characteristics. If two or three of these are present, consider the hypothesis that the patient's symptoms are at least partly attributable to somatization. You can test this hypothesis by directing your interview toward identifying additional features. For example, given a vague symptom that persists despite therapy, you might be particularly careful to explore the symptom's cognitive or emotional meaning ("What do you think is causing this?") and to search for evidence of psychiatric disorders such as major depression.

Helping the Somatizing Patient

What can you do in the interview to help the somatizing patient? Consistent application of good listening and responding skills is the basis of any effective encounter, laying the groundwork for effective therapy. Although difficult, it is necessary to build a trusting relationship, to validate the patient's suffering as a clinical problem, to explain symptoms clearly, and to actively engage the patient in treatment. Clinical Key 12–5 presents a few pointers useful in your encounters with somatizing patients. Somatizers often fragment their health care. Careful attention to the past history may require obtaining the names and addresses of numerous clinicians and sending for the patient's records. A patient who doesn't think it is relevant may not volunteer the names of a cardiologist and dermatologist when seeing you for a gastrointestinal complaint. Try to establish goals, indicating that if a syndrome has been present for a long time, a similarly long period of treatment may be required before it improves or resolves. Remember to devote some time, even if only a couple of minutes, to "healthy talk" in each interaction. This will be difficult at first because the patient may find any topic other than his or her symptoms irrelevant and perhaps suspicious. However, genuine empathic concern may break through the "body" barrier and allow the somatizer to be more open with you. Finally,

TABLE 12–3

CHARACTERISTICS OF PATIENTS AND SYMPTOMS SUGGESTIVE OF SOMATIZATION
1. The symptom's description is vague, inconsistent, or bizarre.
2. The symptoms persist despite apparently adequate medical therapy.
3. The illness begins in the context of a psychologically meaningful setting (e.g., death of relative, conflict with spouse, or job promotion).
4. The patient denies any emotional distress or psychological role of the symptoms.
5. The patient has engaged in polydoctoring, has had polysurgery, or both.
6. There is evidence of an associated psychiatric disorder.
7. The patient has features suggesting a hysterical personality style.
8. Discussion reveals that the patient attributes an idiosyncratic meaning to his or her symptoms.
9. The patient has difficulty describing emotions or inner processes in words.

SOURCE: Adapted and abridged from Lipkin M Jr. Psychiatry and medicine. In: Kaplan H, Sadock B (Eds.). *Comprehensive Textbook of Psychiatry,* 5th ed. Baltimore, Williams & Wilkins, 1987.

CLINICAL KEY 12–5

Interviewing the Somatizing Patient

- In the initial assessment, obtain a complete patient profile, including functional status, occupational history, and family constellation, even though the patient may want to limit the discussion to symptoms.
- Pay particular attention to the sequence and details of the past medical history.
- Examine the patient to avoid missing disease and to validate the patient's concerns by showing that you take the symptoms seriously.
- Establish goals with the patient. In particular, if the patient presents multiple symptoms and concerns, agree on which of them need attention first.
- Sometimes an explicit contract is helpful: you agree to address the patient's concerns systematically, and the patient agrees to accept reassurance if there is no cause for alarm.
- Avoid "vague reference" (see p. 179). Although you may not be sure of a symptom's underlying cause, you can still explain its operation and your plan for treatment in physiological terms, such as "Your intestine feels painful when it is stretched or goes into spasm."
- Speak of the body, not of the mind. Many patients will have been told by clinicians, "It's all in your head." It is generally not useful to explain symptoms as originating in the mind because this approach makes the patient feel that the symptom is not "real."
- When talking about "stress" or "tension," relate those concepts to physiologic parameters (e.g., the autonomic nervous system), which cause the disagreeable sensation or symptom.
- In each encounter, focus some attention on healthy talk (e.g., the patient's strengths and activities), rather than concentrating only on symptoms.
- Schedule regular follow-up visits.

schedule regular, possibly frequent, follow-up visits so that the patient does not need a new or worsening symptom to see you again.

DIFFICULT FEELINGS IN THE MEDICAL INTERVIEW

The patient's feelings or emotions frequently influence the clinical interview and may interfere with communication. The same is true of your feelings. Strong emotions may produce behaviors that prevent you from obtaining accurate information, making good clinical judgments, educating patients, and establishing therapeutic relationships. When such feelings get in the way, you need to identify and acknowledge them so that the interview can proceed successfully. Experienced clinicians find that empathic responses not only help the patient feel understood, but also facilitate the interview by making it more efficient, accurate, and therapeutic. Other basic strategies to help deal with feelings that threaten to subvert the interview include:

- Eliciting the patient's permission, perhaps with a question such as "Is it all right if we go on?" If the answer is yes, show your appreciation. If the answer is no, accept the patient's noncooperation and ask for the reasons in a nonthreatening way, recognizing the patient's right to refuse.
- Indicating your willingness to compromise within limits, such as by asking, "Would it help if I came back in an hour? Rescheduled the appointment? Talked louder? Talked slower?"
- Preparing the way for potentially threatening questions. For example, "You have had a lot of back pain, and from what you tell me, it has also made you quite depressed.... Has it affected your marriage? Your sex life?"
- Trying to remain "in sync" with the patient, particularly when you notice that the patient feels upset or misunderstood. For example, "Just now, as you were describing your pain, you got a very worried look on your face.... Did I say something that upset you?"

Anxiety

Every illness produces at least some anxiety, if not outright fear, in the patient. Common sources of anxiety are feelings of helplessness, fear of pain and disability, inability to accept warmth or tenderness, fear of expressing anger, and, of course, uncertainty about the future. When people are anxious, they tend to intensify their customary ways of coping with the world: a compulsive patient may become more particular and a paranoid patient may become more guarded. Signs of anxiety that may appear in the interview include facial flushing, sweating, rapid speech or silence, cold hands, fidgeting, or even trembling. The anxious patient may be difficult to interview until the anxiety has been discussed. In Clinical Key 12–6, we describe a few ways you might begin to defuse your patient's anxiety.

Consider this example. A 57-year-old woman saw her primary care provider for an annual examination. The thought of an examination, even on a day when she had no worrisome symptoms, made her nervous. Her red lipstick was coated with antacid as she entered the office; she was so distraught that her stomach felt queasy. It was clear (in retrospect) that just showing up for the examination was a major effort. Everything, fortunately, was in order. The clinician had only one prescription:

CLINICAL KEY 12–6

Interviewing the Anxious Patient

- Be unhurried and calm in your manner.
- Sympathize, but remember that too much sympathy may magnify the patient's fears.
- Be specific as to what you expect of the patient; for example, in preparing for a physical examination, tell the patient what clothing should be removed or what position he or she should assume and where.
- Be specific about what is normal or not normal and explain your actions (e.g., "Now I'm checking the size of your thyroid and it feels normal.")
- Tell the patient that anxiety is normal and appropriate; most patients feel this way. It is okay to feel scared.

> Everything is fine. I have only one recommendation, and that is that I'd like you to get a mammogram.
>
> *Oh my God! You mean I've got cancer? Not my breast!*
>
> No, no, of course not. No, I recommend a mammogram for all my patients over the age of 50. It's routine.

As though the clinician were not leveling with her, the woman continued:

> *I couldn't stand to lose a breast; chemotherapy is awful. I already have thinning hair, you know; chemotherapy makes that worse. No, I won't do that—I can't.*

In retrospect, this patient's fragile adaptation to her clinical encounter was shattered by the suggestion of a routine screening test. She evidently thought that the recommendation was particular, not routine, despite her clinician's protests to the contrary. If we look back at how the clinician introduced the idea, we notice a possible contradiction: "Everything is fine ... get a mammogram." For this anxiety-ridden patient, "If 'everything is fine,' why do I need a mammogram?" The clinician might have been able to achieve the aim of getting her to have a mammogram (which, by the way, she never agreed to) by saying:

> Everything is fine. Your exam is completely normal. Just like you come for a Pap test because you know that's routine in all women, we also routinely recommend a mammogram for all women your age. Have you ever had one done?

In this instance, the clinician reassures the patient by specifying the nature of "fine" ("Your exam is completely normal"), framing the screening function of the mammogram in a concrete way (comparing it to the Pap test), and anticipating the woman's worry by explaining the reason for the test before she can spin a fantasy of calamity.

Anger

Although a patient's anxiety may make us sympathetic, we usually find anger more difficult to handle. Patients behave in a hostile manner for many reasons. Often these reasons have nothing to do with us personally but rather relate to the patient's own situation, such as inconsiderate care by previous health professionals, life disappointments, or perceived injustice. What makes one patient depressed may make another patient angry, and the seemingly angry patient may really be depressed. Review the guidelines in Clinical Key 12–7 for coping with anger in the interview as you consider the following examples.

In the first example, the patient responds to an anger-provoking question:

You're just as insensitive as the rest of 'em.

I guess that was a foolish question to ask. Now that I understand you a little better, do you think we could start over?

In another example, a patient was angry after being interviewed in front of a group of students and residents at a psychiatric case conference. She is talking to her clinician following the conference:

CLINICAL KEY 12–7

Interviewing the Angry Patient

- Recognize and acknowledge anger with a statement such as "I can see (hear or feel) that you are angry and frustrated," or, because many people do not like to be accused of being angry, "Waiting so long makes most people angry."
- If you are not sure that what you are hearing is anger, ask, "Are you feeling angry?"
- Accept the anger by continuing to listen, while explaining the situation in a neutral fashion, even though a logical explanation will not necessarily change the patient's feelings.
- Explore contributing factors and identify any underlying feelings, such as fear, hurt, disappointment, or powerlessness.
- Accept the patient's reason even if you do not personally agree with it. Remember that there is always a reason, although it may not be immediately evident.
- If the patient's anger is justifiably directed at you, acknowledge your error. We all make mistakes; you can learn from them and correct them.
- If the anger is not directed at you, help the patient recognize ways he or she can deal with the anger-provoking situations.

I now know what it's like to be poor. I never would have been at that conference if I had my own private doctor. I know what it's like to be a guinea pig. That doctor asked about my early childhood when what I needed was someone to find out what's been going on over the last 10 years and how tough life has been for me so that he could help me. I thought he would be able to give me something to help my nerves right now, not just talk about my grandmother.

Although this patient reminds us of the "entitled demander" (see p. 203), and indeed may be one, she has good reason for being upset. Talking about what she considered ancient history confused and frustrated her. The conference ended apparently without a definite formulation or plan of action, and although the clinician was actually attempting to remedy the situation by having her present at the conference, the patient may not have known that. An explanation and an acknowledgment of her feelings are in order:

It certainly must seem strange to talk about old things when you feel so bad now and want relief. I can understand your frustration. Actually, the reason I wanted to talk with you is to discuss what to do next to get you to feel better. Because Dr. Smith had some good ideas that I think we should try. In fact, he suggested some medication that he thinks will be helpful, and I think so, too.

The other aspect of her anger was a sense of being on display or of being experimented with (perhaps two sides of the same coin). She may have been surprised by the conference format, requiring her to sit in front of a room full of people she had never met before. Someone should have prepared her for what was to occur; if no one did, the clinician can only apologize:

I'm sorry, I guess I didn't really explain very well what was supposed to happen to you. I'm sorry you felt uncomfortable. But I did learn a lot about you that I think will help me to take better care of you.

Okay. What I really need is to feel better.

Depression

Depression may be a manifestation of a psychiatric disorder, a response to recent loss (such as death of a spouse), an expression of a pessimistic approach to life, or a transient feeling state. Major depressive disorder may be the underlying problem in a substantial percentage of patients who complain of fatigue, weakness, lack of energy, insomnia, backache, or headache, but depression as a feeling or response to illness is also common. Depressive characteristics include feelings of worthlessness, hopelessness, apathy, and guilt, together with a profoundly empty and lonely feeling. These are manifest in the patient's manner, tone of voice, posture, and speech: the patient may think slowly and talk little, speak softly and have a "flat" affect, look down or away from you, and be tearful. Sometimes a statement such as "You look sad" or "You look as if all this has gotten you down" gives the patient an opportunity to talk about depressed feelings, thereby facilitating other more "medical" aspects of the history.

Some patients have endured such tragic events that you fear being overwhelmed with sorrow. In such instances, it is appropriate to say that you, too, find the situation sad. In this way you demonstrate your sympathy, compassion, or fellow feeling. You are also a professional, however, and your feelings should be used constructively to help the patient. Consider this example: The patient is a 57-year-old woman who had coronary bypass surgery at the age of 53, followed 2 years later by a left radical mastectomy for aggressive carcinoma of the breast. She is now suffering from metastatic disease and is about to lose her health insurance coverage because her husband's business is failing and they can no longer afford the premiums.

> A lot of bad things have happened to you. You must be a pretty strong person to have endured all this ... How have you managed?
>
> *Well, I have my faith ... and my family has been just wonderful to me.*

Notice how the interviewer acknowledges the feeling content but, instead of getting deep into the tragedy, allows the patient to express her strength and her coping style. This technique serves the dual purpose of keeping both parties from being overwhelmed.

Often the best follow-up questions are simple statements such as "Tell me more about these feelings" or "Tell me more about it," or the use of simple prompters and facilitators such as "Mm hmm" followed by silence to encourage the patient to speak. This technique may uncover information vital to the diagnostic process:

> You look sad. Is it about this chest pain you're having or something else?
>
> *I guess I am sad. My chest has been hurting all week. Well ... see ... I don't know if I can say it ... I get all choked up ... excuse me [trying to hold back tears]. My mother died on Monday. Every time I think about her I get this choked-up feeling in here and it starts to hurt like my angina down into my arm.*

Here the interviewer discovers the crucial connection between an exacerbation of angina and the recent death of the patient's mother.

Although perhaps more appropriate to a consideration of depression as an illness, no discussion of depression is complete without considering how to assess the depth of depression and risk of suicide. Some useful questions are:

- Do you get pretty discouraged (or blue)?
- What do you see for yourself in the future? How do you see the future?

And if answers to these questions indicate a risk of suicide:
- Have you ever thought of hurting yourself? Of doing away with yourself? Of ending your life? Of suicide?
- Are you having any thoughts of hurting yourself? Of killing yourself?
- Did you ever think about how you would do it?

The patient may need a few extra seconds (or even longer) to answer these questions. Far from putting the idea of suicide into their heads, most patients experience relief at the opportunity to talk about their feelings of suicide. Here is an example of an assessment of a patient who is seeing an internist for follow-up of abdominal pain and asthma:

Last time I talked to you, you were feeling pretty bad.
You know, sometimes I scare myself.
You mean ... have you ever tried to kill yourself?
Yeah.
How did you do it? How did you try?
Uh, I turned on the gas once.
What happened?
Somebody, they smelled the gas.
When was that?
That's not the first time I tried to kill myself. One time I climbed up on the bridge.
Uh hmm. What stopped you?
I don't know.
I'm glad you stopped. How are you feeling right now?

The need to assess suicide risk often arises in the context of routine clinical care. Notice how this physician does not shy away from asking specific questions about past and current suicide intent. The physician also reaches out to the patient by sharing genuine happiness ("I'm glad you stopped") that the patient is still alive.

Denial

Denial is a common response to illness. Denial is evident in statements like "This isn't really happening to me," "I can't believe it," and "That wasn't blood I saw in my bowel movement—at least, I don't think it was." In some patients, denial is strong enough to make them ignore or forget symptoms. Alternatively, they may minimize a worrisome symptom and report it as a trivial event: "I had a little pain in my chest, but it only lasted an hour." Only later do you find out that the chest pain was severe and associated with nausea, sweating, and a feeling of impending doom.

Whereas some patients play down symptoms, others deny the emotional impact of a diagnosis or prognosis. At times, it is hard to tell the difference between denial and optimism, such as in the patient with a potentially lethal disease who smiles and says, "I'm a fighter. I know I can beat it." When patients accept bad news (see Chap. 13) with apparent equanimity, it is unclear whether they are realistically "handling it well" or engaging in denial. Denial can lead to serious delays in seeking care, but it may also be a useful mechanism for coping with bad news, so you should handle denial with circumspection and respect. Try to assess the patient's understanding of what is happening. Two useful techniques are:

- Accept denial as the patient's unique and current experience.
- Inform the patient gently and calmly that many people feel differently, including you. For example, you can say, "Most people feel very sad when they hear they have a serious illness," or "I guess I would be worried."

Consider this example of a young woman who came for a "checkup." This was her first visit to a new clinician. On palpating the abdomen, the clinician found a large mass, which later proved to be an enormous uterine fibroid. The patient seemed unaware that it was present, even though it was the size of a 5-month pregnancy. When she was told that a hysterectomy might be necessary, she appeared unconcerned. The clinician needed to find out if this 30-year-old childless woman understood and accepted what a hysterectomy would mean to her, or, alternatively, if she had not internalized the implications of surgery:

You don't seem very concerned at the idea of a hysterectomy.
Well, if I have to have it, that's it.
Do you know what a hysterectomy is?
Well, I guess that's when they take everything out.
Well, actually, it means the removal of the uterus or womb—that's where this fibroid is. Now the tumor is an overgrowth in the muscle, but even though it's not cancer, it may be impossible to remove without removing the uterus. Now your ovaries, which are the glands next to the uterus that make female hormones like estrogen, you've heard of estrogen? Okay, the ovaries would not be removed. [Draws picture.] They would stay, so your hormones would still work right.
But I still couldn't have babies.
That's right, you couldn't have babies. What do you think about that?
I don't know. I guess I never thought much about it, not being married and all, but I guess it hasn't really hit me yet. I'm more worried about the operation itself.

Notice how the interviewer gently probes the patient's knowledge and offers a clear explanation as to what will happen. The patient is not denying the outcome of the surgery but is, perhaps, delaying dealing with it pending resolution of her more immediate fears about the operation itself, and it is reasonable for her to do so.

The Clinician's Feelings

The clinical encounter may be highly charged with emotion. For you as a clinician, just as for the patient, the interaction may bring out attitudes and behaviors that reflect previous experience and relationships. The sicker the patient, and the more helpless and dependent he or she is, the more likely it is that the patient's attitude toward you will reflect previously learned attitudes, styles, and coping behaviors. Sometimes these attitudes are manifest in ways that may appear totally irrational. For example, a patient who has had an angry, competitive relationship with his father may perceive a male physician as a powerful authority and may become antagonistic, sarcastic, and competitive, even though the physician has done nothing that would ordinarily elicit such a response. Similarly, female professionals may encounter seemingly irrational responses based on the patient's early experiences with being mothered. Although you may not be able to figure it out at the time, seemingly irrational behavior often has a reason and constitutes important data about your patient.

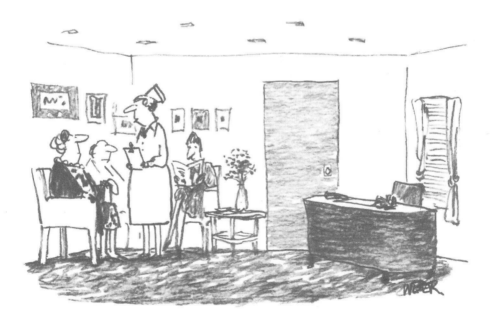

"The doctor will see you now, Mrs. Perkins.
Please try not to upset him."

On the other hand, you have feelings about your patients, sometimes very strong or negative feelings. You may try to hide these emotions because you think they are inappropriate, or believe they will interfere with your objectivity in caring for the patient. Some patients are very likable, others less so, and some perhaps positively unlikable. A few patients will so upset you that their presence on your office schedule threatens to ruin your day. Some will make you angry, and others will make you sad. You will find a few patients so humorous that you wonder whether your response to them is "professional." You may even feel sexually attracted to certain patients and, therefore, feel embarrassed or behave awkwardly.

There are two crucial points to remember about such feelings. First, the patient's behavior pattern probably engenders similar feelings in other people. Therefore, your negative response might be useful clinical information, helping to explain some of the patient's difficulties. Second, your response, particularly if it is strong or exaggerated, probably also represents an interaction with factors in your own life history and personality—so-called *countertransference.*

The best approach to such feelings is first to identify and acknowledge them. Ask yourself, "How is this patient making me uncomfortable? And why?" The answers to the "how" and "why" questions will allow you to identify behaviors in the patient that help your assessment. For example, do you dread seeing this patient because the individual makes too many demands? If all demanding patients seem to put your teeth on edge, you should be self-reflective enough to understand that fear of being exploited or manipulated is a particular problem for you. You can't change your personality, but you can develop support systems that may help you in coping with demanding patients. Alternatively, perhaps you are uncomfortable with patients who are depressed or dying; you are afraid that there is nothing you can do for them. Remember that these are *your* problems, not the patient's.

What can you do for yourself as you struggle with these difficult interactions? Somatizing patients, exaggerated personality styles, and certain feelings hit us in two vulnerable places. First, these patients defy the comfort of mind–body separation. They present the endless problem of "when to say when"; after all, there is always the remote possibility that you have, indeed, missed an occult physical explanation for their symptoms. Second, these patients place a great deal of stress on our already fragile emotions. We often see them as oppositional, demanding, recalcitrant, perverse, or frustrating. One difficult interaction or "dreaded patient" on the morning's schedule can sour your whole day. It may help to share your feelings with helpful colleagues. Health care professionals who get in touch with their feelings and discuss them with colleagues are more likely than others to "survive" difficult interactions. As you become comfortable with these feelings, you may also be able to share them with the patient and so improve his or her self-understanding. The opportunity to create a real connection with your patient can be the basis for a professional intimacy as you learn more about each other over time.

SUMMARY ▪ DIAGNOSING AND TREATING THE "SICK" INTERVIEW

Although we'd like all interviews with our patients to go well, sometimes our best efforts to apply basic skills go awry. When this happens, our ability to get accurate and precise data, as well as our relationship with the patient, may be impaired. We may ascribe too much importance to one symptom, too little to another, or entirely miss a vital point. In this chapter, we explore common sources of interviewing problems including interactive styles, somatization, and feelings. Although it is useful to discuss each as a distinct category, problems rarely occur in pure form, and a number of common approaches are helpful to diagnose and treat the "sick" interview:

- View the problem as one involving the interaction itself rather than only the patient. All patients (and all clinicians) have personality styles and feelings; problems arise when there is a mismatched or exaggerated response by either party.
- Try to diagnose the problem. (Is this seemingly angry patient really depressed? Are these requests reasonable? If not, why not?)
- Observe the basics of good interviewing technique (open-ended questions, time for the patient to respond, use of summaries and interchangeable responses).
- Accept and respect the patient's feelings and coping style.
- Focus on good interactions, which, repeated over time, lead to productive relationships.
- Establish sufficient control over the relationship, which means setting goals, limits, and guidelines. Remember that the patient wants to control his or her frightening feelings and will appreciate a method to deal with them.
- Develop strategies to cope when you feel yourself reacting too emotionally to certain patients or situations. Such strategies will help you maintain your empathic focus on the patient.

References

1. Kahana RJ, Bibring GL. Personality types in medical management. In: Zinberg NE (Ed.). *Psychiatry and Medical Practice in a General Hospital.* New York, International Universities, 1964, pp. 108–123.
2. Groves JE. Taking care of the hateful patient. *N Engl J Med* 1978; 398:883–887.

Suggested Reading

American Psychiatric Association: Somatoform disorders. In: *Diagnostic and Statistical Manual of Mental Disorders*, 4th ed. Washington, DC, American Psychiatric Association, 1994, pp. 445–469.

Balint M. *The Doctor, His Patient and the Illness*. New York, International Universities, 1972.

Block MR, Schulberg HC, Coulehan JL, et al. Recognition and characteristics of depression in primary care practice. *J Am Board Fam Pract* 1988; 1:91–97.

Callahan EJ, Bertakis KD, Rahman A, et al. The influence of depression on physician-patient interaction in primary care. *Fam Med* 1996; 28:346–351.

Coulehan JL, Schulberg HC, Block MR, et al. Symptom patterns of depression in ambulatory medical and psychiatric patients. *J Nerv Ment Dis* 1988; 176:284–288.

Keeley R, Smith M, Miller J. Somatoform symptoms and treatment nonadherence in depressed family medicine outpatients. *Arch Fam Med* 2000; 9:46–54.

Schafer S, Newlis DP. Personality disorders among difficult patients. *Arch Fam Med* 1998; 7:126–129.

Servan-Schreiber D, Kolb NR, Tabas G. Somatizing patients. Part I. Practical diagnosis. *Am Fam Physician* 2000; 61:1073–1078.

Simon GE, VonKorff M, Piccinelli M, Fullerton C, Ormel J. An international study of the relation between somatic symptoms and depression. *N Engl J Med* 1999; 341:1329–1335.

Whooley MA, Avins AL, Miranda J, Browner WS. Case finding instruments for depression. *J Gen Intern Med* 1997; 12:439–445.

CHAPTER 13

Something New and Dreadful

● ● ● ● ●

TELLING BAD NEWS

*There was no deceiving himself: **something new and dreadful** was happening to him, something of such vast importance that nothing in his life could compare with it.*

Leo Tolstoy, *The Death of Ivan Ilych*

Telling bad news is among the most difficult interpersonal situations that clinicians encounter. The idea that one should inform a patient that he or she has a lethal disease is a relatively new one in medicine. As recently as the 1960s, most American physicians routinely misled cancer patients about their diagnosis and, especially, the prognosis of their condition. This paternalistic tradition was based on the belief that the knowledge that they were suffering from a fatal illness would be harmful to many or most persons. Such patients would lose all hope of being cured, the argument went, thus damaging their quality of life and perhaps even shortening their lives because of the loss of the "will to live." The last 30 years have seen a remarkable reversal of these beliefs. We now know that nearly all people in our society desire to know their prognosis and that such knowledge is far more helpful than harmful to them. Of equal importance is the development of greater respect for patient autonomy or self-determination as a fundamental principle of medical ethics. We now have a better appreciation of patients' rights, especially the right to choose (or refuse) treatment. This right demands that patients be given adequate information about their diagnosis and prognosis, as well as the risks and benefits of therapy. Today it is standard practice in the United States for patients to be told bad news.

During the same period, however, another change has taken place: we have come to neglect some of the more positive features of the traditional approach to caring for dying patients. In the past, when there was little that could be done to change the course of fatal illnesses, clinicians emphasized the caring aspects of their role; if they couldn't cure, they could, at least, remain faithful, available, and supportive to dying patients and their families. Witness the traditional images of nighttime house calls and bedside vigils. Now that medicine has enormous power to intervene, we tend to focus almost exclusively on the technical aspects of what we can do for a patient: Can the cancer be cured? Will chemotherapy be beneficial? When the answer to all such questions is negative, we often conclude that our role is finished. We think we can do nothing more. The lack of technical potency makes clinicians feel uncomfortable, so we minimize our interactions with the patient, rather than remaining available and using the therapeutic power of the clinician–patient relationship to provide physical and emotional support.

In this chapter we present an approach to telling bad news that arises from the basic interactive skills featured throughout this book. The first section examines and illustrates a series of personal and cultural barriers that we must overcome to communicate bad news clearly and empathetically. The second section outlines a skill-based approach to improving these difficult interactions. In the third section we consider issues of interviewing in the continuing care of dying patients. The next section takes up the topic of advance directives and how to incorporate discussion about advance directives into routine patient care. Finally, we consider cultural differences in talking about death and dying.

BARRIERS TO COMMUNICATING BAD NEWS

Clinical Key 13–1 lists several psychological and professional barriers that clinicians must overcome to communicate bad news in a clear and effective manner. In this section we describe and illustrate them, partly through the voices of patients.

The Clinician Delays: Denying Defeat

Given the wide array of available diagnostic tests and treatment options, it is perhaps natural that clinicians tend to wait until the last possible minute to tell bad news. In a sense, they convince themselves the news is not really "that bad," at least now. After all, this argument goes, there are additional tests to be done. Perhaps these tests will show that the cancer has not yet metastasized. Why tell the patient the diagnosis before we have the whole picture? Why create useless anxiety? Alternatively, after cancer surgery a clinician might think, "Why discuss the fact that we were unable to remove the whole tumor? Let's wait until the patient is stronger and better able to take the news." This approach essentially denies the reality of terminal illness by postponing

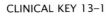

CLINICAL KEY 13-1

Barriers to Telling Bad News

- **Denying defeat:** There is always a chance.
- **Filtering the data:** Professional language disguises the truth.
- **Fear of diminishing hope:** The patient needs the will to live.
- **Keeping your distance:** Having feelings is unprofessional.
- **Disappearing:** There is nothing I can do.

discussion about it simply because certain information about the prognosis is missing. This form of denial obviously flounders on the shoals of respect for self-determination and the doctrine of informed consent: a patient cannot make informed choices about his or her care without knowing what the problem is.

The Clinician Filters the Truth: Confusion Instead of Clarity

When clinicians do give bad news, they often do so obliquely or in a language that the patient doesn't understand, hiding behind disease-specific issues (e.g., the name of the cancer or what the treatment is) rather than addressing the patient's human concerns in simple, clear language. Alternatively, they may use vague language that is literally true ("The tumor isn't responding as well as we would like it to") but does not convey the meaning of the situation. The following example of an interaction with the family of a dying patient illustrates this type of miscommunication[1]:

> Your mother's condition is deteriorating, and we don't expect her to do too well.
>
> *[Family]: Thank you, doctor, we know you are doing your best.*
>
> Well, so far we've been able to keep her blood pressure up with pressors.
>
> *[Family]: That's good, isn't it? At least the blood pressure isn't a problem.*
> *[Clinician leaves.] [Family to each other]: Thank goodness, he didn't say she's dying.*

The use of complex descriptions about *what can be done* to disguise honest discussion about *what it all means* is probably the most common form of miscommunication in caring for dying patients. This type of interchange is illustrated in Leo Tolstoy's *The Death of Ivan Ilych*[2] when Ivan Ilych realizes that "something new and dreadful was happening to him, something of such vast importance that nothing in his life could compare with it."[2(p80)] His doctor blathers on about technical details, such as telling him the problem is a "floating kidney" and then describing just how it became detached and what might be done about it. Later, Ivan Ilych goes to another doctor who tells him that the problem is "a tiny little thing in the caecum," and then proceeds to describe what must be done: "Stimulate the energy of one organ, depress the activity of another." But none of the physicians addresses the most important issue: "To Ivan Ilych only one question mattered: was his condition serious or not?"[2(p75)]

In an essay describing his recovery from a devastating stroke, Robert McCrum[3] wrote about his physicians' retreat into vague language: "... the experts took refuge in a studied vagueness—'probably' I'd be fit in 'about a year'; after six months, it would be 'fairly clear' how much movement would return to my left side; then 'perhaps' my arm would become 'useful.'" The functional outcome after a stroke is, of course, uncertain. But there is an enormous difference between sharing this uncertainty with the patient in an interactive and constructive way and relying on broad terms or qualifiers to create a "studied vagueness."

The Clinician Wills to Live: Not Destroying Hope

This dynamic is well characterized by the Yale surgeon Sherwin Nuland in his best-selling book, *How We Die*[4(p223)]: "Too often physicians misunderstand the ingredients of hope, thinking it refers only to cure or remission. They feel it necessary to transmit to a cancer-ridden patient by inference if not by actual statement, the erroneous assumption that it is still possible to attain months if not years of symptom-free life. When an otherwise totally honest and beneficent physician is asked why he does this, his answer is likely to be some variation of, 'Because I didn't want to take away his only hope.'"

In the past, clinicians justified their reluctance to "tell it like it is" because they thought the truth would harm the patient by taking away all hope and perhaps causing a loss of the will to live. It seemed reasonable then that truthfulness was often at odds with the Hippocratic dictum, "Help, or at least do no harm." We now know this to be false in most cases, yet it is still difficult, when faced with a real patient in a real situation, not to think that perhaps the truth should be watered down or delayed in *this* particular case. There is a sense in which the better the relationship we have with a patient, the more difficult it might be to avoid the "loss-of-hope fallacy." If a patient is important to us, it is easy to imagine many ways in which bad news might cause him or her harm. Alternatively, clinicians who stick to the technical aspects of medicine might have an easier time of it—if you can't imagine a person's life narrative, psychological harm remains simply an abstract concept rather than a real concern. Dr. Nuland illustrates precisely this dynamic when he describes his own intervention in his brother's terminal illness. Even though he was aware that both he and his brother's physicians should be completely truthful about the dismal prognosis, "I did exactly what I warned others against."[4(p226)] Because he loved his brother so much, he confused the hopelessness of curing or ameliorating his metastatic colon cancer with human hopelessness. Not wanting his brother to face the latter, Nuland orchestrated deceptive options, encouraging his brother's belief that additional treatment might arrest the tumor.

The Clinician Is Detached: Maintaining Distance

Health care professionals also have difficulty dealing with the emotional aspects of talking about dying and death. They may not want to confront their own feelings about dying. They may be frightened by the patient's, or a family member's, potentially strong emotional response to the news, and by continuing emotional involvement. They may feel awkward and not know what to say. Clinicians who are extraordinarily skillful at detached, technical aspects of medicine may at the same time be very insecure in dealing with sensitive interpersonal relationships. This leads dying patients to feel emotionally abandoned.

In "Intoxicated by My Illness," a posthumous collection of essays about his experience as a cancer patient, the literary critic Anatole Broyard wrote about the tendency of his physicians to remain detached: "(Some) doctors give you a generic, unfocused gaze. They look at you panoramically. They don't see you in focus.... If he could gaze directly at the patient, the doctor's work would be more gratifying. Why bother with sick people, why try to save them, if they're not worth acknowledging? When a doctor refuses to acknowledge a patient, he is, in effect, abandoning him to his illness."[5(p50)]

Broyard also went on to describe what he desired in a physician treating him during terminal illness—not necessarily a close friend or hand-holder, but someone who was carefully observant, emotionally honest, and insightful: "Now that I know I have cancer of the prostate, the lymph nodes, and part of my skeleton, what *do* I want in a doctor? I would say that I want one who is a close reader of illness and a good critic of medicine."[5(p40)] He wanted most of all to be viewed as a fellow human being, not just as a face in a bed or across a desk: "I would like my doctor to understand that beneath my surface cheerfulness, I feel 'the panic inherent in creation' and 'the suction of infinity'."[5(p42)]

The Clinician Vanishes: Disappearing

When patients become terminally ill, they sometimes find that their clinicians have performed a vanishing act. There are a number of reasons for this. First, if a clinician is oriented toward using office visits only for "medical indications," he or she might feel there is no justification for frequent visits—after all, the patient is not on active treatment. Likewise, the hospital physician or nurse may have plenty of complicated work to attend to and not feel he or she has the time to spend "socializing" in a dying patient's room. Second, terminally ill patients may have difficulty getting around; because house calls are rare nowadays, these patients may find it physically difficult to see their clinicians. Finally, many clinicians find it emotionally difficult to care for dying patients. Oriented toward aggressive therapy and attempts to cure, they are very uncomfortable with the maxim, "Don't just do something; sit there." Thus, they either tell the patient explicitly, or communicate implicitly, "There is nothing more I can do."

EMPATHY AND INTERACTION IN TELLING BAD NEWS

Setting the Stage

The first step in effectively communicating bad news (see Clinical Key 13–2) is to prepare yourself for the encounter and to select an appropriate setting. In the hospital, this means choosing a relatively quiet time to sit by the patient's bed, a time when you don't have to jump up and finish rounds or answer pages. Some patients prefer the presence of a spouse or other family members; others prefer to receive the news on their own. The old practice of informing the patient's family first and then deciding whether the patient should be told is disrespectful and paternalistic. It is also a breach of physician–patient confidentiality. When a patient is elderly or very ill, it often seems natural to speak with a family member first about diagnosis or prognosis. In some such cases, this may be appropriate because it is clearly consistent with the patient's wishes, but you should make it clear that the patient has a right to know. These generalizations pertain to our general American culture, in which self-determination is a paramount moral and legal value. In certain other cultures, dying persons expect their families to play a larger role in managing

CLINICAL KEY 13–2

How to Communicate Bad News in the Clinical Setting

Set the Stage
- Choose a quiet setting.
- Give the news in person, not by phone.
- Allocate adequate time for discussion.

Tell the News
- Use simple, clear language.
- Avoid the temptation to minimize the problem.
- Assess the patient's emotional state.
- Express sorrow for the patient's situation.

Continue the Interview
- Assess how the patient feels after receiving the news.
- Reassure the patient of your continued availability.
- Communicate a plan for care if not cure.

their care, to the extent that sometimes it is not culturally appropriate to give bad news directly to the patient. We will discuss these issues again at the end of this chapter.

Giving bad news over the telephone is almost always a bad decision. Consider the following example[6]:

> [By telephone]: The bad news is that you have a brain tumor. The good news is that we think it's a meningioma, which means it'll be easy for us to get to.
>
> *[Long pause.] What, what are you saying? I don't know what you mean.*
>
> I mean it's a probably a benign tumor on the outside of your brain, so we can remove it by surgery.
>
> *Uh, I don't know what to say.... Can I come in and talk with you about this?*
>
> Okay, yes, we can do that. Call Judy. Let's make an appointment for next Tuesday.

This physician's flip "good news/bad news" opening demonstrates his insensitivity to the human dimension of his message. He seems to believe that having a meningioma is a wonderful opportunity for the patient, certainly nothing to become upset about. When the patient requests a meeting, this physician blithely suggests a future appointment and asks the patient herself to set it up ("Call Judy"). He has neither allowed adequate time for discussion of the news today—after all, the patient can't suspend her feelings until next week—nor assessed the patient's emotional state to determine what needs to be done right now.

How could this situation have been handled better? First, the physician or his staff could have called to arrange a prompt appointment to discuss the test results. Second, as we discuss in the next section, he could have approached the topic in a direct and emotionally appropriate manner without minimizing the issue or hiding behind euphemisms.

Telling the News

It is usually good to preface your remarks with a clear statement like "I'm afraid I have bad news." The patient will already know by your behaviors (e.g., an intake of breath, an uncharacteristic hesitation) that something is wrong; in fact, your selection of a quiet place or invitation to a family member will broadcast that you are about to say something difficult. It is best to avoid the natural temptation to tiptoe up to the main point by beginning with small talk or side issues. You can better help the patient by spending the entire time explaining the situation, answering the patient's questions, and providing emotional support. There is also a risk that, if you begin slowly, you will end up by minimizing the problem, stopping at half-truths, or leaving important facts unexplained. Here is an example of a physician beginning to tell bad news in a clear, straightforward way[7]:

> Good morning, Mr. Lee. How are you feeling today?
>
> *Better than I did a week ago.*
>
> I'm glad of that. We have some very serious matters to discuss regarding your health. Do you feel ready for this discussion?
>
> *Well, I want to know.*
>
> It's hard to ever be ready for bad news. This is not easy. I need to let you know that we got the results of your test back.... As we had feared, the lump is a malignant tumor, cancer.

In this case the physician moves almost directly from "We have some very serious matters to discuss..." to "It's hard to ever be ready for bad news." Her one intervening question is, "Do you feel ready for this discussion?" An important aspect of this type of encounter is assessing the patient's emotional state, both directly by specific questions and indirectly through paralanguage and nonverbal cues (see Chap. 2). The clinician should acknowledge the difficulty of the situation and adjust the pace and form of the presentation based on an assessment of the patient's emotional needs. It is appropriate to express sorrow for the patient's pain. This may involve not only verbal expressions of concern, but also nonverbal evidence of solidarity, such as maintaining good eye contact, reaching out and touching the patient's hand or sleeve, or even shedding tears.

Continuing the Interview

As the interview progresses, it is important for the clinician to monitor both the patient's understanding of the information and his or her emotional response to the news. With regard to understanding, patients who have just received bad news are unlikely to remember complex information about diagnostic strategies or treatment options. Thus, it is usually best to stick to the major points, reiterate them, offer to answer questions, and arrange for your continued availability, including a prompt follow-up appointment. Often however, there are one or more specific tasks that need to be done relatively quickly, such as further diagnostic studies to delineate the extent of disease, or urgent radiation therapy in the case of threatened spinal cord compression. In such cases, it may be necessary to discuss technical issues at the same time that you are breaking the bad news. To help facilitate the patient's retention of information, follow the guidelines suggested in Chapter 16 (p. 272). Other useful suggestions to consider include:

- If the patient agrees, encourage at least one other family member to participate in the interview.

- Illustrate your major points with charts and drawings.
- Make an audiotape of the interview for the patient to keep and review at home.
- If available, lend the patient videotapes that describe the condition and relevant tests or treatments.

At all stages of the interview, you should check the patient's understanding and invite questions. At the end, summarize and recheck.

Patients' emotional responses may vary greatly. Some may be very calm and cool, focusing entirely on technical details. This reaction (or lack of reaction) is likely to relieve the anxious physician, who then might conclude that his or her patient is coping exceptionally well. However, extreme calmness suggests that the person either hasn't really understood the news, or hasn't emotionally "connected" with it. It might be useful for the physician to draw attention to this lack of response: "I notice you are taking this situation very calmly, but in my experience many people react differently."

Other patients might display anger and hostility. One of the authors cared for a middle-aged man who had, in a period of weeks, developed facial flushing, shortness of breath when lying down, and other symptoms of the superior vena cava syndrome. This indicated that a tumor was compromising the venous return from the upper part of his body. Because it took 2 weeks to accomplish the diagnostic studies and arrange a mediastinoscopy, which ultimately revealed that he had non-Hodgkin's lymphoma, the patient responded to the news with angry comments about what he perceived to be a delay in diagnosis. Why hadn't we acted more quickly? Why wasn't the hospital more efficient? In such cases it is always best to acknowledge the anger without minimizing it or trying to explain it away—for example, "I know this is devastating news. I understand your feelings and I do want to help." Some patients will combine anger with denial, challenging the diagnosis or demanding a second opinion. Again, the clinician should acknowledge the shocking nature of the news and support the patient in obtaining another opinion ("I think that's a good idea, do you have someone in mind?") if he or she so desires.

INTERVIEWING IN PALLIATIVE CARE

In many cases, bad news ushers in a period of intensive therapy that leads to remission or cure. For others, therapy to alter the course of the disease will be ineffective and treatment should be directed to symptom relief. The care of terminally ill patients presents continuing difficulties for clinicians. The barriers of avoidance, partial truth, emotional distance, and so forth tend to make it more and more difficult to face a patient as "medical" options available become fewer. In the interview it is important to communicate a plan for continued care, even when remission or cure is impossible. This plan should be specific to the patient's needs and renewed as appropriate at each contact; for example:

- "No matter what happens, I'll do my best to see this through with you.... I won't abandon you."
- "I want you to know I'll continue to be available. You can always call me if you have questions or problems.... I'll get back to you."
- "My goal is for you to be as comfortable and functional as possible. We have good medications to help us do that. You and I will work on this together."

The emotional barriers we encounter to telling bad news do not disappear when your patients have reached the terminal phase of illness. If anything, unless you make a conscious commitment to addressing your patients' emotional and spiritual needs, denial, detachment, and disappearance can become even stronger. During this phase, clinicians sometimes increase their sensitivity and supportiveness concerning the patient's physical problems, while totally avoiding the issue of emotional or existential suffering. Addressing the physical symptoms is extremely important, and it is a complex medical task that often requires specialized knowledge and skills. But pain and nausea are examples of only the somatic or physical component of the dying person's suffering.

Clinical Key 13–3 presents a number of questions that you might use to let the patient know you are interested in hearing about their existential concerns. Clinical Key 13–4 suggests some further questions to explore the more specifically spiritual concerns of the dying patient.

CLINICAL KEY 13–3

How to Initiate a Conversation about End-of-Life Care

- "What concerns you most about your illness?"
- "How is treatment going for you (and your family)?"
- "As you think about your illness, what is the best thing that might happen?"
- "What is the worst thing that might happen?"
- "What has been most difficult about this illness for you?"
- "What are your hopes (expectations, fears) for the future?"
- "As you think about the future, what is most important to you?"

Adapted from Lo B, Quill T, Tulsky J, 1999. Discussing palliative care with patients. *Ann Intern Med* 1999; 130:744–749, at p. 745, with permission.

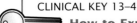

CLINICAL KEY 13–4

How to Explore Spiritual Issues in End-of-Life Care

To Open the Topic

- "Is faith or spirituality important to you during this illness?"
- "Has faith (spirituality, religion) been important to you at other times during your life?"
- "Do you have someone to talk to about religious (spiritual) matters?"
- "Would you like to explore religious matters with someone?"

To Initiate Further Discussion

- "What do you still want to accomplish during your life?"
- "What might be left undone if you were to die today?"
- "What is your understanding about what happens after you die?"
- "Given that your time is limited, what legacy do you want to leave your family?"
- "What do you want your children and grandchildren to remember about you?"

Adapted from Lo B, Quill T, Tulsky J, 1999. Discussing palliative care with patients. *Ann Intern Med* 1999; 130:744–749, at p. 746, with permission.

ADVANCE DIRECTIVES

An advance directive is a written statement ("living will") or an explicit arrangement with another person (health care proxy or durable power of attorney) that permits a patient's wishes regarding treatment to be honored, even when the patient loses his or her decision-making capacity. The Patient Self-Determination Act is a Federal law requiring that hospitals and certain other health care facilities inform patients about advance directives. The idea is to give patients the opportunity to formulate their own treatment goals and to express them, or to appoint a surrogate decision maker prior to the possibility of losing their decision-making capacity during that hospitalization or a subsequent one. A seriously ill patient just admitted to the hospital is generally not physically or psychologically prepared for a thorough discussion about health care choices near the end of life, however. Likewise, physicians and other health professionals dealing with a patient's acute, overwhelming illness are not likely to set a high priority on explaining advance directives and their meaning. **Thus, the best time to interview patients regarding advance directives is during their ongoing outpatient care, particularly in the primary care setting.**

With whom should you raise the topic of advance directives? First, it is useful to include a question about whether or not a patient has a "living will" or has designated a health care proxy in every initial medical history on a new adult patient. If you use a structured questionnaire as a method of obtaining some initial data, these questions may be included on the questionnaire. The patient profile should include information about the person's health beliefs and values, and the existence and character of an advance directive fits appropriately in that segment of the medical history. Advance directives should be explored further with patients who have serious chronic or progressive illnesses.

Telling bad news is not an event that occurs at one point in time; it is a process that may extend over several visits and several conversations. An important component of this process is a thorough discussion of the patients' beliefs and values about life-sustaining treatments under various circumstances. The patient should receive information about written advance directives and health care proxies, with particular emphasis on the appropriate legal mechanism in your state. Written information and the required legal forms should also be available in the clinician's office.

When initiating a discussion of advance directives, you should set the stage by clearly stating the issue, rather than making any assumptions about the patient's knowledge or asking pointed questions about treatment. Consider these three examples of clinicians asking patients about end-of-life decisions:

- "Now we need to talk about Living Wills. You ought to consider signing a Living Will because if you become incompetent later in this illness, we need to know what you would want us to do, let's say, if we had to put you on a breathing machine."
- "As I said, there is nothing more we can do to stop the disease from progressing, so we are going to be faced with some tough questions sooner or later. For example, if your heart stops, would you like us to do what we can to try to start it up again?"
- "Now we need to talk about what kinds of treatment decisions you would like somebody to make for you if you are no longer able to make your own decisions. What I'm thinking about is something we call a Living Will or a Health Care Proxy. You've probably heard about Living Wills. They are written statements that tell us what you would like us to do or not to do, let's say, if your illness reaches the point where we have to put you on a breathing machine and there is no hope that you will recover. A health proxy is just a person whom you designate now to speak for you and to make all your medical decisions for you if you become so ill you can't make your own choices. Lots of people have both Living Wills and Health Care Proxies. Would you like to discuss more about this now?"

In the first case, the clinician assumed that the patient would know what a "Living Will" and "incompetent" mean, and failed to explain the terms or put them in perspective. The second clinician jumped immediately to a very specific question about cardiac pulmonary resuscitation, after beginning on a very negative note: "there is nothing more we can do...." The third clinician, however, was careful not only to set the stage for discussing the issue, but also to allow the patient to decide whether the discussion should continue at that point. She was explicit about the meaning of Living Wills and Health Care Proxies and indicated they were not incompatible. Also, she did not frame her reference to "breathing machine" as a leading question. The exchange might continue in this way:

> *I don't know, doctor, I've heard about Living Wills, but I'm not sure I know enough about them.*
>
> Well, I can give you a brochure that I think will answer a lot of your questions about Living Wills, and also it tells how to designate someone you trust to make decisions for you. I can also give you the form for designating a proxy, so you can see what it looks like.
>
> *OK, but ... I don't know, talking about this makes me feel like it's all over, you know, like there's no hope.*
>
> I can understand why you would feel that, but it really means nothing of the sort. There's a lot we can do for you and a lot you can do for yourself.... And you and I will work together on this. I'll respect your decisions every step of the way. That's really why I bring the issue up now ... to make sure that we can continue respecting your choices and values if something happens and you can't tell us at the time. I guess you could call it a type of preventive medicine.

A major point in this dialogue is the physician's attempt to diffuse the patient's understandable anxiety when confronted with the issue of advance directives. In this case, she makes sure that the patient understands that he is not "signing over" his participation in decision making, but is rather extending his participation beyond the point it would normally end. Unlike the clinician in the second example, she is also alleviating the patient's feeling that "Living Will equals nothing-more-we-can-do."

CULTURAL CONSIDERATIONS

In Chapter 10 we explored the topic of cultural sensitivity in the interview and suggested some concrete approaches. In this section we deal briefly with cultural differences in the way people handle (or hear) bad news about their own health, or the health of loved ones. The first and most important point to make, though, is the need to avoid cultural stereotypes. Each patient is a unique person with his or her own history and life trajectory. Never assume that a Hispanic patient will behave according to some generalized Hispanic pattern, or an African–American patient will necessarily approach health care decision making by expressing a "traditional" African–American attitude. The key is to know your patient as a person who has his or her own, unique life narrative.

Cultural sensitivity will assist you, however. First, it should help you minimize your own cultural blind spot. Remember that most of what we have said thus far about talking with the dying patient is, in fact, heavily grounded in our own cultural values of self-determination, independence, and privacy. When we employ practices like truthfulness, informed consent, and confidentiality, we demonstrate our respect for a person by acknowledging his or her autonomy. In other cultures, autonomy may be balanced by or even secondary to more communal values when it comes to sensitive topics like death and dying. For example, the dying patient's family may be expected to play a prominent decision-making role, and will shoulder major responsibility for providing nurture and hope. Second, remember that individual patients will almost always try to handle their serious illnesses in ways that seem best to them. Their approaches or strategies will reflect cultural values *in some way,* but you cannot predict *precisely what values,* or even precisely what culture, without listening carefully to your patient.

Telling Bad News Is Sometimes Bad News

One of us was taking care of a 56-year-old Chinese woman with ovarian cancer. A few weeks earlier she had been working at her usual job as a hospital nurse and was feeling "perfectly normal." Suddenly, she developed abdominal pain and swelling. After the diagnosis was made, we sat down to tell her the bad news, only to find that the patient, whom we assumed was quite acculturated after living and working in the United States for many years, was uncomfortable and inarticulate. She avoided eye contact. She asked no questions. Her only comment was that, in fact, she thought her symptoms were caused by benign fibroid tumors. It was evident that our attempting to share the name of her diagnosis—even tentatively—caused extreme anxiety. The conversation went on:

> I can see that you don't feel like talking right now. You're tired. I know you had trouble sleeping last night.
>
> *It's okay, though, doc. I think I'll sleep, just as long as I get that Restoril along with the morphine.*
>
> Yea, I'll make sure of that. Uh, is there anyone else I should talk to?
>
> *[Pause] Ling. You should talk to Ling first—I think she's coming in later after work. She'll know what to do.*
>
> Well, I could have them page me. Uh, shall I try to come here and talk with her in your room?
>
> *No, it's okay. I'm tired.*

This patient was a medically sophisticated nurse. Notice that she uses the correct names of her medications. Notice also that she is no shrinking violet. She indicates exactly what she wants—for Ling to handle the medical information: "She'll know what to do." In fact, Ling was an older sibling who was far less educated and more traditional than the patient was. She had emigrated from China with their mother only 2 or 3 years earlier. Ling subsequently assumed a maternal role, arranging for our patient's medical care and handling her affairs. She indicated that the patient should not be told the prognosis because it would result in her losing hope and "dwelling on negative things."

Traditional Navajo people believe that talking about death or dying will lead to grave harm. Such behavior may hasten a person's death either by attracting malevolent spirits or by making the person more vulnerable to spirits already causing the illness. Either way, saying the words will make it so. Navajos also avoid talking about the dead or visiting places where someone has recently died. For Navajo culture, the question is not so much "To whom do you reveal the bad news?" but "In what way might you speak about end-of-life issues at all?" This cultural feature is particularly difficult when it comes to the question of withholding or withdrawing life-sustaining therapy. To provide culturally appropriate care, some clinicians have found it effective to initiate discussion about end-of-life decisions by couching the whole scenario as a story or a hypothetical event affecting other people:

> I've heard it said that some people, when it comes to using a machine to breathe for them—this is if they ever get so sick that they can't breathe on their own—what I've heard is that these people won't agree to be hooked up to the breathing machine. What do you think about that?

To many Americans this type of statement would be beating around the bush. To a Navajo family it may serve as a point of entry into a complex discussion, much of which the clinician would consider tangential if she understood the language. In this culture, however, both group consensus and avoidance of direct speech about death are important values.

SUMMARY ▪ COMMUNICATING BAD NEWS

We began this chapter by exploring five barriers to communicating bad news to patients (see Clinical Key 13–1). Clinicians tend to deny to themselves that the situation is as bad as it is and, therefore, delay telling the news. They often use vague or complicated language. They believe that patients will lose hope once they know the truth about their prognosis. Clinicians also become emotionally distant and disappear. To provide good care for terminally ill patients, these barriers must be overcome.

Before telling bad news, the clinician should set the stage by providing a comfortable environment and allowing sufficient time (see Clinical Key 13–2). It is usually best to begin with a preparatory but direct statement like "I'm afraid I have bad news to tell you." Verbal and nonverbal expressions of sorrow and support are appropriate. As the interview progresses, the clinician should monitor the patient's understanding and emotional response, realizing that it is difficult for persons to take in and process so much significant information at one time. Good continuing care for the critically ill and dying patient demands that the clinician be both emotionally and physically accessible. At the same time, he or she should recognize that the suffering of dying patients is multidimensional. Appropriate palliative care involves giving patients the opportunity to talk about emotional, existential, or spiritual suffering (see Clinical Keys 13–3 and 13–4), as well as about their physical functioning.

Advance directives help ensure that patients' wishes are respected even if they lose decision-making capacity. A question about a living will or health care proxy should be part of every initial medical interview. The topic of advance directives should be explored further with patients who suffer from serious chronic, progressive, or terminal illness. The subject requires a direct and clear explanation, followed by willingness to answer questions and provide emotional support.

Finally, dying and death are sensitive topics. Telling bad news must always be considered in its cultural context. Because respect for autonomy is paramount in contemporary Western culture, our "default" position emphasizes forthrightness and truthfulness. However, it is important to recognize that in our multicultural society patients and families will bring other values to the table, requiring us to individualize our approach. Cultural sensitivity *does not* mean that we should create stereotypes of cultural practices; it *does* mean that we should pay careful attention to the needs and desires of our individual patients.

References

1. Campbell ML. Breaking bad news to patients. *JAMA* 1994; 271:1052.
2. Tolstoy L. *The Death of Ivan Ilych*. New York, Bantam Books, 1981.
3. McCrum R. *My old and new lives. The New Yorker*, March 1996.
4. Nuland SB. *How We Die*. New York, Alfred A. Knopf, 1994.
5. Broyard A. *Intoxicated by My Illness*. New York, Clarkson Potter Publishers, 1992.
6. Lind SE, Good M, Seidel S, Csordas T, Good BJ. Telling the diagnosis of cancer. *J Clin Oncol* 1989; 7:583–589.
7. Miranda J, Brody RV. Communicating bad news. *West J Med* 1992; 156:83–85.

Suggested Reading

Block MR. The bad news. *JAMA* 1987; 257:2952.
Lo B, Quill T, Tulsky J. Discussing palliative care with patients. *Ann Intern Med* 1999; 130:744–749.
Poulson J. Bitter pills to swallow. *N Engl J Med* 1998; 338:1844–1846.
Ptacek JT, Eberhardt TL. Breaking bad news. A review of the literature. *JAMA* 1996; 276:496–502.
Tulsky JA, Fischer GS, Rose MR, Arnold RM. Opening the black box: How do physicians communicate about advance directives? *Ann Intern Med* 1998; 129:441–449.

CHAPTER 14

A Great Many Remedies

●　●　●　●　●

TALKING WITH PATIENTS ABOUT COMPLEMENTARY AND ALTERNATIVE MEDICINE

*If **a great many remedies** are suggested for some disease, it means the disease is incurable.*

Anton Chekhov, *The Cherry Orchard*

Complementary and alternative medicine (CAM) is among the most rapidly expanding areas of clinical practice. It is likely that a large percentage of your patients will have tried some form of unconventional therapy for their health problems, and many will be using CAM concurrently with orthodox clinical treatment. Yet these patients may be reluctant to tell you about their experiences. In this chapter we discuss the context and importance of talking with patients about their use of complementary medicine. The first section presents a brief background, rationale, and lexicon. Next, we consider some guidelines for talking about the "alternatives." The final section suggests an approach to taking the next step, negotiating a care plan. Negotiation is covered in more detail in Chapter 16.

CONSIDER THE CONTEXT

At the beginning of the 20th century, scientific (or allopathic) medicine had many competitors for patients' allegiance. Osteopathy, chiropractic, homeopathy, and naturopathy were all popular, and immigrants, pouring into the country from all over the world, brought their own folk or traditional forms of healing. Allopathic medicine was already considered the orthodox standard for health care, but its benefits in comparison with many of these other forms of treatment were unclear. Scientific understanding of physiology and pathology had progressed rapidly in the late 19th century, but therapeutics was still in its infancy. Great clinicians like Sir William Osler were known for their abilities to make accurate diagnoses and prognoses, but they could do little to cure disease. However, the remarkable scientific and technologic developments of the last century markedly changed that picture. Although cure of chronic degenerative disease remains elusive, there is no question that contemporary medical and surgical interventions can prevent, cure, or favorably alter the course of much human illness.

Thus, many clinicians today are surprised that CAM is among the most rapidly growing sectors in health care. Orthodox clinicians have tended to believe that only people with poor access to standard health care or with certain religious or cultural beliefs sought out "unorthodox" forms of treatment for their health problems. These practitioners thought that the success of scientific medicine would cause alternative systems to wither away. In fact, in the middle of the 20th century there was evidence that this disappearance was occurring. Mainstream medicine progressively marginalized alternative forms of health care, use of these systems stabilized or declined, and the popular stereotype of "quack" therapy developed. As we enter the third millennium, however, the picture has once again dramatically changed.

In the early 1990s, Eisenberg and his colleagues[1] conducted a telephone survey of a large sample of adults in the United States. They found that 34% had used at least one form of unconventional therapy in the preceding year. This treatment was usually for chronic, non–life-threatening conditions. Interestingly, 83% of those who used alternative therapy for a serious medical condition also employed standard treatment from a medical doctor, and nearly three-quarters of these persons had not informed that doctor about the unconventional therapy. In a more recent national sample, Astin[2] found that 40% of respondents had used unconventional therapies in the preceding year. Likewise, investigators surveying patients in large family practices in the northwestern United States found that half of the patients had used alternative treatment, but only half of these patients had told their family practitioner.[3] These and other recent studies highlight two important points:

- Perhaps a majority of your patients will have at least tried some form of unconventional treatment for their illness.
- Most of these patients will not spontaneously tell you about their experience with alternative medicine.

DEFINITION, PLEASE

The terminology for characterizing this field is difficult and confusing. Originally, the most frequently used term was "alternative medicine." Patients use many of the therapies to *complement* rather than to *replace* standard medical care, however, so the term "complementary" was subsequently introduced. Nowadays, these two descriptors are often employed together in the combined term, "complementary and alternative medicine" (CAM), which is the name that the National Institutes of Health adopted for its division that supports research in these fields. The terms "integrative medicine" or "integrative health care" are also sometimes used to capture the idea that many of these therapies favor the combined use of a number of different approaches to address a given health problem.

It is also difficult to determine what criteria differentiate standard or mainstream therapies from CAM. You may think the issue is fairly uncomplicated. "Well," you might say, "mainstream medical treatments are those accepted by allopathic doctors, proven by state-of-the-art clinical trials, and supported by scientific rationale, whereas unconventional medicine is rejected, unproven, and unscientific." However, widespread *acceptance* is not a reliable criterion. Who would have thought 20 years ago that peptic ulcer disease (an accepted psychosomatic condition) was actually caused by a bacterial infection? Likewise, the requirement that treatment be *proven* by clinical trials is an unrealistic standard. Although clinical trial methodology has been around for 50 years, the content of much of contemporary practice has not been tested. In the last 10 or 15 years, there has been an explosion of interest in evidence-based medicine (EBM). This salutary movement has taught health care professionals ways of evaluating the strength of evidence supporting the treatments they prescribe. EBM has also demonstrated in many cases how little rigorous evidence of efficacy there is for many commonly used therapies.

Perhaps *scientific rationale* is a better criterion than the others are, but it also leaves loopholes. Sometimes treatments that work do so for reasons different than we think. For example, chiropractic adjustment might be effective in relieving back or neck pain even if the putative rationale for its effectiveness (spinal subluxation) is incorrect. Likewise, Western scientists who reject the physiological theory underlying acupuncture often accept this ancient therapy as useful. Moreover, it is likely that some herbal preparations contain active pharmacological agents that in the future will become the basis for "standard" medications. This situation has happened in the past and will happen again. Digitalis is an example that comes quickly to mind.

In sum, there is no bright dividing line between standard medicine and CAM. Rather, the line tends to be fuzzy and the practices overlap. For example, acupuncture is now an accepted treatment in many pain clinics. Likewise, whether vitamin treatment is an example of CAM or standard practice depends largely on who prescribes it and what he or she claims it will accomplish. The same can be said for various nutritional plans, exercise programs,

TABLE 14-1

SELECTED FORMS OF CAM AND RELATIVE FREQUENCY OF USE	
Frequency	**Form of Therapy**
Higher prevalence	Relaxation techniques
	Chiropractic
	Massage
Medium prevalence	Spiritual healing
	Herbal medicine
	Imagery
	Lifestyle diets
Lower prevalence	Energy healing
	Homeopathy
	Acupuncture
	Hypnosis
	Megavitamin therapy

Adapted in part from Astin JA. Why patients use alternative medicine. Results of a national study. *JAMA* 1998; 279:1548–1553; and Eisenberg DM, Kessler RC, Foster C, Norlock FE, Calkins DR, Delbanco TL. Unconventional medicine in the United States. Prevalence, costs, and patterns of use. *N Engl J Med* 1993; 328:246–252.

and relaxation techniques. Table 14-1 presents the relative frequencies of some of the types of CAM identified in two national surveys in the 1990s. For our purposes, however, there is no need to use a strict definition of CAM. We are interested simply in the patient's behavior and beliefs regarding therapy, *any therapy,* whether it is considered alternative or mainstream, and how to talk with patients about their concerns and beliefs.

WHO USES CAM?

Why do people choose CAM? Many health care professionals used to believe, and some still believe, that poor education, lower socioeconomic level, and failure to understand the benefits of scientific medicine correlate with use of CAM. This is certainly not the case; in fact, the converse is largely true. Go to any library or bookstore and you will find shelf after shelf of books on herbal medicine, reflexology, spiritual healing, and holistic medicine. Table 14-2 summarizes characteristics of the patient and the situation that correlate with greater use of CAM. Several commonly held beliefs are evident—a fear of invasive medicine, a desire to make one's own decisions, and a general appreciation for "wholeness" or holistic health care. Likewise, patients with chronic and recurrent problems may seek additional help from CAM. In a recent study of arthritis patients seeing rheumatologists, investigators found that two-thirds had used CAM and most continued to do so.[4]

TABLE 14–2

FACTORS ASSOCIATED WITH PATIENT USE OF COMPLEMENTARY AND ALTERNATIVE MEDICINE
Characteristics of the Patient
• Higher socioeconomic group
• Desire to avoid toxicity or invasiveness of conventional therapy
• Preference for high personal involvement in decision making
• Dissatisfaction with attitudes and practitioners of conventional medicine
• A particular healing system as a part of a patient's cultural heritage
• Belief in the importance of a holistic health philosophy
• A transformational experience that changes one's view of life and illness
Characteristics of the Condition or Situation
• Failure of conventional therapy
• Failure of diagnosis
• Serious or chronic illness with poor prognosis
• Acute or chronic conditions for which conventional treatment is lacking or ineffective
• Certain specific medical problems: anxiety, back pain, chronic pain, urinary tract problems.

Dissatisfaction with conventional medicine might occur because of incorrect diagnosis or ineffective conventional treatment or it may arise from process or interactive issues—clinicians don't have the time to listen, they convey negative attitudes, they don't give adequate explanations, they don't "connect" with the patient. Patients may have such experiences with several different clinicians before they simply give up conventional medicine. Dissatisfaction breeds dissatisfaction. Among the subgroup of persons who rely primarily on CAM rather than standard medicine, a large percentage express distrust of and serious dissatisfaction with conventional physicians.[2]

For the most part, the rising popularity of CAM is not based on deeply held beliefs. On the contrary, today's alternative medicine movement has a pragmatic flavor. Although clinicians find it surprising, patients are usually the best judges of what works for them. People seek out acupuncture, chiropractic, homeopathy, megavitamins, and other forms of complementary therapies simply because they are looking for something that works. A given person might try homeopathy one month and megavitamins the next, even though the belief systems underlying these therapies are totally different and perhaps incompatible.

Some patients do seek care based on deep cultural or religious beliefs, but we've found it risky to jump to conclusions based on a person's religion or ethnic group. For example, one of us once encouraged an elderly Chinese woman to consider traditional Chinese approaches for treating her illness. She had diabetes and heart failure, complicated by an episode of major depression. Another internist had prescribed Prozac with no success—she said the drug gave her the "jitters." She also explained that psychiatrists were "for the birds." Her symptoms included insomnia, poor concentration, malaise, and terrible self-esteem. She identified herself as a housewife who had not worked outside the home for many years, having relied on her (now absent) college-professor husband to support the family. She felt that her husband had left her because she was "worthless" and didn't "know how to do anything." Several features—her age, her traditional lifestyle (not working outside the home), and her negative attitude toward psychiatry—suggested that traditional Chinese medicine might be just the "right cup of tea" for her.

However, she was offended by a referral to a Chinese Holistic Health Center near her home. She proceeded to give a stern lecture about her awareness that Western medicine was better. "You can't get rid of me that easy," she said, "I need your help." This response could have been avoided if we had explored her beliefs and expectations regarding her illness before jumping to a plausible, but unwarranted, conclusion. In fact, traditional Chinese medicine might have benefited this bereaved (over the loss of her husband) woman—but it couldn't help her unless she believed that it was worth trying.

LEARNING ABOUT CAM IN THE CLINICAL INTERVIEW

How do you find out where your patient stands on CAM? Clinical Key 14–1 presents some guidelines for inquiring about your patient's use of alternative health care.

Introduce the Topic

The first step is to introduce the topic of CAM as part of your standard medical interview, whether in the context of health maintenance and preventive medicine, or when evaluating a patient with a specific problem. After the

---

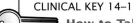

CLINICAL KEY 14–1

How to Talk to Patients about Complementary and Alternative Medicine

- Ask as part of your standard medical interview, "What else are you doing to take care of your health?"
- Give permission for patients to raise the topic.
- Listen for "nondisclosing" clues.
- Check with patients regularly regarding their explanatory models.
- Seek more information from patients and other sources.
- Become familiar with local patterns of use.
- Be frank about what you do not know.

patient tells you about any medical treatment he or she has had, you might ask, "And what else are you doing to take care of your health?" or "What have you tried so far?" These are rather nonspecific queries, and patients will often use the opportunity to tell you about their dietary or exercise programs. In some cases these programs will be related to alternative therapies; in many cases, they won't be. (Exercise and diet history and use of over-the-counter medications are, of course, important in themselves.)

Give Permission to Talk

Your acceptance of these particular "what elses," as indicated by your active listening and facilitative responding (p. 13, pp. 25–29), may encourage the patient to tell you more. Useful follow-up questions are "What about other types of practitioners or other types of health care?" or "Have you seen anyone else about this problem?" This approach gives patients permission to talk about their alternative therapies if they wish to do so. In some cases they will not, perhaps because they are embarrassed or because they are uncertain about your reaction.

Nondisclosing Clues

A nondisclosing clue is a verbal or nonverbal indication that the patient has something to say that he or she is *not* telling you. Listen carefully for nondisclosing clues, which may appear in almost any part of your interview.

Here is an excerpt from an initial interview between a general internist and a young woman with a 9-month history of fatigue, poor concentration, and repeated respiratory infections. For most of that time, she had been able to maintain her busy schedule as a corporate attorney, but in recent weeks the condition "laid me low" and forced her to severely limit her workload. She has already described the narrative of her illness, including the fact that she has sought help from two doctors: an endocrinologist, who "put me through a lot of blood tests and told me there is nothing wrong," and an Urgent Care doctor, who "keeps giving me antibiotics."

> And what else have you been doing for your health?
>
> *I can tell you I've read every book I can get my hands on about it.*
>
> You mean about your health problem?
>
> *Yeah, chronic fatigue ... or there's other names for it, too. Most of them say it's a problem with the immune system.*
>
> So you've been told that you have chronic fatigue syndrome.
>
> *No, actually, the doctors told me that I was depressed, or one of them did, Dr. X. He tried to give me Prozac, which was ridiculous. Dr. Y at the Urgent Care, she doesn't say anything, just that I should slow down.*
>
> Gee, not having any answers must drive you up the wall. Feeling so terrible all the time and just not knowing.

> *There has to be something. I'm not imagining this.*
>
> And what about other practitioners? I mean, other types of health care?
>
> *Well, I went to this chronic fatigue specialist, I think he started out as a chiropractor and nutritionist, but now he specializes in chronic fatigue. And he put me on this regimen to build up my immune system, you know, vitamins, and some other stuff, herbs, like St. John's Wort. It's pretty complicated.*
>
> And how's it going?
>
> *Uh, it's only been a month or so, but I think there's improvement, I mean it's hard to tell.*

Note how the patient initially responds by telling the doctor how many books she has read about her condition. No doubt she has also scoured the Internet for additional information. What is her conclusion? "Most of them say it's a problem with the immune system." It seems unlikely that a patient with her education and personality would have been satisfied to remain for 9 months solely with two doctors who are neither helping to relieve her symptoms nor providing her with a good explanation of her problem. These features—her job, her personality, and the fact that she read so much—are *nondisclosing clues* that she might well have sought alternative treatment. The clinician continues with an empathic response tailored to the patient's need to get to the bottom of things, "Gee, not having any answers must drive you up the wall." Perhaps this additive response (see p. 28) helps her develop sufficient trust to bring up the chronic fatigue specialist that she is currently seeing. The clinician evidently accepts the additional data, although the tone and nonverbal features of his response ("And how's it going?") could make a big difference in how the interview proceeds.

At this point the internist is left with more questions than answers. Why is the patient seeking his help? At first she said her symptoms had worsened in the last month, but now she says, "I think there's improvement" from her new regimen of vitamins and herbs. The internist can now pursue several paths. He could gently confront his patient with this discrepancy and ask for clarification, "I'm a bit confused here. You said earlier that things are steadily getting worse, but now it sounds as if the vitamins might actually be helping...." Another possibility would be to avoid an explicit confrontation, but, after completing the history, go back to the basics of who, what, when, where, and why. "What leads you to come to me now? What would you like me to do for you?"

The Patient's Explanatory Model

Before pursuing the issue either way, it would be useful to learn a bit more about this patient's *explanatory model*. She has already explained that her previous doctor thought she was depressed and that "most of them" (authors of books about chronic fatigue) think it is an immunological problem. But she has not spelled out her own belief. This may be difficult to pin down for two reasons: she may not yet be willing to trust this new clinician with her private thoughts on the matter, or those thoughts may not be entirely clear or consistent, even to the patient herself.

Let's consider another example. A middle-aged man with hypertension comes to see a new doctor for an initial evaluation and checkup. He explains that in the past he had taken a prescription for his blood pressure, but it had run out and he had not refilled it:

> *I don't believe in eating chemicals.*
>
> You mean you don't like to take medicines? Not even for your high blood pressure?
>
> *Well ... I used to take a lot of different things, but they never seemed to help. My doctor kept changing them, you know, adding new ones. The pressure never budged, and then I found out it was only high when he checked it, or his girl checked it. So I said, why do I need all this aggravation?*
>
> So you don't take any medications now?
>
> *Naw. No chemicals.*
>
> So not even aspirin or something for headache?
>
> *Naw. I don't get headaches since I started this stuff called feverfew, it's an herb.*
>
> Feverfew? Isn't that....
>
> *It's natural, perfectly organic.*
>
> Do you take any other organic pills or herbs?
>
> *Yea, my wife gets a lot of stuff from the health food store. We go to Vitamin Central.*
>
> Do you know what all of it is?
>
> *Yeah, well, there's vitamin E and zinc and.... I'm telling you, doc, the stuff is all natural.*

In this case the patient obviously believes that "natural" or "organic" substances are not "chemicals." Chemicals can hurt him, but natural substances like vitamins and herbs will not hurt him. This belief probably played a role in his decision to discontinue his antihypertensive medication. It may have also been responsible, at least in part, for his dismal medical experience—"a lot of different things" that "never seemed to help." Finally, it highlights the question of why the patient is now seeking a new doctor. Sure enough, the man had selected this particular doctor from a panel of available internists because the insurance company's book indicated that the doctor was board certified in preventive medicine, as well as internal medicine. The patient indicated that to him preventive medicine signified vitamins, herbs, and other forms of "natural" therapy, pointing out that many chiropractors and other practitioners who focus on such therapy advertise themselves as specialists in preventive medicine.

What are the clinician's options at this point? Note how he observes basic skills of interviewing by demonstrating respect for the patient's approach, despite his concern about the patient's high blood pressure. It appears that to gain this patient's trust, the clinician must either avoid prescribing antihypertensive medications or teach the patient that in some cases "chemicals" are beneficial. Such teaching will require a better understanding of why he thinks drugs are unnatural and harmful in the first place. Simply telling him the facts (e.g., "herbs contain chemicals, too, you know") is unlikely to help. It will be more useful to explore the basis of his belief (see Chap. 10) and then to negotiate a mutually acceptable plan (see Chap. 16).

Seek More Information From Patients and Other Sources

The hypertensive patient we just met takes feverfew for his headaches, along with unspecified doses of vitamin E and zinc. The previous patient with chronic fatigue is evidently on a complex regimen of vitamins and herbs, including St. John's Wort. What do you know about these herbs? What are they supposed to do? What are their potential side effects? Likewise, is there anything you should ask about the chiropractor–nutritionist–chronic fatigue specialist? Should you obtain more detail about the specific course of treatment he or she has prescribed? Does it include spinal adjustment? Or colonic cleansing? Or visualization? You should seek more information from two sources:

- **From the patient.** Learn the specific form of alternative treatment, its frequency and characteristics, and what the objective is. Learn what the patient believes is the mechanism of action. If there are vitamins, minerals, or herbs involved, learn the approximate dosages.
- **From other sources.** Try to find out the potential risks and benefits of your patient's CAM therapy.

Find Out About Local Patterns of Use

The relative frequencies of CAM use shown in Table 14-1 are based on data from two large national surveys. CAM availability and use in your community, or among patients in your practice, will vary depending on demographics, illness characteristics, media attention, and location.

It's Okay To Say You Don't Know

If patients trust you with information about their CAM use, they might ask what you think about it. Do you approve or not? Or patients might bring in magazine articles, Internet printouts, or brochures about the "latest fantastic cure for insomnia" or "We guarantee a 20 lb. weight loss in 20 days, or your money back." If your patient has cancer and is considering forgoing indicated primary chemotherapy in favor of macrobiotics, your reply may be "This form of treatment doesn't seem logical or make physiological sense." But often the relative risks and benefits will be less obvious. It is reasonable to tell the patient that you do not know. In this context you should:

- Indicate the rationale for medical treatment.
- Indicate the specific expected benefits and risks of medical treatment.
- Help the patient to formulate his or her questions about the type of CAM therapy being considered.
- Encourage the patient to request satisfactory answers to these questions from the CAM practitioner.
- Make it clear that you are willing to see the patient again and to continue to discuss the matter.
- Agree to disagree, while maintaining respect and open communication.

WORKING WITH THE ALTERNATIVES

Once the clinician is aware that his or her patient is using CAM, there are three important questions to consider:

- Are the alternative therapies dangerous?
- Do they prohibit medical care that is necessary?
- Can I work within the patient's belief system to provide good medical care?

Consider the following example. At a subsequent visit to your office, the patient with chronic fatigue brings copies of lab work performed by her holistic practitioner. She shows you a hair analysis in which the magnesium level is low and a test for reactivity to candida (a type of yeast commonly found in the environment) is positive. She goes on:

> *He said that the magnesium was because of my diet and he recommended some changes there, but he wanted you to prescribe an antibiotic for the candida allergy. He said the first thing to do is to clear it up, and it might take a long time. Sometimes people have to take antibiotics for months.*

But you don't actually have an infection.

> *He said there's no obvious infection, yes, but I'm extra-sensitive to it … like I react to the spores in the air, which activates my immune system all the time.*

The CAM practitioner has given this patient an explanation of what she needs—unfortunately, from you. "Isn't this a good example of interprofessional cooperation?" you might ask. The chronic fatigue specialist is treating her "holistically" for an overactive immune system and you have to do your part by prescribing an antibiotic to suppress the offending agent (candida). The problem, however, is that you do not believe there is a scientific basis for the concept of candida allergy as a cause of chronic fatigue, and you wish to avoid using a potentially harmful antifungal agent. Although you also want to avoid criticizing a CAM practice, the CAM practitioner has put you on the spot by using a medical test inappropriately and suggesting a course of medical treatment. How can you decline while remaining empathic and respectful of the patient? Our clinician might respond:

> I think I understand what your chronic fatigue doctor explained to you, and I know it sounds reasonable. But the thing is, I don't think you actually have a yeast infection. Infection means that the germs get into your tissues and your body tries to fight them off. You see, these yeasts are everywhere, on the skin and so forth, and everybody has a certain amount of sensitivity to them. So lots of people have positive tests whether or not they have chronic fatigue. But that's not what's causing your illness. And, unfortunately, the antibiotics for candida have a lot more side effects than the antibiotics we use every day for sinus infections or strep throats....

He might go on to explain the side effects and other risks of antifungal agents. There are two crucial factors in this interchange. The first is the clinician's tone and manner, his nonverbal and paralanguage communication, and the words he says. He wants to maintain trust and support the patient, while at the same time explaining why he disagrees. Unfortunately, he has no "magic bullet" alternative to prescribe, so it is especially important that he convey his ongoing concern for her. Second, he must give her the opportunity to ask questions and to discuss the point until she understands his explanation.

In most cases you will not actually be asked to participate in the CAM therapy. Instead, you will have to judge whether the CAM therapy is consistent with the treatment you propose, and if not, what you should do if you believe it poses risks to your patient. Here is an example of an elderly woman, blind from glaucoma, who was undergoing chelation therapy, as well as taking standard medical treatment for cerebrovascular and heart disease. Chelation involves intravenous administration of ethylenediaminetetraacetic acid (EDTA), an agent that binds calcium and other cations in the blood, thus removing them from the body when EDTA is excreted in the urine. Chelation is effective in treating lead poisoning, for example, by removing certain heavy metals from the body, but there is no credible evidence that it removes calcium from plaques in the arteries. Moreover, it requires repeated intravenous treatments that may be dangerous and are definitely expensive. Chelation for atherosclerosis is considered unacceptable medical therapy. In this example, the patient has already explained to her new physician that she has been suffering for several months from "creeping numbness" in both legs. Her previous physician conveyed the impression that this symptom was not serious. The new physician has helped the patient become comfortable enough to explain her interpretation of the problem and what should be done about it:

> You had this creeping numbness, and they didn't seem to know what to do about it?
>
> *Well, no, and then after the stroke, my back actually.... I told you about what the doctor said. He said it wasn't important, that it had already happened.*
>
> That your back had already collapsed?
>
> *Well I didn't understand, I thought that it meant my backbones would fall down. I was talking to Dr. Smith about it, but he wouldn't do a thing. I mean, it didn't seem to bother him at all. And then my bitter fear for my legs. Then, it actually came to the point where my legs were just like a couple of logs. I would try to sleep at night and turn over and I would drag my legs.*
>
> Is that what made you afraid?
>
> *I was afraid. Well, I explained to Dr. Smith. 'Look, Dr. Smith, there are people that lose the use of their legs and they go and use a wheelchair, but you got to have eyes to guide the wheelchair and I don't have that, so what am I going to do?' But it was like talking to the wall. Once he got very angry. 'Do you think that if there would be something that would help you, I wouldn't do it for you?' Well, as if it was a sin for me to be concerned about myself. So anyway, well, the situation was really awful, I was really fretting my mind all the time. I just lost the use of my eyes, next I lost the use of my legs, then what to do?*

The patient had osteoporosis and vertebral compression fractures. Evidently she had tried first to attribute her leg numbness to the "collapsed" back, but her physician vetoed that explanation and never provided an alternative. Moreover, he seemed to ignore both her symptom and her growing anxiety about it.

> So what did you think, though? I mean, where did the numbness come from?
>
> *Well, then I decided to go to Dr. Brown and he said 'I'll chelate you and you'll have no more strokes.' So that's when I made up my mind to go to the chelation and I did, and it's better.*
>
> Do you mean Dr. Brown said the numbness was related to the stroke?
>
> *Well, that's the only thing that made sense. Blockage of the arteries. That's what I thought. So chelation must help.*
>
> You were afraid to tell me about this, too, weren't you?
>
> *Well, you should have seen Dr. Smith. He got mad. I felt so sick that time, he got so mad ... actually I don't know what was the matter with him. Like he was ready to get a nervous breakdown or something. [Long pause] The thing is, it's so cruel. It's so cruel. Maybe the chelation does do some good, and if it does then why deprive a patient, just because of politics, that's not right. You come to Dr. Brown's office and it's always*

filled with chelating people, you know. So, once I heard this woman telling, not to me, to others, about a friend she knew. How his legs were so bad they turned black and his doctor advised him to have them amputated. Well, that's a horrible prospect! But somebody told him about chelation, so he went and did it, and slowly the color came back in his legs. He started to be okay and he went back to work. This is hard to believe. And when he went to his doctor to show him, the doctor's response was, 'If it was up to me I would still amputate.' It's hard to believe such extreme cruelty.

And your legs are better now?

Yes, well, the numbness is still there, I can notice it, but it's not as bad, really, and I'm not afraid of it.

Notice that the patient makes the assumption that her numbness is due to "blockages" and infers that chelation will help. Her experience at Dr. Brown's chelation center is quite positive; unlike Dr. Smith, Dr. Brown seems to know what he is doing. Moreover, she heard a miraculous testimonial of chelation's effectiveness. Had the new physician not made her comfortable and shown interest in her beliefs, he would not have learned that she attributes the problem to calcium deposits ("Where did the numbness come from?") and had sought out chelation. Nor would she be able to discuss her fears ("You were afraid to tell me about this, too, weren't you?").

The clinician is faced with a patient who has spent much time and money on a form of treatment that orthodox medicine considers worthless. Earlier physicians had let her down, both by saying there was nothing to be done despite her "bitter fear for my legs" and by becoming angry when she told them about chelation. The main point from this clinician's perspective is that she feels better, her symptoms are largely resolved, and no academic discussion of quackery will alter that fact.

What does a respectful, empathic clinician do next? Consider the three questions posed at the beginning of this section:

- **Are the beliefs really dangerous?** In fact, chelation does carry some risk because it involves repeated intravenous injections of a chemical. It is also costly.
- **Do they prohibit medical care that is actually necessary?** The patient seems willing to accept standard medical treatment, provided the clinician pays attention to her symptoms. Or, perhaps more importantly, pays attention to *her*.
- **Can I work within the patient's belief system to provide good medical care?** This patient may well be amenable to decreasing or discontinuing her reliance on CAM if she becomes aware of a desirable alternative. The next step would be to arrive at a mutually acceptable course of action through the process of negotiation, which we discuss in Chapter 16.

SUMMARY ■ TALKING ABOUT CAM

CAM is a rapidly growing component of the health care system. In primary practice, it is likely that nearly half of your patients have used or are using CAM, although most of them will not initially tell you about it. Highly educated, self-directed persons who are concerned about the invasiveness and toxicity of conventional medicine are likely to seek out CAM, as well as those who are dissatisfied with conventional practitioners, particularly if they have chronic, ill-defined, or poorly treatable conditions. A common theme in these patients' stories is that allopathic physicians simply don't take the time to listen to them.

You should introduce a discussion of CAM by including relevant questions in your standard interview, as well as by giving the patient permission to broach the topic, listening carefully for nondisclosing clues. To enlarge and clarify the discussion, ask about the patient's explanatory model and request specific information about the type of CAM therapy used. Differentiate clearly between what you know and what you do not know about a given therapy and support the patient in efforts to obtain answers to important questions about benefit and risk.

- Is the alternate therapy really dangerous?
- Does it prohibit necessary medical care?
- Can you work within the patient's belief system to provide good care?

If the answer to the last question is "yes," the next steps include negotiation and education.

References

1. Eisenberg DM, Kessler RC, Foster C, Norlock FE, Calkins DR, Delbanco TL. Unconventional medicine in the United States. Prevalence, costs, and patterns of use. *N Engl J Med* 1993; 328:246–252.
2. Astin JA. Why patients use alternative medicine. Results of a national study. *JAMA* 1998; 279:1548–1553.
3. Elder NC, Gillcrist A, Minz R. Use of alternative health care by family practice patients. *Arch Fam Med* 1997; 6:181–184.
4. Rao JK, Mihaliak K, Kroenke K, Bradley J, Tierney WM, Weinberger M. Use of complementary therapies for arthritis among patients of rheumatologists. *Ann Intern Med* 1999; 131:409–415.

Suggested Reading

Druss BG, Rosenheck RA. Association between use of unconventional therapies and conventional medical services. *JAMA* 1999; 282:651–656.
Lazar JS, O'Connor BB. Talking with patients about their use of alternative therapies. *Primary Care* 1997; 24:699–711.
Kaptchuk TJ, Eisenberg DM. The persuasive appeal of alternative medicine. *Ann Intern Med* 1998; 129:1061–1064.
Kaptchuk TJ, Eisenberg DM. Varieties of healing. 1: Medical pluralism in the United States. *Ann Intern Med* 2000, in press.
Kaptchuk TJ, Eisenberg DM. Varieties of healing. 2: A taxonomy of unconventional healing practices. *Ann Intern Med* 2001, in press.
Sierpina VS. *Integrative Health Care: Complementary and Alternative Therapies for the Whole Person.* Philadelphia, F.A. Davis Company, 2001.

CHAPTER 15

The Sum of All the General Rage

● ● ● ● ●

MALPRACTICE AND THE CLINICAL INTERVIEW

*He piled upon the whale's white hump **the sum of all the general rage** and hate felt by his whole race from Adam down....*

Herman Melville, *Moby Dick*

A few years ago, the issue of malpractice prevention would not have been addressed in a textbook on clinical interviewing skills. Clinicians then thought (as many still do) that there are two ways of trying to avoid negligence suits. The first, of course, is minimizing clinical mistakes, but we all know that a lawsuit may follow an adverse outcome even if no mistakes are made. The second approach is practicing "defensive medicine"—that is, making some of your medical decisions on the basis of perceived liability risk rather than on the basis of good clinical judgment. Usually this approach involves excessive diagnostic testing. For example, an emergency medicine physician might routinely order computed tomography scans on patients with head injuries, even if the clinical circumstances do not warrant the scan. Similarly, an internist or neurologist might order a magnetic resonance imaging scan on all patients with headache, knowing, of course, that very few such scans are clinically indicated.

Studies of malpractice claims have repeatedly demonstrated two remarkable findings, however:

- **Defensive medicine *does not* prevent malpractice suits.** If a patient has a bad medical outcome, the fact that the clinician ordered inappropriate tests does not reduce the risk of a lawsuit. The best policy, in fact, is to follow clinical guidelines or the standard of care.[1,2]
- **Good clinician communication *does* prevent malpractice suits.** A patient who feels that the clinician listens to and understands him or her is not likely to sue that person, even if there is a bad outcome.[1,2]

In other words, good communication is the *real* defensive medicine. Because this finding is so consistent and striking, malpractice insurance carriers now sponsor seminars on communication skills. Clinicians who complete these seminars often receive discounts on their malpractice insurance premiums (a sure sign that this training works!). An empathic, compassionate approach with good interactive technique leads to better diagnosis and therapy and also enhances patient satisfaction. Satisfied patients generally do not sue. In fact, if an adverse outcome occurs, the strongest predictor of a malpractice action is a pre-existing poor clinician–patient relationship.

These findings have implications for clinical interviewing. In this chapter we focus on specific aspects of the clinician–patient encounter relevant to malpractice prevention: earning trust through mastering basic skills, building a negligence-free relationship, achieving truly informed consent, communicating with other members of the health care team, and keeping good records.

EARNING TRUST THROUGH MASTERY OF BASIC SKILLS

Some clinicians, especially older ones, believe that patients don't trust health care professionals the way they used to. These clinicians express nostalgia for a time when patients were silent, faithful, appreciative, undemanding, and trusting. Although such a time probably never existed, it is true that we live in a culture in which people have particularly high expectations of health care and assert themselves when they feel betrayed, injured, or abandoned. Nowadays you have to *earn* a patient's trust and satisfaction. The mantle of professionalism no longer gives you immunity from being questioned, contradicted, or sued.

Let us be clear about the role of *competence*. Because medicine and other aspects of health care are technical fields, there is a widespread belief in our culture that technical competence is what makes a good clinician. But the concept of "technical competence" is only considered applicable to the machines and procedures of high technology. The other technical aspects of clinical practice—for example, the clinical skills this book discusses—are either not considered fundamental to good practice or are redefined as nontechnical personal qualities that are nice but not essential. This line of reasoning concludes that "good bedside manner" is desirable but secondary. After all, you often hear people ask, would you rather have a pleasant, communicative surgeon, or a competent one?

When it comes to medical negligence issues, we submit that technical competencies in *both* spheres—your scope of clinical practice and your interactive skills—are paramount. We assume that you will make every attempt to avoid errors of scientific knowledge and judgment. Our concern here is with the *other* sphere of technical competence. The evidence indicates that "interactively competent" clinicians engender trust and satisfaction in their patients, and they experience fewer negligence suits.

Exactly what does this mean? Levinson and colleagues[3] compared primary care physicians who do not get sued to those who do. They found that both groups demonstrated similar performance in strictly informational aspects of the encounter—that is, asking relevant questions ("What can you tell me about the chest pain?") or providing information ("This medication may make you constipated.") However, they found that the clinicians who do not engender claims engage more often in the behaviors listed in Clinical Key 15–1. Facilitative responses give patients permission to talk and to tell their story in their own way (see pp. 25–29). These responses demonstrate that the clinician cares about what they have to say and, by implication, cares about them. Likewise, inquiries about the patient's beliefs suggest that the clinician is taking the patient-as-person seriously. Orienting statements demonstrate respect and help establish realistic expectations of the visit and, by extension, of the therapeutic enterprise. For example, here is a segment from the interview of a 70-year-old man who is seeing a new primary care physician for the first time:

CLINICAL KEY 15–1

Interview Behaviors of Primary Care Physicians Who Don't Get Sued

- Facilitative responses—paraphrases, mirrors, and statements like "Tell me more about that"
- Inquiries about what the patient thinks or understands about the problem
- Interpretive statements
- Orienting statements—instructions about the flow of the visit ("First I'll examine you and then we'll discuss the possible causes.")
- Orienting statements—transitions ("Now I'd like to find out about how your health has been in the past.")
- Humor and laughter

SOURCE: Levinson W, Roter DL, Mullooly JP, Dull VT, Frankel RM. Physician-patient communication. The relationship with malpractice claims among primary care physicians and surgeons. *JAMA* 1997; 277:553–559 at p. 557.

> Okay.... Well, I think I have some idea now of your major concerns. What I'd like to do next is have you step over here [indicates examination table] and I'll take a look at you from head to toe. While we're doing that, you can give me some more details.
>
> *There was something else I wanted to apprise you of ... but I can't think of it.*
>
> Not to worry, it may come to you and when I'm done with the exam I'll give you time to collect your thoughts and see if you have any questions. How does that sound?
>
> *It sounds good.*
>
> [The clinician conducts and finishes the physical examination.] Okay.... That's all we'll do today. Let me step out for a few minutes while you get dressed. That will give me a chance to review the files you brought in. Then I'll come back and we'll make a plan.

Finally, laughter and humor indicate warmth, friendliness, and a personal connection between clinician and patient, helping the patient perceive himself or herself as a real person as opposed to a "case."

BUILDING BLOCKS OF A NEGLIGENCE-FREE RELATIONSHIP

In a general sense, this whole book is about avoiding malpractice litigation. Look at Clinical Key 15–2, which summarizes four ways in which the interview serves as a tool in clinical practice. Remember that these functions overlap considerably. For example, it would be difficult, if not impossible, to master the interview as a diagnostic tool or an instrument of healing without first inspiring the patient's trust.

Let us now focus the discussion on additional behaviors that seem to be lacking in clinicians who are often sued. Clinical Key 15–3 summarizes these negligence-deflecting behaviors, which we will review in detail.

Listen to What the Patient Says and Doesn't Say

Consider these comments by dissatisfied patients:

- "My last doctor never listened to me. There wasn't time.... I was always in and out of his office, like an assembly line."
- "The thing about Doctor Jones, he's got his own spiel.... You have to do it his way or else."
- "I just couldn't get a word in edgewise."
- "Doctor Adams just didn't understand me."

These statements share a high level of frustration and probably anger. The patients didn't feel that they were getting their message across; thus, they couldn't connect with their clinicians. No wonder they sought new clinicians.

CLINICAL KEY 15–2

The Interview as a Tool for Malpractice Prevention

- Develop the interview as a **trust-building tool:** empathy, respect, and genuineness bring you closer to the patient (see Chap. 2).
- Develop the interview as a **diagnostic tool:** the more you listen, the more you will learn (see Chaps. 3–6).
- Develop the interview as a **relationship-building tool:** good conversations make good relationships (see Chaps. 2, 5, and 10–14).
- Develop the interview as a **therapeutic tool:** good clinicians make good healers (see especially Chaps. 12–16).

CLINICAL KEY 15–3

Building Blocks of a Negligence-Free Encounter

- Listen to what the patient says and doesn't say.
- Avoid trivializing or demeaning the patient.
- Acknowledge the patient's level of concern.
- Strive for transparency in your reasoning and recommendations.
- Be clear about what you know and what you don't know.
- Never make promises you can't keep.
- Be available to the patient.

If one of them had a bad outcome or missed diagnosis, he or she might believe that Dr. Adams or Dr. Jones was negligent. What behaviors prevent this kind of frustration?

Allow enough time. The first patient experienced a treadmill-like environment. He didn't feel he had time to explain anything, which at first frustrated him and later, perhaps, prevented him from trying to do so. Although the actual time you spend with a patient may be limited, there is no excuse for not listening actively and completely during the time you have. If you do so, the patient is likely to experience the encounter as lasting longer (*perceived time*) and to feel understood.

Keep quiet. In the second and third cases, the clinicians evidently had their own agenda, rather than the patient's agenda, in mind. They may have been friendly or reassuring, but they took over the conversation. Remember to allow patients time to state *their* concerns, even those concerns that don't surface in the first few seconds of the interview.

Keep listening not only to what is said, but also to what isn't said. When the patient says, "Dr. Adams just didn't understand me," we only learn the outcome, not the specific problem. Dr. Adams may have thought she was doing a good job taking care of the patient's verbal complaints, but the patient didn't feel safe enough to express her real concern. The nonverbal cues, the hand-on-the-doorknob phenomenon, the seeming magnification of mild or simple health problems—all these slipped past Dr. Adams, who was focused solely on addressing the explicit concerns.

Avoid Trivializing or Demeaning: Acknowledge the Patient's Level of Concern

Next, consider these tortured outbursts:

- "Who does he think he is? He just walks in with this high and mighty air about him, like he's God or something. He doesn't even sit down. He just says, 'Well, the good news is your tests are normal. So it's not your heart. It must be in your head.' Like I'm making it all up."
- "So she told me to take Naprosyn for 2 more weeks. I've been taking Naprosyn a month now and I'm in pain. I can't get out of bed in the morning. And she tells me it can't be that bad, I should have more patience."

The first doctor demeaned the patient's assessment of her illness, turning her into a "psycho" or "crock," because to most people symptoms that are "in your head" are less real than symptoms that are "in your body." The doctor thinks the patient should be happy because she doesn't have cancer or hypothyroidism, but he ignores the fact that she is suffering from symptoms that she doesn't understand.

The second doctor trivialized the patient's experience. The patient has disabling symptoms that the medication is not helping. After a month there is little reason to believe the same drug will lead to a major improvement. Nonetheless, the doctor says, "It can't be that bad." Of course, it can—it *is* that bad! Why wasn't this doctor listening? Maybe she had a preconceived notion that the patient was dramatizing his symptoms. Maybe she couldn't think of any better treatment. Maybe she was just having a bad day. In any case, she lost her patient's confidence.

To avoid demeaning or trivializing, address your patient's level of concern with interchangeable, empathic responses. The concern is real, even if *you* believe it is unwarranted. Moreover, in some cases it will turn out that *you are wrong*—the first patient might have occult cancer, and the second might have an unusual form of arthritis that you failed to diagnose. If so, you might end up with a lawsuit as well as a dissatisfied patient.

Strive for Transparency

By "transparency" we mean that the patient should be able to visualize or understand your reasoning. Consider this explanation given by a cardiologist:

- "OK, Mr. Marsden, what we have here is a lesion in the left anterior descending artery, looks like about a 90% occlusion, and then there's a 100% occlusion of the first perforator. We need to send you to the hospital as soon as possible."

Several behaviors facilitate transparency. First, *don't use jargon.* Clinicians often speak opaquely. Because so much of our time and energy is invested in the culture of medicine, medical terms trip lightly off our lips. Words like "occlusion" seem perfectly clear and natural to us, and certainly more precise than "blockage." We may not take the time and trouble to translate.

Second, *explain how and why you came to the conclusion.* Another aspect of clinical transparency is to explain your conclusions or recommendations. Mr. Marsden's cardiologist couches his explanation in medical jargon—it sounds ominous, but Mr. Marsden has no way of judging specifically what it means for him. The recommendation is blunt—"You need to go to the hospital as soon as possible." Why? For what purpose? What's the danger if I don't go? How long will I be there? Are there any alternatives? The doctor needs to explain more and in a way that Mr. Marsden understands. We discuss this question of transparency in more detail in the section on informed consent, but remember that we should always be eliciting informed consent when we expect patients to follow our instructions.

Finally, *remember that conversations with patients are always, in a sense, cross-cultural and, as such, may result in misunderstanding.* Sick people live in the culture of illness, vulnerability, and fear. Clinicians live in the culture of health, technique, and knowledge. Thus, even an encounter between a middle-class African-American doctor and a middle-class African-American patient is a cross-cultural experience. The language and culture discrepancies often manifest themselves as misunderstandings about what was said or not said during an encounter. Sometimes a clinician who thinks that she has completely explained the benefits, risks, and alternatives to a procedure or treatment will discover later that the patient had absolutely no idea what she was talking about.

Be Clear about What You Know and What You Don't Know

Consider the following excerpt:

- "So she kept telling me it was my heart.... She had me on the patch and three or four different pills—headaches, weakness, you wouldn't believe it. So I said they just seem to make me sicker, and what about the burning and the sour taste? But, no, she said it was definitely my heart, but I probably couldn't have more heart surgery, since I already had a quadruple bypass."

This patient was experiencing several chest symptoms. Because of his past history of severe coronary artery disease, the cardiologist was treating him medically for angina, despite features also consistent with gastroesophageal reflux (for example, he often developed the pain when lying down). Without a referral, he went to a gastroenterologist suggested by a friend and was discovered to have severe inflammation of his lower esophagus, secondary to chronic reflux. Why didn't the cardiologist at least consider this possibility, especially when the antiangina treatment wasn't working? We don't have enough information to answer that question, but the case highlights two issues about diagnosis and disclosure. First, if you believe there are possible competing diagnoses, let the patient know. For example, "Given everything we know about your condition, I'm pretty sure this is angina. Let's increase your medication and see. If by any chance it doesn't get better, then we might have to do some other tests." Second, if you *don't* believe there are possible competing diagnoses, ask yourself why. Are you missing something? Have you closed your eyes prematurely to additional data? Are you sure you understand the whole picture? Naturally, in many cases you will have a high degree of certainty, but you should always keep your eyes open for conflicting or unexpected features and share these with the patient. ("Here's what I'm thinking ....")

Admit your errors. When it comes to medical mistakes, honesty is almost always the best policy. It is also an extraordinarily difficult policy. Most of us are tempted to avoid the pain and embarrassment of admitting a clinical error by arguing that the error was trivial or the patient is better off not knowing. We also firmly believe (and sometimes are willing to admit) that fear of malpractice litigation influences our decision. The truth is that patients have a right to know if they are the victims of medical error.

Never Make Promises You Can't Keep

Listen to this patient, who has suffered for years from debilitating back pain:
- "The doctor said if I had the operation everything would be okay, my back would be fine, no more pain, no more painkillers. So I had the operation and it's been hell ever since, why it's worse than it was before."

Clinicians commonly hear stories like this. Nonclinicians do, too—at cocktail parties, in the elevator, at the supermarket, on the bus. Wherever you go, you encounter people who are dissatisfied with their medical care, often because of what they consider a broken promise. Surgery is one example. Whether or not the surgeon actually said, "Everything will be okay" is a moot point. The patient feels betrayed.

Medicine is fraught with uncertainty. We want to help our patients, and sometimes in the process of providing encouragement, we say the equivalent of "Everything's going to be all right," even if the diagnosis or prognosis is unclear. In the case of back surgery, patients must be selected carefully and, even then, the outcome (relief of pain and disability) varies greatly. If this middle-aged man's orthopaedic surgeon actually said "No more pain, no more painkillers," he was taking a risk that turned out to be unwarranted. However, patients often can't relate to statistics; they are looking for definitive answers. Thus, some patients will interpret a clinician's vague assurance as a clear-cut promise, and others will listen to a jargon-filled explanation, which they can't understand, and decide that it means whatever they want it to mean. When the prediction proves false, these individuals will be convinced that their clinician misled them.

Avoiding promises you can't keep is part of informed consent (discussed later) and requires that you present the benefits (including the probability of success) and risks (including the probability of side effects or adverse outcomes), along with alternatives and your assessment of them. This conversation needs to be in clear, understandable language. The patient whose back surgery was unsuccessful might have been satisfied had his surgeon presented the procedure in this way:

> ... Now that I've explained what the surgery is and what we're trying to accomplish with it, I want to emphasize an important point. The back problem that you have is very complicated. We don't fully understand the relationship between slipped discs—which you definitely have— and the severe back pain, which you also definitely have. Sometimes people continue to have back pain even after surgery. So I want to tell you that we can't promise anything. That's important to realize—it's tough, but it's true. All I can say is that in my professional judgment, surgery is the best choice we have right now. I think it will give you the best chance of relief, but remember it's still a "chance" of relief, not a sure thing.

Be Available

The following patient's experience is, unfortunately, not uncommon:

- "I'd call his office time and again and they'd say 'We'll give him the message, Joyce,' and then I'd wait, but he'd never call back. Finally, things really reached a head. I couldn't take the pain any more, I was desperate, and then I got short of breath ... but I simply couldn't get through to him. He never called back. Finally, this other doctor called and he didn't seem to know what he was talking about...."

If you are a trainee just entering clinical practice, your responsibility for patient care is limited and you are unlikely to face the on-call situation described by this patient. However, professional availability is an attribute that begins at the beginning—in your clinical interview and the initial clinician– patient encounter. The patient needs to be taken seriously and to sense that you are *available* to her as a person, that you will respond to her anxieties and concerns and that you will *not* hold yourself distant and aloof. Similarly, if you are helping to care for a patient in your role as a trainee, your availability should be sustained over time, whether during a hospitalization, a clerkship, or a preceptorship. In this case, you have a responsibility to explain to the patient the characteristics and limits of your availability: "I'll come to see you every day, Mr. Jones, but I'm a student and I won't be here on night call."

Most patients understand that their clinicians can't be on call 24 hours a day, 7 days a week. The issue here has to do with your overall pattern of responsiveness to the needs of patients. Many malpractice claims arise out of unanswered phone calls, or from inappropriate recommendations made by an on-call clinician whom the patient doesn't know and who is unfamiliar with the case. This is a complex topic, but here are a few basic guidelines on availability:

- Return patient calls promptly whenever it is feasible.
- If another clinician (e.g., a nurse, physician assistant, or nurse practitioner) screens calls and responds to some of them, explain the system to your patients and reassure them that you are available if needed.
- If you encourage patients to call at a certain time of day, make sure your patients are aware of that time.
- Clarify what patients should expect on nights and weekends.
- If you are going to be away, make appropriate arrangements for coverage and inform patients who seem likely to have problems during your absence.

INFORMED CONSENT

We assume patient consent in many aspects of health care. When patients answer our questions during the interview, submit to a physical examination, take prescription drugs, or allow themselves to be stuck by needles or penetrated by x-rays, their actions constitute implied consent. However, more invasive procedures and more specialized therapies pose sufficient potential risk to patients that clinicians must obtain explicit consent before performing them. This consent must be an informed judgment based on adequate information about benefits, risks, and alternatives. We cannot fully examine here the moral and legal doctrine of informed consent or the controversies about how truly "informed" consent can be in medical practice, especially when it involves desperately ill patients and complex treatments. Nevertheless, you often will be required to obtain informed consent. And sometimes when bad outcomes occur, you might be required to provide evidence that the patient was, in fact, adequately informed about whatever he or she consented to. The following guidelines should be of some help.

The Process

Informed consent is an interactive process, not a form or a piece of paper. Typical consent forms present the information in formal, bureaucratic language. They require that the patient (and a witness) sign them to indicate an informed and voluntary agreement. Such forms can serve as an outline to guide discussion, but the patient's act of signing this paper does not in itself constitute informed consent. And although it does serve as evidence, the signed consent form is not necessarily sufficient proof of informed consent in court. The legal doctrine of informed consent demands that the consent process include four distinct elements, as shown in Clinical Key 15–4.

Because informed consent is a process, it requires skillful patient–clinician interaction. Katz[4] employs the metaphor of conversation to describe the process. If possible, he says, we want to continue a given conversation until each party has attained its goal. In this case, the clinician's goal is for the patient to understand the relevant information and to make an informed choice. Brody[5] extends this metaphor by recommending a standard, which he calls the "transparency" standard of consent, for judging when these goals are met. According to Brody, the clinician obtains an adequate informed consent when a reasonably informed person participates in the medical decision to the extent that he or she wishes. In turn, "reasonably informed" means that (1) the clinician discloses the basis on which the proposed treatment or alternatives were chosen, and (2) the patient is allowed to ask questions suggested by the disclosure of the clinician's reasoning, and the clinician answers those questions to the patient's satisfaction. In other words, the clinician reveals his or her thought process so that it is transparent to the patient and then encourages questions. For example, a physician prescribing a blood pressure medication might say:

> I know you're concerned about your blood pressure, so let me tell you what I'm thinking. We know that we can reduce the risk to your health by treating your blood pressure, and we know that there are a number of very safe and effective medicines that have been used for many years. In your case the blood pressure isn't too high, we'd call it "mild," and you don't have any other serious health conditions, so we'll begin with a "mild" pill that you can take just once a day and that usually doesn't have many side effects. So here's what I'd like to recommend for you.... [Names the medication and possible side effects.] So what do you think?

CLINICAL KEY 15–4

Elements of Informed Consent

- **Information:** The patient should be provided with information that a "reasonable person" would want to know about the nature of the procedure, benefits, risks, and alternative courses of action.
- **Understanding:** The patient must understand the information provided.
- **Voluntariness:** The patient's decision must be freely made, without evidence of coercion.
- **Competency:** The patient should be capable of making an autonomous medical decision in the particular setting.

The important issue here is that consent is obtained in the context of a conversation during which the clinician gives clear explanations and assesses the patient's understanding. Although we often think of informed consent only in the context of explaining risky procedures, consent is a part of the most ordinary patient interactions. Such a conversation may lead to negotiation and compromise (as we discuss later) if the patient objects to proposed procedures or treatments; the conversation also usually has the potential of being reopened at a later time. The therapeutic core qualities of empathy, genuineness, and respect (see Chap. 2) build trust and thereby facilitate the consent process, an important component of malpractice suit prevention.

Barriers to Informed Consent

Some barriers to informed consent (see Table 15–1) inhibit strict adherence to all the necessary elements. Not all omissions arise simply from patient ignorance or lack of clinician cooperation. One problem is that some patients think decision making ought to be in the hands of professionals and these patients defer to the clinician's judgment. They opt out of the formal decision. Nonetheless, most patients desire to be thoroughly informed about what is going on. Caregivers should not confuse ready acceptance of a diagnostic test with disinterest in its purpose and characteristics. Another problem is that the medical care process often confuses patients because there are many decisions to be made at different times, and often a variety of people are responsible. It is difficult to focus on one decision or one issue. You have an excellent opportunity to help your patients by listening to their concerns and by encouraging and then answering their questions. Informed consent may also be compromised when different members of the health care team inform the pa-

TABLE 15–1

BARRIERS TO INFORMED CONSENT
Nature of Medical Decisions
Treatment decisions tend to evolve over time, rather than being quick and clear.
Often numerous, related decisions must be made.
The decision-making process often involves numerous people.
Patient Characteristics
The patient wants information but believes the actual decision is the clinician's task.
The patient does not know which clinician is responsible.
The patient fails to "hear" because of conflict or denial.
Clinician Characteristics
Clinicians do not understand the rationale for patient involvement.
Clinicians do not take time to explain issues clearly to the patient.

SOURCE: Based on Lidz, CW, et al. Barriers to informed consent. *Ann Intern Med* 1983; 99:539–543.

tient differently. Mixed and conflicting messages may have grave consequences for patient understanding, impair the patient's quality of care, and (if the outcome is poor) raise questions about possible malpractice.

COMMUNICATION WITHIN THE HEALTH CARE TEAM

Modern medical treatment is often extremely complicated. In the case of cancer, for example, treatment may require the interaction of primary care doctors, oncologists, surgeons, radiation therapists, and other clinicians. Cardiovascular, respiratory, neurologic, and psychiatric disorders each involve a different array of specialists. Nowadays, even patients who have relatively minor health problems may engage the services of a team of professionals—for example, a family physician, a gynecologist, a dentist, a chiropractor, and a massage therapist. Communication among these professionals is important. When the illness is severe, or different therapies may interact to cause risk of harm, communication is even more important. If a clinician is unaware of important clinical information because he or she has not communicated with a consultant or other member of the health care team, that may be negligence. Likewise, poor communication among team members often leads to mixed messages for the patient. Even if all parties share the same facts, different ways of presenting those facts may confuse the patient and make it appear that the clinicians disagree. Guidelines for communication among professionals were presented in Chapter 7 (pp. 125–126).

KEEPING GOOD RECORDS: DOCUMENTATION, DOCUMENTATION, DOCUMENTATION

The Clinical Record

Written communication can sometimes be almost as important as the clinician–patient interaction itself in preventing malpractice suits. When patients experience bad outcomes, they or their families sometimes question the clinician's diagnosis or treatment, even when they are otherwise satisfied with the care they received. In other cases, they might be unable to remember critical aspects of the story, like a recommendation you made or a treatment you prescribed at a certain point in time. They might believe incorrectly, for example, that you failed to follow appropriate guidelines.

The clinical record helps you remember what actually happened and when it happened, which is likely to be useful in explaining and discussing the situation with the patient. Moreover, the record serves as crucial documentation that can be used to ascertain the quality and appropriateness of your patient care. Thus, your chart entries are of great importance. Table 15–2 presents a convenient mnemonic—the five Cs—to remind you that clinical progress notes should be contemporaneous, clear, comprehensible, concise,

TABLE 15–2

THE UNIMPEACHABLE CLINICAL RECORD		
The Record Entries Should Be	**Which Means**	**To Accomplish This, You Should**
Contemporaneous	Written or dictated during or shortly after the patient visit	Set aside time to create your notes between patients.
		Organize a private "space" for writing or dictation.
Clear	Legible, uncluttered	Think before you write.
		Use a standard format or form.
		Dictate when possible.
Comprehensible	Logical and accurate representations of your clinical thinking and judgment	Think twice before you write.
		Read over before you finish and sign.
		Use a standard, step-by-step approach in your thinking.
Concise	To the point, with no excess verbiage	Keep your goal in mind. Remember the reader.
Complete	Inclusive of all the essential issues and aspects of the clinical situation	Ask yourself, "Who is this patient? What is the problem? What can be done? Have I explained it?"

and complete. The third column of this table presents some useful guidelines for achieving each "C" in your own practice. Here are a few additional pointers specifically aimed at liability prevention:

- Always write (or dictate) your notes promptly, so that you don't forget any details of the interaction before documenting its content.
- If you do not receive a consultant's report in a reasonable period of time, ask for it.
- Although it is important to be concise, be sure to include all relevant information regarding differential diagnosis, reasons for diagnostic tests, or reasons for treatments you prescribe. (This is another aspect of transparency in your thinking.)
- If a patient declines a test or treatment that you recommend, document not only the refusal, but also your explanation to the patient and possible remedial measures ("Will bring this up again at next visit," or "Patient asked to think about it and will give me a call.")
- Use nonjudgmental language when a patient does not follow your recommendation (e.g., the word "declines" is preferable to "refuses" or "fails.")
- If a declined test or treatment is particularly important, revisit the options with the patient within an appropriate period.

What a Difference Some Notes Make

"Delay of diagnosis" is a frequent claim on malpractice suits. It occurs when a patient seeks help for a condition that eventually proves to be a serious illness (usually cancer), but for one reason or another the diagnostic process takes a long time. For example, a woman might present to her gynecologist with a lump in her breast. The doctor orders a mammogram, which appears to show that the lump is a manifestation of fibrocystic disease, rather than malignancy. What to do next? The doctor might recommend a repeat mammogram in 2 or 3 months. Let's say the patient returns in 3 months, has a mammogram and ultrasound as recommended, and the lump proves to be cancer. She then undergoes definitive treatment, but the cancer is very aggressive and in a year or so she develops metastases. Some such patients might question the gynecologist's original diagnostic plan. What if she had had the ultrasound and a biopsy when she first went to see him? If the cancer had been discovered earlier, perhaps she could have been cured. In her pain and anxiety, the patient may blame the doctor for the bad outcome, claiming that the diagnosis was inappropriately delayed.

The crucial factor here is whether the physician followed accepted clinical guidelines in waiting 3 months before repeating the test or ordering other tests. If he did, there is no basis for a suit—he was practicing state-of-the-art medicine, which in this case is evidence-based. On the other hand, if the standard clinical guidelines recommended an immediate ultrasound, then he may well have been responsible for a delay in diagnosis. Whether the delay actually contributed to the patient's bad outcome is a moot point. The cancer may have been so aggressive that earlier diagnosis would not have prevented its spread. However, the combination of a clinical mistake (failure to follow standard practice) and a bad outcome is usually considered by juries to be prima facie evidence that the mistake resulted in the outcome.

What would have happened if the doctor's recommendations were correct, but the patient had not returned in 3 months? Let's say she waited 6 or 8 months, then went back to the gynecologist because the breast lump had gotten bigger. A similar scenario followed—she proved to have cancer, which by that time had spread to her lymph nodes and bones. If this patient subsequently decided to sue her doctor, a great deal would depend on (1) written documentation in the chart of the original conversation and recommendation and (2) possible evidence of measures that the doctor might have taken to remind her of the need for a follow-up mammogram. The office note should specify what was said and how it relates to the standard practice or clinical guideline. It should also indicate the manner of follow-up, such as a prescription for a repeat mammogram in 2 or 3 months and a follow-up office appointment. For something so important, there should also be evidence of a "tickler file" or some other method of initiating contact with the patient if she misses the follow-up appointment. For example, the office might send a standard reminder letter to patients who miss repeat mammograms or Pap smears, or an office staff member might even leave a telephone message inviting the patient to call for another appointment.

If the diagnostic plan was both reasonable and clearly documented, there would be no basis for a "delay of diagnosis" suit. But if the doctor had forgotten to write down the plan, or to document its importance, the suit becomes an issue of the doctor's word against the patient's. She is, after all, the person who has suffered a misfortune. The doctor's word—no matter how sincere it is—may not convince a jury of her peers.

On the Record

No matter how careful you are, you will sometimes make mistakes while writing in the clinical record. Your mind might wander and soon you find yourself jotting down the wrong material—an incorrect observation or plan, for example, or perhaps a correct observation, but placed in the wrong patient's chart. More frequently, if you dictate your notes, you will identify errors of transcription. Sometimes, too, you might change your mind in the process of recording a note. Suddenly, the clinical data "click" into a different pattern. Aha! You want to pursue a new course of action, but you have already written a paragraph outlining your original plan. What should you do?

It is tempting to pursue either the *snuff-it-out* or the *throw-it-out* approach. *Snuff-it-out* means that you take a pen and carefully scribble over your sentences so that they disappear in a pool of blue or black lines, or at least can no longer be understood. By all means, suppress the temptation to snuff it out. Defacing the medical record raises serious doubts about your truthfulness when the record is used as evidence in malpractice litigation. The *throw-it-out* approach is also inappropriate, perhaps even worse, because it may require you to rewrite not only the present clinical entry, but also other entries on the page you toss out. Here are some guidelines for correcting errors in the health care record:

- Strike through the incorrect passage with a single line, so that the original writing can still be read and understood.
- Make your corrections.
- If the correction is word, a date, or a short phrase, enter it above or in the margin of the incorrect entry.
- If the correction is longer, enter it in the text below the incorrect material as a continuation of the note.
- Date your corrections. (This obviously should be the same date as the original entry.)
- Explain clearly why you are correcting the entry.

SUMMARY ■ AVOIDING MALPRACTICE CLAIMS

The best way to prevent malpractice suits is to practice with a high degree of technical competence: competence in the skills of clinical interviewing and clinician–patient interaction, as well as competence in your sphere of professional practice. By becoming an empathic, respectful practitioner who listens well and responds appropriately, you will generate trust and satisfaction among your patients. To avoid malpractice claims, pay particular attention to the following guidelines:

- Listen to what the patient does and doesn't say.
- Avoid trivializing or demeaning the patient.
- Acknowledge the patient's level of concern.
- Strive for transparency in your reasoning and recommendations.
- Be clear about what you know and what you don't know.
- Never make promises you can't keep.
- Be available to the patient.

In addition, pay careful attention to informed consent. Employ a transparency standard for evaluating the information you provide and your patient's response. Likewise, look closely at your communication with other health professionals involved in a patient's care. Make sure they know what you are doing and you know what they are doing. Don't expect information simply to fall into place; seek it—by letter, phone, e-mail, or fax. Finally, remember that documentation is essential. Make your progress notes contemporaneous, clear, comprehensible, concise, and complete. Also document your attempts to follow up on missed appointments or tests. When you make a mistake writing in the patient's record, correct the mistake carefully and transparently enough so that others can understand what you are doing and when you are doing it.

References

1. Lichtstein DM, Materson BJ, Spicer DW. Reducing the risk of malpractice claims. *Hosp Pract* 1999 (July 15); 34:69–72, 75–76, 79.
2. Vincent C, Young M, Phillips A. Why do people sue doctors? A study of patients and relatives taking legal action. *The Lancet* 1994; 343;1609–1613.
3. Levinson W, Roter DL, Mullooly JP, Dull VT, Frankel RM. Physician-patient communication. The relationship with malpractice claims among primary care physicians and surgeons. *JAMA* 1997; 277:553–559.
4. Katz J. *The Silent World of Doctor and Patient*. New York, The Free Press, 1984.
5. Brody H. Transparency: Informed consent in primary care. *Hastings Cent Rep* 1989; 19:5–9.

Suggested Reading

Beckman HB, Markakis KM, Suchman AL, Frankel RM. The doctor-patient relationship and malpractice. *Arch Intern Med* 1994; 154:1365–1370.
Bogardus ST, Holmboe E, Jekel JF. Perils, pitfalls, and possibilities in talking about medical risk. *JAMA* 1999; 281:1037–1041.
Lidz CW, et al. Barriers to informed consent. *Ann Intern Med* 1983; 99:539–543.
Shapiro, RS, Simpson DE, Lawrence SL, Talsky AM. Sobocinski KA, Schiedermayer DL. A survey of sued and nonsued physicians and suing patients. *Arch Intern Med* 1989; 149:2190–2196.

CHAPTER 16

Not Through Argument but by Contagion

● ● ● ● ●

EDUCATION AND NEGOTIATION

*The faith that heals, heals **not through argument but by contagion**. But to heal, faith must have substance. A speculative balance of probability is not enough. The faith that heals must have deep roots in the personality of the healer.*

W. R. Houston, *The Doctor Himself as a Therapeutic Agent*

Among the outcomes of an initial clinician–patient encounter, we pay particular attention in this text to data collection and hypothesis generation and testing—the diagnostic function of clinical interviewing. However, we also set the stage for relationship building. Therapeutic relationships are built on a series of single encounters. Each clinician–patient interaction has the potential to influence the way the patient behaves, thinks, and feels.

You influence **behavior** by asking patients, for example, to undertake diagnostic studies, follow a regimen of medication, return for follow-up visits, stop smoking, or start exercising. When patients change their behavior in these ways, we say that they are compliant, adherent, actively involved in their health care, or "good patients." Clearly, the best diagnoses and plans in the world are useless without patients' cooperation. Second, you influence how patients **feel**. As a result of positive encounters, patients may feel less lonely, less anxious, less depressed, or more able to cope with their problems. Negative encounters may lead to increased anxiety, anger, and greater feelings of confusion or powerlessness. The patient may walk away relieved or sorely distressed. Finally, you influence the way patients **think.** Through education and negotiation, they may change their concepts of what illness is and what should be done about it. They may learn to understand themselves differently. These three types of influence are interdependent and in practice often occur together. Each encounter may either add to or subtract from the burden of suffering. This influence is what Michael Balint had in mind when he taught that "the doctor is the drug."[1]

In other words, your treatment of the patient is not just the medication or intervention you prescribe. The drug is only a small part of the influence you have on the patient and the healing process. Even as you complete your initial interview and physical examination, you bring other influences to bear in managing the patient. You may simply be ordering further diagnostic studies while explaining your preliminary findings and expecting the patient to return. Even so, you want to maximize the probability that the patient actually obtains the studies, follows your advice, and returns to your office. You also want to do what you can to make the patient feel better starting today, rather than next week or next month. If possible, you want to reduce anxiety and relieve suffering in some way. A skillful interview grounded in respect, empathy, and genuineness (see Chap. 2) is the first step in enhancing your patient's active participation in health care and reducing the suffering caused by needless anxiety and uncertainty.

How do you maximize the chance that your influence will be positive or beneficial? In this book, we are concerned with the technical skills of medical interviewing. Your employment of those skills has multiple effects. Good technique maximizes objectivity and precision, and facilitates good clinical decision making. At the same time, good technique influences the patient to follow your advice and to leave your office with a sense of well-being and relief. Sick persons seeking medical help are frequently in a crisis situation, a time when seemingly small interventions have significant outcomes. Among all these possible outcomes, relevant ones cluster into beneficial or harmful groups, as shown in Figure 16–1. In other words, **any clinician–patient interaction is likely to influence the suffering of a sick person.**

Most treatment requires active patient cooperation. Unless the patient is comatose, it is difficult to imagine a medical care situation in which the behavioral component of therapy is not significant. Although "compliance" is a common term in medical parlance, it has two drawbacks. First, the word suggests that the clinician's orders are uniquely right and that any patient who fails to be 100% compliant will have a less-than-successful outcome. Second, it suggests a passive, plastic patient rather than an active, participating one. To some extent, the word "adherence" escapes the second connotation, but still implies the first. The patient must adhere, albeit actively, to the clinician's correct regimen. Rather than using either of these terms, we prefer to talk simply

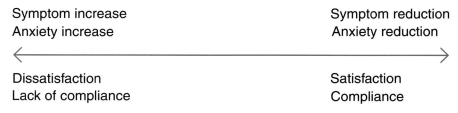

FIGURE 16–1   Possible outcomes of the clinician-patient interaction.

about the patient's cooperation with regard to treatment and instructions and to consider how clinicians themselves influence that behavior.

This chapter deals with how clinicians influence patients in the course of everyday clinical interactions. We show how these interactions are learning experiences that can be used to encourage personal responsibility and behavioral change. In Chapter 11, we presented simple steps to enhance patient understanding in the office. In this chapter we discuss in more detail what works in conveying information, not only with regard to instructing patients but also with regard to establishing appropriate expectations about the illness and its treatment. Then we consider the art of negotiation and its component skills and behaviors, concluding the chapter with an extended example of clinician–patient negotiation.

EDUCATION: CONVEYING THE INFORMATION

Why don't patients follow their clinician's instructions? Clinical Key 16–1 lists a number of factors that might explain so-called noncompliant behavior. Although each of these factors plays a part at least some of the time, studies indicate that the cognitive factor is critical and often present even when other factors also play a role. Patients frequently do not remember much of what is said to them. Simply put, people can't do what a clinician recommends if they can't remember it. Investigators agree that patients, on average, initially remember 50% to 60% of the information that clinicians give them, and subsequently retain about 45% to 55%.[2] Interestingly, neither the intelligence nor the age of the patient seem to be important factors in how much is remembered. Even writing down the information, which would seem to be a fail-safe method, does not, in fact, necessarily lead to better cooperation or increase the amount of information remembered. Of note, patients who have a moderate level of anxiety about their problems are more likely to remember than if they have either very high (paralyzing and distracting) or very low (nonmotivating) anxiety levels. So the first step in ensuring patient involvement, conceptually at least, is to make sure that the patient understands what you are saying and remembers it. How do you do that? Consider the following example:

CLINICAL KEY 16–1

Factors in "Noncooperation"

- **Personality**—The patient's personality structure precludes cooperation.
- **Psychodynamics**—Defense mechanisms, such as denial, prevent cooperation.
- **Interpersonal dynamics**—Emotional issues arising from the clinician–patient interaction prevent cooperation.
- **Economics**—The patient cannot afford the prescribed treatment.
- **Culture and Beliefs**—The patient's beliefs about the illness interfere with cooperation.
- **Cognitive factors**—The patient simply doesn't understand what is to be done and why.

So we're going to treat your hypertension with this diuretic and....

My hyper-tension? But I don't feel tense....

... We'll see how things go and we'll keep adding drugs until we get things in control.

I don't know, with my job and all, I can't afford not to be sharp....

This example is not unlike the one presented in Chapter 11 (p. 178), and it is easy to see the clinician's errors. Not only the words but also the style of this segment of the interaction suggest a range of behaviors and missed opportunities. We are left wondering whether the clinician, who must have taken the patient's blood pressure (we hope several times) during the interaction, has been silent all this time, thereby raising the patient's anxiety by saying nothing about blood pressure until the very end, then using the word "hypertension," which seems common enough but can be misunderstood by even the most well-educated patient. The clinician is rushing to a discussion of treatment before even explaining the diagnosis. She is also vague about what the patient can expect, thereby increasing uncertainty and anxiety. Note, too, that the use of the word "drug" in relation to the word "hyper-*tension*" appears to leave this patient, a high-powered attorney, completely confused. He associates "drug" with "sedative" or "tranquilizer," and expresses his fear of becoming less "sharp" in his work.

Consider how the clinician might have facilitated better understanding by adopting the measures listed in Clinical Key 16–2. The following transcript suggests how the same clinician might, on a better day, share her findings and arrive at a plan with the patient:

CLINICAL KEY 16–2

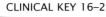 **How to Enhance Patient Understanding**

- Use words and phrases the patient is likely to understand.
- Be concrete and specific about the nature of the problem, the treatment, and expected outcome.
- In particular, give the name, purpose, mechanism (in lay terms), schedule, and duration of any prescribed medication.
- Inquire about how much the patient understands.
- Ask the patient to repeat explanations and instructions.
- Give corrective and supportive feedback.
- Encourage questions.
- Write down instructions for the patient.
- Provide instructional material, like brochures and printed handouts.
- Refer the patient to specific web sites for further information.

Well, as I mentioned during my exam, when I take your blood pressure it is repeatedly high.

Yeah, you said that and it's making me kinda worried.

Well, we consider normal anything under 140 over 90 [writing this out and showing it to the patient], and yours is 160 over 105.

Uh huh, umm.

Another word for high blood pressure is "hypertension," even though it has nothing necessarily to do with tension or feeling tense. It just means that your body has re-set your blood pressure at a higher level, like a thermostat. What I'd like to do next is explain to you what this means, what are some of the options we have to treat it, and then give you time to ask questions so I'm sure you understand. Okay?

This time the clinician has done a number of things to influence the patient by better transfer of information. The patient may well be more satisfied than in our first example and go home less anxious and confused about his condition. In addition, the clinician anticipated one of the common errors in patient understanding ("it has nothing to do with tension"), not only laying the groundwork for the proposed plan of treatment, but also making it easier for the patient to reveal other possible misconceptions he might have.

NEGOTIATION

Although patients cannot follow your advice unless they understand and remember it, they may also reject your advice because they disagree with it. Your knowledge of the patient's personal and cultural beliefs about illness and healing (see Chaps. 10 and 14) will help you to view the situation from the patient's perspective. You then have several options. You can modify your therapeutic plan to accommodate the patient's health beliefs, attempt to modify the patient's beliefs through education or persuasion, or negotiate a therapeutic alliance, which involves some "give" on both sides. Negotiation, using discussion and compromise to arrive at a settlement of some issue, is a method of conflict resolution that respects the values of all parties. In practice, negotiation is a way of optimizing patient cooperation and is a sign of respect for the patient's autonomy. Toward the end of a clinical encounter, you have hypotheses about the patient's illness, but you may remain uncertain about why the patient is ill or what the course of the illness will be. Your goals are to influence behavior, decrease anxiety, and increase the patient's sense of mastery over the problem. How can you accomplish this in the clinical interview?

Clinical Key 16–3 summarizes the process of negotiation. In a successful clinical encounter, you reach agreement with the patient in four different areas:

- Agreement on what the clinical information really is
- Agreement on the nature of the problem
- Agreement about what can or should be done
- Consent for procedures or treatments

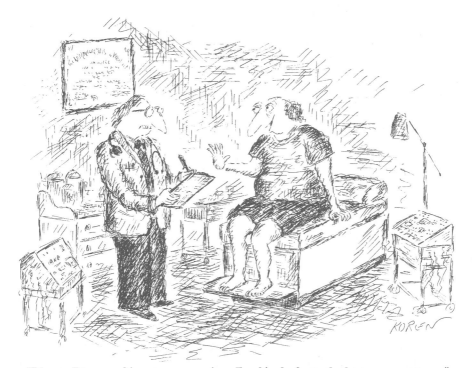

"Please, Doc—nothing too aggressive. I'm kind of attached to my symptoms."

CLINICAL KEY 16–3

Negotiation Skills in the Clinical Interview

- Begin with the core qualities of respect and empathy.
- Provide the patient with enough information and opportunity to ask questions (see Clinical Key 16–2).
- Elicit the patient's perspective.
  - Goals
    What would you like to happen?
    What do you think will happen?
  - Suggestions
    How do you think we should handle this?
    How do you think we should proceed?
  - Preferences
    Of the alternatives, which do you think will work best?
    Are there other alternatives we haven't discussed?
- Help the patient weigh burdens and benefits, including tradeoffs between quality and quantity of life.
- Consider your recommendations in light of the patient's beliefs and goals.
- Modify your plan of action insofar as is possible to incorporate the patient's perspective.
- Formulate an agreement with the patient on the nature of the problem and what should be done about it.

The characteristics of your patient, your own traits, and the qualities of the relationship may facilitate or may hinder reaching agreement. It is important to understand the patient's comprehension, decision-making processes, beliefs, and environment to have the greatest positive influence on the patient's behavior. These components restate in different terms the familiar themes of respect, empathy, communication skills, and acknowledgment of the patient's beliefs and expectations. You influence patients more when you respect them, communicate well, and understand "where they're coming from."

In day-to-day practice, education and negotiation occur together and may take only a few moments. For example, here is a middle-aged patient with bronchitis returning to see the clinician because of increased coughing:

It's going on 8 days now, doc. I was better 2 days ago, but then the coughing started up again yesterday. I'm not bringing up that thick, yellow stuff any more—it's dry, hacky—but I'm still coughing a lot. What about an antibiotic?

Well, here's what I think is happening. It sounds to me as if you've turned the corner, the infection has cleared up, but your throat is still raw and irritated. Things are healing.

Well, I do feel better... it's just this cough.

> Do you think you can hang in there another 24 hours? Just use the cough medicine. Then if you're not clearly improving we'll go with an antibiotic.
>
> *That sounds good. Should I call you around this time tomorrow?*

In this case the patient has already told the clinician that his wheezing is gone and his cough is no longer productive. Overall, he feels better. Moreover, the fever is down and on physical examination his chest sounds clear. Yet, the patient quite reasonably interprets his dramatic (but dry) cough as a sign of worsening infection. Thus, he believes that he needs an antibiotic. The clinician first reframes the situation—the dry cough represents healing rather than continued infection. The patient can accept this interpretation because it accords with other data ("Well, I do *feel* better"). The clinician then presents a counterproposal—let's see how it goes for the next 24 hours. The patient, who is now less frightened, accepts the plan, at least in part because he recognizes the clinician's logic and concern.

The next example is from an interview with a 71-year-old patient who has chronic obstructive pulmonary disease and bronchospasm. Although she has wheezing throughout both lungs, because this condition is chronic she does not experience herself as being ill:

> *I smoked my last cigarette that day I had those tests.*
>
> I'm really glad you're not smoking. And I know how hard it is for you.
>
> *I'm determined this time. I don't want to be sick.*
>
> I really would like you to be on an inhaler ... it's not good for you to be wheezing all the time.
>
> *But don't I sound better to you? I haven't smoked at all, I think I'm better, I'm not a medicine person.*
>
> Well, not smoking will definitely be better for you. It will be a big help. Still, your lung condition has been going on a long time. There's a lot of inflammation and spasm in your bronchial tubes. You know how short of breath you get.
>
> *But I believe that everything will heal naturally if I just give it a chance. I mean, by not smoking.*
>
> Well, here's what we can do. Let's agree to wait and see how it goes, provided you call me if you have any trouble breathing, any cough or wheezing. How's that? [The patient nods.] How about we recheck things in 3 months?
>
> *Okay, that's good. You'll see, my lungs will be clear as a bell.*
>
> Okay, 3 months. And keep up the good work.

This patient is convinced that her health will improve if she stays away from cigarettes. She is experiencing a sense of mastery ("I'm determined this time") that leads her to interpret the situation in a favorable light ("But don't I sound better to you?"). The clinician knows that her patient has reversible bronchospasm and, in fact, would have less wheezing and better exercise tolerance if she were to use an inhaler regularly. She explains this to the patient in simple, understandable terms, while reiterating the long-term benefits of not smoking. However, the clinician also realizes that the patient's sense of empowerment is a critical factor in her self-image. Thus, the clinician proposes an alternative program that combines monitoring (return visit) and potential crisis intervention ("call me if you have any trouble...") with respect for the patient's values and strong motivation.

We end this chapter with a more extended case example, which demonstrates the interactive nature of clinical problem solving. The case illustrates negotiation both in the "give-and-take" bargaining and the "maneuver to find a path" senses of the word. The patient is a 25-year-old woman who came to her family physician's office with the complaint of a severe and persistent vaginal itch. She expressed her distress and summarized her problem in an opening statement that we encountered previously in Chapter 3 (p. 52):

> *Well, I have a terrible vaginal itch, and I don't know whether it's from vaginitis or whether it's the urinary tract infection, you know ... ah, my regular doctor treated me for vaginitis first....*
>
> That was Doctor X?
>
> *Uh huh, then I, um, got a urinary tract infection, then the vaginitis came back, but during the whole ordeal I've never got no relief.*

We learn several important things about this patient from her opening statement: she is suffering ("terrible," "ordeal," "no relief"), she is medically sophisticated ("vaginitis," "urinary tract infection"), and she is not necessarily well educated ("I've never got no...").

The physician performs an examination and checks a specimen of vaginal secretion under the microscope, finding that the infection is clearly caused by *Trichomonas vaginalis* and can be easily and effectively treated with a single dose of eight pills. At this point, both patient and physician agree on the nature of the problem: it is a *Trichomonas* infection. To the patient, the end of her suffering is in sight. The physician begins to write out a prescription. But on seeing the name of the drug, the patient makes an unexpected comment:

> *Flagyl. You don't have any ... there's nothing else you can take besides Flagyl, huh?*

Until this point, it seems as though the physician has made not only an accurate diagnosis but also a correct decision about therapy, with which the patient will be happy. But the patient, instead of being grateful for the expertise, is not satisfied. The negotiation begins:

> It's the best for it.
>
> *Okay, but I might ... well, I'll try it.*

It is easy to imagine a scenario here in which the physician simply says "fine," and the patient is left to her own doubts about the drug, perhaps taking it, perhaps not. But the physician, listening to her hesitation, replies:

> What's the problem?
>
> *I think I was allergic to that.*
>
> Why do you think that?
>
> *Because I remember taking Flagyl before, and it did something ... I think I broke out in hives or something.*
>
> Really?
>
> *But I'll try it. If I break out I'll let you know, but I think I did.*
>
> That's a worry ... let me look at the record. It says here that you were sensitive to ampicillin and sulfa ... now could it have been ... Oh, it does say Flagyl....
>
> *I think it was just hives. Maybe I've outgrown it.*
>
> I don't want you to take it if you had hives from it.
>
> *Well, maybe I'll have ... I'll have outgrown it 'cause I think it's been a while back.*
>
> [Still looking through the chart.] Yeah, it does say Flagyl.

The patient actually begins with an interpretation ("allergic") of some past event associated with the drug. The two then exchange information, together trying to verify or refute that interpretation. The patient provides supporting evidence with the descriptive term "hives," while the physician searches for other evidence by going through the patient's chart. (She is new to this physician, but had previously been seen in the same clinic.) This is more than a simple discussion of evidence, however, as we can see both patient ("I'll try it") and physician ("I don't want you to take it....") apparently on the verge of decisions, albeit opposite ones. Perhaps, seeing the physician's concern and despite her willingness to risk hives, the patient offers a new interpretation to the data ("Maybe I'll have outgrown it"). The physician then offers:

> What we could do is we could treat your husband and we could treat you with something else, but ...
>
> *Well, if that's the best, I want that.*
>
> ... most of the "something elses" aren't as effective.
>
> *Well, I'll take Flagyl. It can only break me out in hives a day like ... it'll probably go away in the morning.*
>
> I would be kind of worried about that before prescribing it for you because you could get an even more serious reaction to it.

Data have been exchanged ("I was allergic"), verified ("hives," written record), and now reinterpreted ("I've outgrown it"). The patient, echoing the physician's "It's the best," rejects the notion of "something else" by reversing the implication of concession in her earlier statement on taking Flagyl ("Well, I'll try it"). In the context of the physician's earlier statement, "something else" would have to be judged decidedly inferior. We are tiptoeing on a threshold-of-risk boundary: take Flagyl and get rid of the itch but risk an allergic reaction, or take something else and avoid the reaction but risk not curing the itch. Much of what the patient says in subsequent statements suggests that she places a higher value on getting rid of the itch than on avoiding an allergic reaction. She acknowledges that there is a risk involved but discounts it ("just hives"); the physician, on the other hand, emphasizes that the risk is more than what the patient says ("You could get an even more serious reaction").

The decision has become problematic, and we begin to see patient and physician engage in a dialogue regarding risks and benefits. Lacking the data necessary to value or weigh the risks, the physician returns to a discussion of the evidence, by turning again to the written record to find the supporting data for the diagnosis of allergy, while the patient in turn supplies additional details pointedly aimed at discrediting her own report of an allergic reaction:

> Uh, let me see what Dr. X said about that.
>
> *I don't even think that Dr. X was here when I had that.*
>
> Dr. Y? Dr. Z? ... because that may be why you've been treated with all this other stuff.
>
> *But they, I remember I told them it did that to me, it might notta been that.*
>
> But it does say you're allergic to it.
>
> *That's cause I told him that.*
>
> I've never heard of anybody being allergic to it but it's....
>
> *That's what I'm saying, it's....*
>
> ... certainly possible.
>
> *Probably what happened was I broke out in hives in reaction to other things.*

It is remarkable that the patient understands that the source of the data in question—or rather the interpretation in question—is herself ("cause I told him that") and that she may not be the most reliable interpreter of the evidence. Perhaps, if she is the source of the original interpretation, she can also be the source of a new interpretation. In the end the physician is persuaded—to some extent. Note the ensuing discussion in which various outcomes are valued and a decision is reached:

> Well, I'll tell you what I want you to do. Since you have taken a lot of drugs because of all these urinary infections....
>
> *That might be why it's never left.*
>
> Uh hum....
>
> *So I'd rather take the Flagyl.*

> Well I'll tell you what I want you to do.
>
> *... it won't be your fault....*
>
> Well, I'm still the one that prescribes it. Let me tell you what I'd like you to do. I'd like you to take one pill out of your eight as a test dose. OK? And if you have no reaction to it, then we will hope it is safe to take the rest, though we can't know for sure.
>
> *Um hmm.*
>
> Today, just one, see what happens, and if you have no reaction to it at all, then tomorrow take the remaining seven. OK?
>
> *OK.*
>
> OK? So if you are allergic we'll know.
>
> *Yeah, I'll get hives (ha ha).*
>
> Well, let's just be on the safe side, let's use a test dose ... OK? Because *Trichomonas*, while it's uncomfortable, it can't kill you, so you know....
>
> *It can drive you mad.*
>
> I know, but the point is that we don't want to do anything that would be harmful to your health.

Although there was a lot of back-and-forth maneuvering, the physician takes ultimate responsibility for the decision ("I'm still the one that prescribes it"), but the decision is clearly influenced by the value the patient places on getting rid of the itch ("It can drive you mad"). The patient took the medication, had no reaction, and got rid of the itch. It is not difficult to imagine a different situation with a patient who, perhaps, had suffered more from hives. In that case, the negotiation would have resulted in a different outcome, such as the prescribing of a somewhat less effective therapy.

SUMMARY ■ INFLUENCING THE PATIENT

In this chapter we addressed the question of how you **influence** the patient's behavior and feelings through the clinical interview. We divided this influencing skill into components for the sake of discussion, although in practice they often flow together. The patient's **understanding** and **recall** of information must serve as a basis for any behavioral influence you might have. The patient cannot cooperate unless he or she knows what to do and how to do it. Moreover, the patient is not likely to be motivated to cooperate unless he or she knows why something is to be done and how it works. Finally, we discussed the role of **negotiation** in achieving an effective therapeutic outcome. Respect for the patient and knowledge of his or her beliefs helps you to influence the patient when you engage in a process of negotiation, the **give-and-take of ideas and feelings that allows you to arrive at a mutually agreed-upon plan of action**.

References

1. Balint M. *The Doctor and His Patient and the Illness*. New York, International Universities Press, 1972.
2. Ley P. Toward better doctor-patient communication. Contributions from social and experimental psychology. In: Bennett AE (Ed.). *Communication Between Doctors and Patients*. Oxford, Nuffield Provincial Hospitals Trust, Oxford University Press, 1976, pp. 77–98.

Suggested Reading

Beckman HB, Frankel RM. The effect of physician behavior on the collection of data. *Ann Intern Med* 1984; 101:692–696.

Buetow S. Four strategies for negotiated care. *J R Soc Med* 1998; 91:199–201.

Cegala DJ, Marinelli T, Post D. The effects of patient communication skills training on compliance. *Arch Fam Med* 2000; 9:57–64.

Fins JJ. Approximation and negotiation: Clinical pragmatism and difference. *Cambridge Quarterly of Healthcare Ethics* 1998; 7:68–76.

Heaton PB. Negotiation as an integral part of the physician's clinical reasoning. *J Fam Pract* 1981; 13:845.

Krueter MW, Chheda SG, Bull FC. How does physician advice influence patient behavior? Evidence for a priming effect. *Arch Fam Med* 2000; 9:426–433.

O'Mara K. Communication and conflict resolution in emergency medicine. *Emergency Medicine Clinics of North America* 1999; 17:451–459.

CHAPTER 17

The Hunt Is On

● ● ● ● ●

THE MEDICAL
INTERVIEW AT WORK

*Time after time I have gone out into my office in the
evening feeling as if I couldn't keep my eyes open a moment longer.... But once I saw the patient all that would disappear. In a flash the details of the case would begin to
formulate themselves into a recognizable outline, the diagnosis would unravel itself, or would refuse to make itself
plain, **and the hunt was on.** Along with that, the patient
himself would shape up into something that called for attention, his peculiarities, her reticences or candors. And
though I might be attracted or repelled, the professional attitude which every physician must call on would steady me
and dictate the terms on which I was to proceed.*

William Carlos Williams, from *The Autobiography*

Throughout this text we maintain that most of the information you need to
make appropriate diagnoses and to take care of your patients comes from
the clinical encounter. For the sake of convenience and to create manageable
pieces to learn, we have artificially dissected the interview into component parts
as though the information presents itself in a linear fashion—chief complaint before patient profile, for example. But we don't interview congestive heart failure
or sexual problems, we interview persons; and interviews—like persons—are
rarely neat and linear. Interviews tend to be messy, with information coming at

you in the opening moments that you may need to "file" in several places, perhaps in the present illness, family history, and other active problems, as for the patient who begins: "I'm a diabetic but I'm worried about this terrific headache I have because my father had a stroke when he was my age."

As you gain experience, you will be less distracted by what may, at first, seem like endless tangents that threaten to get you off track. Your mind is very busy not only following the flow of information, but keeping track of how the patient's story is turning into a diagnosis, what questions you need to ask, what details need clarification, and whether you are developing rapport with the patient.

Figure 17–1 illustrates how the medical interview works as a continual feedback loop of information, thinking, and technique that refines and remodels itself throughout the interaction with the patient. Elements of process or technique allow the clinician to obtain certain data (content), which ultimately are organized into the traditional sections of a medical history. Even in the earliest phases of the interview, however, the clinician formulates hypotheses that influence the continuing process of data collection. A central concern of clinical practice is differential diagnosis, formulating hypotheses

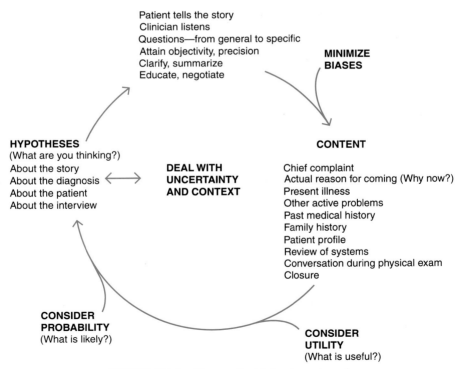

FIGURE 17–1   The medical interview at work.

about the patient's disease process. However, the accuracy of differential diagnosis depends on a set of preliminary hypotheses about the quality of the story itself and about the patient: Did X happen before or after Y? Is the narrative plausible? Does the patient exaggerate or minimize symptoms? The clinician generates hypotheses about the patient's personality and interactive style: What sort of coping style does he or she have? What might one expect in terms of adherence to treatment recommendations or behavioral change?

Finally, when problems arise in the interview, one must also consider hypotheses about the clinical encounter itself: What is going wrong here? Why do I feel so frustrated or uncomfortable? Why is the patient so angry? And because we encounter patients who may annoy us, or worry us, or confuse us, we are always trying to minimize bias, consider utility (can the problem be fixed?) and probability (is the diagnosis likely?), and deal with uncertainty.

We close this text with a slightly altered transcript (to protect the patient's privacy and to shorten the length) taken from a real interview of a new patient by a medical resident. We have annotated the transcript to illustrate some of the skills and thought processes that have been presented throughout this book and summarized in Figure 17–1. We hope this interview provides opportunity for analysis and reflection as you develop your own style and techniques.

This 32-year-old woman comes into the clinic for a "checkup."

Transcript	Comments
It's good to meet you. I guess the best place to start is to ask you what brings you here today.	Greeting, opening.
Well, I haven't had a physical really since 5 years ago, since my son was born.	
I am going to be writing some things down on paper here, okay? Is there any particular reason why you chose *now* to come in?	Acknowledges note taking. Open-ended question. Probe for iatrotropic stimulus, chief complaint.
I figured I kept putting it off and putting it off. I'd make appointments and put them off. There was no particular reason. I just felt as though it was time, I suppose.	
Nothing is bothering you at this point?	Additional probe for actual reason for coming.
No, it's just that I am overweight, that's all. I go up and down, up and down.	

So that was your major concern, the weight problem?	Summary statement and interchangeable response. Agenda setting.
Yeah.	
Can you tell me about that?	Open-ended question. Listening.
Well, I've always been big. All the women in my family are big. It's never slowed me down or anything, but I would like to just like firm up, maybe my thighs and my stomach. From after having children I don't know, they say everything takes time, you don't put it on right away, but I guess I'm impatient.	
How much do you weigh right now?	The doctor inquires in detail about the symptom—what, how much, when, why?—developing accuracy and precision and hypotheses about the diagnosis and the patient.
I don't basically know. Last time I weighed myself I weighed 200 pounds and that was like about 2 months ago.	
Say a year ago, what did you weigh?	What happened first, what next?
A year ago I weighed about 230 pounds.	
230 pounds? So you have actually lost 30 pounds between then and now?	The doctor checks back with patient, confirming data.
Yes.	
Have you been on a diet?	A closed question, perhaps pursuing a hypothesis (e.g., could the patient have lost weight because she has become diabetic?)
No.	
How have you lost the weight?	
I don't know. In the last, I'd say the last 6 months or so to a year, I've been getting to the point I'd go all day without eating. I'm real active. I'm very active.	

Can you tell me about the activity?	Open-ended question with topic specified.
Well, I do a lot of tennis. I have dance class. It seems like I don't want to stop to fix anything when I'm working in the house. I won't stop to fix anything to eat. I'll just keep on going.	
Is that a conscious effort on your part, to try to lose weight?	Closed-ended and, perhaps, a leading question with a vague response.
Yeah, something like that.	
What did you used to consider your normal weight?	A series of closed questions, still dealing with the weight issue.
I always weighed about 140 pounds.	
How many years ago was that?	
When I was 18.	
When would you say that you had gained the majority of weight between then and now?	
When I had my second child.	
What do you think it was between then and now that's made you gain the weight?	Open-ended question with, perhaps, a surprising response.
Nerves made me do a lot of eating. Then a lot of marital problems.	
Do you want to discuss that a little bit more?	Open-ended question, leading to further exploration of possible emotional causes for weight change. But leaving it up to the patient as to whether this topic is too intimate for her to discuss right now.
Oh, it was just a thing, me and my husband were—just like any other marriage I guess—good times, bad times—but more bad times than good. I had gotten to the point that I felt as though, I got all these children, what am I worth? You know, that kind of depressed me a little bit and I started gaining all that weight. After I had my last child I don't know, something just hit me, and I came up out of that.	Listening.

When was that?

Five years ago.

So, how would you describe your general mood now?

Open-ended question, topic specified, taking advantage of the fact that the patient has raised the topic of mood.

Fine.

You don't feel anything is wrong?

And not just taking "fine" for an answer.

No. I very seldom—last time I got depressed was one day about 2 months ago 'cause there wasn't no jobs and that's about it. But depression, I can't remember at all when I last felt depression. I feel good about myself, good about my surroundings, 'cause you know you are only doing the best you can.

What do you think has brought about that change?

Well, after me and my husband had separated about 3 years ago I got to the point, well, the children have to depend on me now, because I was doing a lot of depending on him.

So since then you have generally felt better about yourself.

A summarization of the patient's statement and additive response.

Yeah.

Can you describe your eating habits over the past several years?

Getting back to the chief complaint. More specifics about dietary habits. Part of the history of the present illness even though most often part of the patient profile.

Okay, well, I eat breakfast. I eat sometimes a large breakfast and during the mid-day I'll drink tea, eat some fruit, drink milk. I drink a lot of milk. I love milk. I might sit down and eat dinner about—lunch, I don't even worry about lunch 'cause I never see it. I eat dinner about 6 or 7 o'clock in the evening. In the last couple months I stopped snacking

Listening to the details. Time for the interviewer to think and plan and "size up" the patient.

on a lot of sweets. Before I used to crave them at a certain period of the time, mostly when it was my menstrual period, I'd crave a lot of sweets. Lately I just don't even care for sweets too much. But I still drink a lot of milk, as long as it's cold, I'll drink a lot of milk.

So you eat basically two meals a day.

Checking back about important data, summary statement but also something the patient herself may not have realized and, therefore, an additive response.

Yeah, sometimes one.

Now besides this weight problem, which seems to be improving, do you have any other complaints?

The doctor asks about other active problems—perhaps an iatrotropic stimulus as yet unmentioned.

None whatsoever.

None whatsoever?

With a mild confrontation (using a mirror or reflective response) the doctor elicits a new concern— edema.

Yeah—now, weird as it might sound, now my ankles—on my right leg, my ankle will not swell up, but my left leg swells up. And I was taking water pills there for a while from a doctor.

How long has this been going on?

Beginning of specific, closed-ended questions defining and categorizing causes of edema. It might have been better for the interviewer to respond, "Tell me more about that."

I'd say for 3 months.

When is the ankle swelling worse? Is it during the morning when you wake up?

No, during the evening.

As the day wears on?

Yeah, as the day wears on.

When you wake up in the morning, has it gone down?

Yes.

Have you been short of breath?

No.

How many pillows do you sleep on?

Now a series of questions that suggest the interviewer is working through some hypotheses about what's causing the edema. Perhaps the interviewer should have introduced this section with a transitional statement such as "Now I'm going to ask you a series of questions about specific symptoms you might have had."

One.

Do you ever wake up in the middle of the night gasping for air?

No.

How many times do you go to the bathroom at night?

About once.

And that's your only other major complaint at this time?

Keep asking until you're sure there's nothing else.

Yes.

Have you had any change in bowel habits?

Beginning of some review of systems (ROS)-type questions probing specifically for symptoms of thyroid disease, pursuing another hypothesis about the weight and edema.

No.

Constipation? Diarrhea?

No.

Change in your voice?

Yeah, my voice has gotten heavier.

Is it clear what the patient means by "heavier"?

How long has that gone on?

I'd say in the about the last year and a half.

Any change in your skin or your hair?

No.

Do you ever feel hot in a room where everyone else is cold or cold whenever everyone else is hot?

I can't stand heat. I cannot stand heat at all. Summertime I stay in the house until the evenings. I've always been like that. Cold weather I love.

Okay. I'm going to ask you a lot of routine questions.

Do you have any drug allergies that you are aware of?

Transition to and beginning of past medical history.

No.

Note the patient's "no" then "yes" that she does have a drug allergy.

Any medications that you are taking?

No. I'm allergic to penicillin.

What does penicillin do to you?

Note the clarification—what does "allergy" mean?

I broke out in hives.

Do you know of any medical problems that you have had in the past?

No. I have low blood. I'm anemic. I used to take iron pills there for awhile. That was about 10 years ago, then I just stopped because they made me feel tired.

Another "no" then "yes."

How's your pep and energy been?

Some ROS type questions as clinician appears to be ruling out another current active problem.

Fine.

Any other illness or operations that you remember?

No.

You mentioned that you have children. Tell me about your family. [Patient describes her family and their health status.] So you have four children. Any problems with any of your pregnancies? [Patient describes.]

Transition to and beginning of the "social history," but notice how much you already know about this person from the manner in which the present illness inquiry is conducted.

Are you fortunate enough to have a job right now?	Notice how well this question is put (respect).
No, not right now.	
What's a typical day like for you?	
[Patient describes typical day.]	
What type of work did you do in the past?	
I've done various things. I drove a bus, did maintenance work, cashier in a store.	
How long have you been unemployed?	
For about 2 months now.	
Any prospects?	
No, just a lot of applications in. That's about it.	
How does that feel? You must be upset.	Occupational history question. Unsuccessful attempt at additive response. Patient has not yet revealed her feelings about this situation.
Not really. Something will come up. Something's bound to come up.	
So you are optimistic?	Successful interchangeable response.
Yeah.	
Did you say you smoked cigarettes? How much do you smoke?	Transition to new topic.
I smoke—a pack will last me about 2 days.	
How long have you smoked?	
I've been smoking since I was 16.	
Drink any alcohol?	
No.	
Have you ever?	
Yes, I stopped drinking when I was 18.	
Why was that?	
I was pregnant with my first child.	
Do you use any other type of drugs?	

No.

I'm just going to run through a bunch of questions now. Have you had any headaches recently?

Transition to and beginning of formal ROS.

No.

Trouble with your eyes or your vision?

In one eye. This one jumps. It's the left one. That's been about 3 months now.

What do you mean by jumps?

Attempt at establishing precise meaning.

It gets to quivering. I don't know whether it's nerves. I used to say something's going to happen.

Do you ever see double out of that eye?

ROS-type questions continue.

No. Once in awhile when I come in from a different room area. Like this one will kind of dart and then it will clear up and my vision gets together.

Any difficulty hearing?

No.

Any bleeding through your nose, mouth, lips, and gums? Difficulty swallowing?

No.

I asked you about shortness of breath before. How about wheezing?

Wheezing, yes, sometimes.

When do you have the wheezing?

At night when I sleep.

Do you take anything for that?

No, not really.

Do you get up, or does it just go away?

Sometimes I'll get up and drink some water and that's it.

How often do you get that?

Every night during the night.

So every night you wake up feeling like you're wheezing and then you get up and have a drink of water?

Yes, almost every night.

Coughing any blood up at all?

No.

Any fever, chills, or sweats?

No.

Belly pain?

No.

Lumps or bumps anywhere in your breasts or under your arms?

No. [Interruption at door.]

What was I asking you, about belly pains?

Yes.

No belly pains?

No.

Diarrhea or constipation?

No.

Any blood in your stools?

No.

Tell me about your menstrual periods.

I guess they're normal, they come regular.

Any pain or bleeding between periods? Are they heavy?

No, nothing like that.

Do you have any sexual problems or concerns about birth control?

Well, I'm not doing anything right now.

Okay, just a few more questions. Any swelling of any of your joints or joint pains? Anywhere on your body?

Just my ankles.

Okay, we already talked about that. Any rash?

Summary statement.

Clinician asks patient to help get back on track after an interruption.

No.	
I think that's about all the questions I have for now. Do you have any questions for me? Is there anything else we need to cover?	Inviting the patient to have the last word.
No.	
Well, we've gone over a lot of stuff. Let's do your physical exam and then we'll make a plan. I'll step out and I'll review your old records while you put this gown on. I'll be back in a few minutes. Does that sound okay?	Transition to physical exam and letting the patient know what to expect.

The clinician went on to complete the evaluation of this patient, who turned out to have venous insufficiency as the cause of her pedal edema and reactive airway disease exacerbated by smoking.

She did not have hypothyroidism or any other endocrine disorder. She and her clinician began working together on a program of weight loss and smoking cessation.

We wish you good listening and learning.

Suggested Reading

Epstein RM. Mindful Practice. *JAMA* 1999; 282:833–839.

Sledge WH, Feinstein AR. A clinimetric approach to the components of the patient-physician relationship. *JAMA* 1997; 278:2043–2048.

APPENDIX

Questionnaires to Assist History-Taking

● ● ● ● ●

TABLE A–1

SELF-RATING DEPRESSION SCALE

The patient is asked to read the following 20 statements and rate each on a 1-to-4 scale: 1 = none or a little of the time; 2 = some of the time; 3 = good part of the time; 4 = most or all of the time. To calculate the total score, the clinician first inverts the patient's reported scores ("4" becomes "1," "3" becomes "2," and so forth) for the 10 questions that are positively worded (numbers 2, 5, 6, 11, 12, 14, 16, 17, 18, 20). The resulting values for the 20 questions are then added to produce a cumulative score. For information on scoring, see Corcoran, K, and Fischer, J: *Measures for Clinical Practice*, ed. 3. The Free Press, New York, 2000, pp. 695–696.

1. I feel down-hearted, blue, and sad.
2. Morning is when I feel the best.
3. I have crying spells or feel like it.
4. I have trouble sleeping through the night.
5. I eat as much as I used to.
6. I enjoy looking at, talking to, and being with attractive women/men.
7. I notice that I am losing weight.
8. I have trouble with constipation.
9. My heart beats faster than usual.
10. I get tired for no reason.
11. My mind is as clear as it used to be.
12. I find it easy to do the things I used to.
13. I am restless and can't keep still.
14. I feel hopeful about the future.
15. I am more irritable than usual.
16. I find it easy to make decisions.
17. I feel that I am useful and needed.
18. My life is pretty full.
19. I feel that others would be better off if I were dead.
20. I still enjoy the things I used to do.

SOURCE: Adapted from Zung WK. A self-rating depression scale. *Arch Gen Psychiatry* 1965; 12:63–70. Copyright 1965, American Medical Association. Reprinted with permission.

TABLE A-2

MICHIGAN ALCOHOLISM SCREENING TEST (MAST) QUESTIONNAIRE

Question	Points
1. Do you feel you are a normal drinker?	2
2. Have you ever awakened the morning after some drinking the night before and found that you could not remember part of the evening before?	2
3. Does your spouse (or parents) every worry or complain about your drinking?	1
4. Can you stop drinking without a struggle after one or two drinks?	2
5. Do you ever feel bad about your drinking?	1
6. Do friends or relatives think you are a normal drinker?	1
7. Do you ever try to limit your drinking to certain times of the day or to certain places?	0
8. Are you always able to stop drinking when you want to?	2
9. Have you ever attended a meeting of Alcoholics Anonymous (AA)?	5
10. Have you gotten into fights when drinking?	1
11. Has drinking ever created problems with you and your spouse?	2
12. Has your spouse (or other family member) ever gone to anyone for help about your drinking?	2
13. Have you ever lost friends or girlfriends or boyfriends because of drinking?	2
14. Have you ever gotten into trouble at work because of drinking?	2
15. Have you ever lost a job because of drinking?	2
16. Have you ever neglected your obligations, your family, or your work for two or more days in a row because you were drinking?	2
17. Do you ever drink before noon?	1
18. Have you ever been told you have liver trouble? Cirrhosis?	2
19. Have you ever had delirium tremens (DTs), severe shaking, heard voices, or seen things that were not there after heavy drinking?	2
20. Have you ever gone to anyone for help about your drinking?	5
21. Have you ever been in a hospital because of drinking?	5
22. Have you ever been a patient in a psychiatric hospital or on a psychiatric ward of a general hospital where drinking was part of the problem?	2
23. Have you ever been seen at a psychiatric or mental health clinic or gone to a doctor, social worker, or clergyman for help with an emotional problem in which drinking played a part?	2
24. Have you ever been arrested, even for a few hours, because of drunk behavior?	2
25. Have you ever been arrested for drunk driving or driving after drinking?	2

Score points for negative answers to questions 1, 4, 6, and 8 and positive answers to all other questions. A score of 5 or more points is highly suggestive of alcohol abuse.

SOURCE: Selzer ML. The Michigan Alcoholism Screening Test: The quest for a new diagnostic instrument. *Am J Psychiatry* 1971; 127:1653–1658. Copyright 1971, the American Psychiatric Association. Reprinted by permission.

TABLE A–3

TRAUMA SCALE FOR ALCOHOL ABUSE
Since your 18th birthday:
1. Have you had any fractures or dislocations of bones or joints?
2. Have you been injured in an automobile accident?
3. Have you injured your head?
4. Have you been injured in an assault or fight? (Excluding sports)
5. Have you been injured after drinking?
One point for each positive response. A score of 2 or more suggests alcohol abuse.

SOURCE: Reproduced with permission from Skinner HA, Holt S, Schuller R, et al. Identification of alcohol abuse using laboratory tests and a history of trauma. *Ann Intern Med* 1984; 101:847–851.

Index

An "f" following a page number indicates a figure; a "t" indicates a table.